AF777866

Dedicated to the memory of

Harry L. DeLozier,

a gentle person of high intellectual and ethical integrity with a commitment to quality post-graduate education

Sandostatin® in the Treatment of Gastroenteropancreatic Endocrine Tumors

Consensus Round Table, Scottsdale (Arizona), March 22, 1987

Editor: T. M. O'Dorisio

With 43 Figures and 22 Tables

Springer-Verlag Berlin Heidelberg New York
London Paris Tokyo Hong Kong

Professor T. M. O'Dorisio, M. D.
The Ohio State University
College of Medicine
Department of Endocrinology
410 West 10th Street
Columbus, Ohio 43210
USA

ISBN 3-540-50715-9 Springer Verlag Berlin Heidelberg New York
ISBN 0-387-50715-9 Springer Verlag New York Berlin Heidelberg

Library of Congress Cataloging-in-Publication Data

Sandostatin in the treatment of gastroenteropancreatic endocrine tumors: consensus round table, Scottsdale (Arizona), March 22, 1987 / editor, T. M. O'Dorisio.
p. cm.
Bibliography: p.
ISBN 0-387-50715-9 (U.S. : alk. paper) : (Germany)
1. Octreotide acetate–Testing–Congresses. 2. Gastrointestinal system–Tumors–Chemotherapy–Evaluation–Congresses. 3. Pancreas-Tumors–Chemotherapy–Evaluation–Congresses. 4. Endocrine glands-Tumors–Chemotherapy–Evaluation–Congresses. I. O'Dorisio, Thomas M.
[DNLM: 1. Intestinal Neoplasms–drug therapy–congresses.
2. Pancreatic Neoplasms–drug therapy–congresses. 3. Somatostatin-therapeutic use–congresses.
4. Stomach Neoplasms–drug therapy-congresses. WI 149 S218 1987]
RC271.025S26 1989
616.99 ' 433061–dc 19
DNLM/DLC 89-4250
for Library of Congress CIP

This work is subject to copyright. All rights are reserved, whether the whole or part of the material is concerned, specifically those of translation, reprinting, reuse of illustrations, broadcasting, reproduction by photocopying machine or similar means, and storage in data banks.
Under § 54 of the German Copyright Law, where copies are made for other than private use, a fee is payable to Verwertungsgesellschaft Wort, Munich.

© Springer Verlag, Berlin Heidelberg 1989
and Sandoz Medical Publications, Basle 1989
Printed and bound by Edwards Brothers, Inc., Ann Arbor, Michigan.
Printed in the United States of America.

Product Liability: The publisher can give no guarantee for information about drug dosage and application thereof contained in this book. In every individual case the respective user must check its accuracy by consulting other pharmaceutical literature.
The use of registered names, trademarks, etc. in this publication does not imply, even in the absence of a specific statement, that such names are exempt from the relevant protective laws and regulations and therefore free for general use.

2127/3335-543210 – Printed on acid-free paper

Table of Contents

Abbreviations

AC	adenylate cyclase
AMP	adenosine monophosphate
ANF	atrial natriuretic factor
APUD	amine precursor uptake and decarboxylation
ATP	adenosine triphosphate
b.i.d.	bis in die (twice a day)
BSA	bovine serum albumin
cAMP	cylic adenosine monophosphate
CCK	cholecystokinin
CGRP	calcitonin gene-related peptide
CNS	central nervous system
CT	computed tomography
CTX	cyclophosphamide
CZT	chlorozotocin
DNA	desoxyribonucleic acid
DOX	doxorubicin
DTIC	dimethyltriazenoimidazole carboximide
EC	enterochromaffin
EDTA	ethylenediaminetetraacetic acid
EGF	epidermal growth factor
EP	end-point evaluation
5-FU	5-fluorouracil
GDP	guanosine diphosphate
GEP	gastroenteropancreatic
GH	growth hormone
GI	gastrointestinal
GIP	glucose-dependent insulinotropic peptide
GRF	growth hormone releasing factor
GRP	gastrin releasing peptide
GTP	guanosine triphosphate
HAO	hepatic artery occlusion
hCG	human chorionic gonadotropin
5-HIAA	5-hydroxyindoleacetic acid
ICC	islet cell cancer
IQR	interquartile range
IRI	immunoreactive insulin
LHRH	luteinizing hormone releasing hormone
MEN I	multiple endocrine neoplasia syndrome type I
NC	no change
NMR	nuclear magnetic resonance
PG	progression
PHM	peptide histidine methionine
PP	pancreatic peptide
PRL	prolactin
RG	regression
RIA	radioimmunoassay
SGOT	serum glutamic-oxaloacetic transaminase
SMS	Sandostatin
SRIF	Somatostatin (somatotropin release inhibiting factor)
STZ	streptozotocin
t.i.d.	ter in die (three times a day)
TSH	thyroid-stimulating hormone
VIP	vasoactive intestinal peptide
WDHA	watery diarrhea, hypokalemia, achlorhydria
WDHH	watery diarrhea, hypokalemia, hypochlorhydria
WDS	watery diarrhea syndrome
ZES	Zollinger-Ellison syndrome

Authors' Addresses

Stephen R. Bloom, M. D.
Department of Medicine
2nd Floor – Francis Fraser Laboratory
Royal Postgraduate Medical School
Hammersmith Hospital
Du Cane Road
London W12 0HS (Great Britain)

Jean Alain Chayvialle, M. D.
Institut National de la Santé
et de la Recherche Médicale
U 45 "Physiopathologie Digestive"
Hôpital Edouard-Herriot
5, Place d'Arsonvale
69437 Lyon Cédex 3 (France)

Michael J. Dunne, M. D.
Department of Health
AIDS Unit
Richmond House
79, Whitehall
London SW1A 2NS (Great Britain)

Richard Elton
Sandoz Pharmaceuticals Corporation
Route 10
East Hanover, New Jersey 07936 (USA)

B. Eriksson, M. D.
Ludwig Institute for Cancer Research
Uppsala Branch
University Hospital
75185 Uppsala (Sweden)

Sheldon Fine, M. D.
Ontario Cancer Institute
The Princess Margaret Hospital
500 Sherbourne Street
Toronto, Ontario M4X 1K9 (Canada)

Timothy Fletcher
Clinical Research Unit London (CRUL)
Sandoz House
98, The Centre
Feltham, Middx TW13 4EF (Great Britain)

Timothy S. Gaginella, Ph. D.
The Ohio State University Hospital
College of Medicine
Division of Gastroenterology
410 West 10th Avenue
Columbus, Ohio 43210 (USA)

Klaus Gyr, M. D.
Department of Internal Medicine
Kantonsspital
University of Basle
4410 Liestal (Switzerland)

Pamela Hofker
Sandoz Pharmaceuticals Corporation
Route 10
East Hanover, New Jersey 07936 (USA)

Guenter J. Krejs, M. D.
Professor and Chairman
Department of Medicine
Karl Franzens University
Auenbruggerplatz 15
8036 Graz (Austria)

Larry M. Kvols, M. D.
Division of Medical Oncology
Mayo Clinic
200 First Street, S. W.
Rochester, Minnesota 55905 (USA)

Steven W. J. Lamberts, M. D.
Academisch Ziekenhuis Rotterdam,
Dijkzigt
Dr Molewaterplein 40
3015 GD Rotterdam (The Netherlands)

Ingrid Norheim, M. D.
Department of Internal Medicine
University Hospital
751 85 Uppsala (Sweden)

Thomas M. O'Dorisio, M. D.
The Ohio State University
College of Medicine
Department of Endocrinology
410 West 10th Street
Columbus, Ohio 43210 (USA)

Kjell Öberg, M. D.
Ludwig Institute for Cancer Research
Uppsala Branch
University Hospital
751 85 Uppsala (Sweden)

Janos Pless, M. D.
Sandoz Ltd
Pharma Division
Preclinical Research
Lichtstr. 35
4002 Basle (Switzerland)

Jean-Claude Reubi, Ph. D.
Sandoz Research Institute
Monbijoustr. 115
3007 Berne (Switzerland)

Uri Sagman, M. D., F.R.C.P. (C)
Ontario Cancer Institute
The Princess Margaret Hospital
500 Sherbourne Street
Toronto, Ontario M4X 1K9 (Canada)

Joseph Shui, Ph. D.
Sandoz Pharmaceuticals Corporation
Route 10
East Hanover, New Jersey 07936 (USA)

Gareth Williams, M. D.
Department of Medicine
University of Liverpool
P.O. Box 147
Liverpool L69 3BX (Great Britain)

Hubert F. Woods, M. D.
The University Department
of Pharmacology and Therapeutics
Royal Hallamshire Hospital
Glossop Road
Sheffield S10 2JF (Great Britain)

Nomenclature

Sandostatin®
Octreotide INN, BAN
Octréotide INN (F)
Octreotida INN (Span.)

1. Prologue

T. M. O'Dorisio

The Ohio State University, College of Medicine, Columbus, Ohio, USA

The overall purpose of this volume is to inform the practising physician and medical scientist of the impact that Sandostatin is having on clinically expressed endocrine tumors of the gastroenteropancreatic (GEP) system.

The book opens with preclinical observations: the pharmacokinetics and pharmacology of this remarkable prototype agent are addressed by Dr J. Pless, a pioneer and major developer of Sandostatin.

Scholarly, textbook-style chapters on the various aspects of the symptomatic endocrine tumors of the GEP system include up-to-date reviews of the carcinoid tumor by Dr H. F. Woods and colleagues and of VIPoma, insulinoma, glucagonoma, gastrinoma and GRFoma by Dr T. S. Gaginella and colleagues. These reviews are embellished by short communications from Drs K. Gyr, S. Lamberts, T. M. O'Dorisio, J. A. Chayvialle and G. Williams. In conjunction with the longer review chapters, these short communications give the reader an in-depth appreciation both of the established knowledge on symptomatic GEP endocrine tumors and of Sandostatin's partial mechanism of action.

A comprehensive chapter by Dr L. Kvols and his colleagues on anatomy, therapeutic strategy and treatment – specifically surgery, cytostasis, hepatic embolization and Sandostatin – is presented together with two short communications by Drs U. Sagman and K. Öberg. These authors address therapeutic strategies for symptomatic endocrine tumors of the GI tract, which include Sandostatin and such peptide agents as interferon.

Drs M. Dunne, R. Elton and colleagues present for the first time the combined European and USA clinical experience with Sandostatin. The data have been standardized in two ways. First, the commonly accepted diagnostic classification and laboratory evaluation has been used to group the patients with symptomatic GEP endocrine tumors. Secondly, in order to standardize the clinical response to Sandostatin therapy from the two independent data bases (representing data from 350 physicians), a common set of mutually exclusive and inclusive criteria of response has been established.

The consensus section of the book reflects the sequence of both the longer presentations and brief communications at the round table meeting in Scottsdale, Arizona. It begins with the universal view that Sandostatin is the most important agent for the treatment of clinically expressed GEP endocrine tumors to emerge since the stabilization of insulin in 1921 and the description of the Zollinger-Ellison syndrome in 1955. The section includes an explanation, incorporating information on the clinical effectiveness of Sandostatin, of the need for agreement on issues such as side effects, tolerance (escape phenomenon) and tumor-specific treatment precautions (to avoid, for instance, worsening hypoglycemia in insulinoma). These issues are addressed by comments and direct quotes from the authors of the short communications. The final section briefly addresses the future directions for Sandostatin. It suggests that we are only now recognizing the unique and multifaceted potential of this novel peptidomimetic agent.

The book closes with an exhaustive list of publications on the use of Sandostatin arranged in general categories. The list includes works not only on GEP endocrine tumors but also on pituitary tumors and on other uses of Sandostatin published to date. Sandostatin treatment of pituitary tumors is the subject of another recent text. It is hoped that these references, as well as the full-length chapters, short communications, and consensus discussion, will provide the dedicated practising physician and medical scientist with the practical information needed in order to use and study this sophisticated peptide analog. It has been a personal pleasure and honor to take part in this round table discussion on this model prototype agent and to act as editor of the exciting discussion that follows.

The Editor personally acknowledges the uncommon extra efforts of Drs. Richard L. Elton, Carol A. Bainbridge, and Louis D. Boyajy, and Ms. Pam Hofker of Sandoz Research Institute (USA) and Ms. Doreen Curtin, and Nancy J. Vobecky of Sandoz Pharmaceuticals for demanding and sustaining the necessary high scientific integrity of Sandostatin both in the pre-clinical and clinical phases of research and marketing. The Editor expresses as well his deepest appreciation to Sue, Joel, Rachelle, and Nathan for their consistent and, often, sacrificing support for the many hours of lecturing and editing required to bring this book and its relevant message to the Clinician/Scientist.

2. Chemical Structure – Pharmacological Profile of Sandostatin®

J. Pless

Sandoz Ltd, Preclinical Research, Basle, Switzerland

With the help of more and more sophisticated detection methodology the list of interesting neurotransmitters and factors seems to grow daily. Somatostatin is not a newcomer; it belongs to the 'establishment', since its discovery goes back to the 70's [2]. It soon became evident that, in spite of its highly attractive biological profile, the naturally occurring 14 or 28 amino acid molecule is not a good candidate for therapy in man because of its short half-life.

This is not an unusual situation in peptide medicinal chemistry. In most cases the naturally occurring substance is rapidly degraded in vitro and in vivo. The task of the medicinal chemist, valid for the peptide, is therefore to attain

- activity equal to or higher than the native hormone
- metabolic stability against degrading enzymes
- long duration of action
- increased selectivity for growth hormone (GH) inhibition compared with insulin
- reduced size, simple synthesis

and only one of these, namely the GH/insulin selectivity, is specific to somatostatin.

One would like at least to maintain the same biological activity in the analog or if possible even surpass it. For the design of more stable peptides one needs 2–3 fundamental pieces of information, such as the site of enzymatic degradation (Fig. 1), in order to strengthen the metabolic resistance of the cleavage sequences. In the case of somatostatin (SRIF) the answer was already available a long time ago [5].

The most dangerous cleavage can occur after Trp 8 because a rupture leads to completely inactive fragments. Aminopeptidase attack at the N-terminal is less important since – as we shall see later – sequences which are 1 or 2 amino acids shorter are as potent as the intact molecule. The usual trick to prevent or slow down enzymatic degradation is the replacement of an L-amino acid by its D-isomer. Fortunately the systematic replacement of L- by D-amino acids demonstrated that this exchange at position 8 is not only well tolerated but also leads to an enhanced GH-inhibitory potency [3] (Fig. 2).

The most exact information on the 3-dimensional structure of any given molecule can be obtained by x-ray analysis. Unfortunately peptides in 99% of the cases do not do us the favour of crystallizing; they are notoriously amorphous compounds. This is a pity since, if only we had the conformation of the peptide, we would be in a position to detect which amino acids are essential in the chain, the so-called active site, and which are those parts of the molecule where one could introduce modifications. If crystals are not

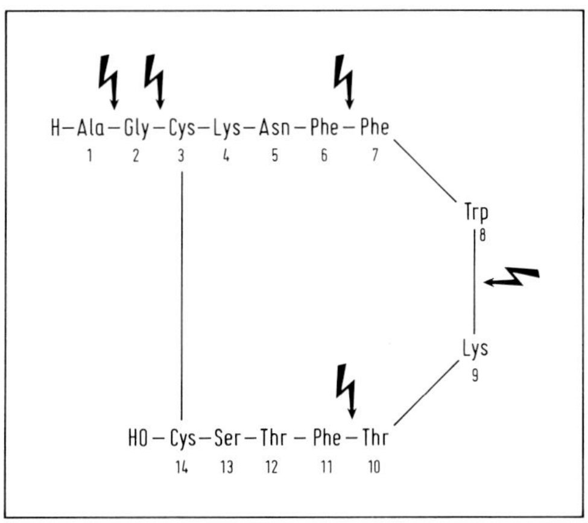

Fig. 1. Sites at which natural somatostatin is enzymatically cleaved

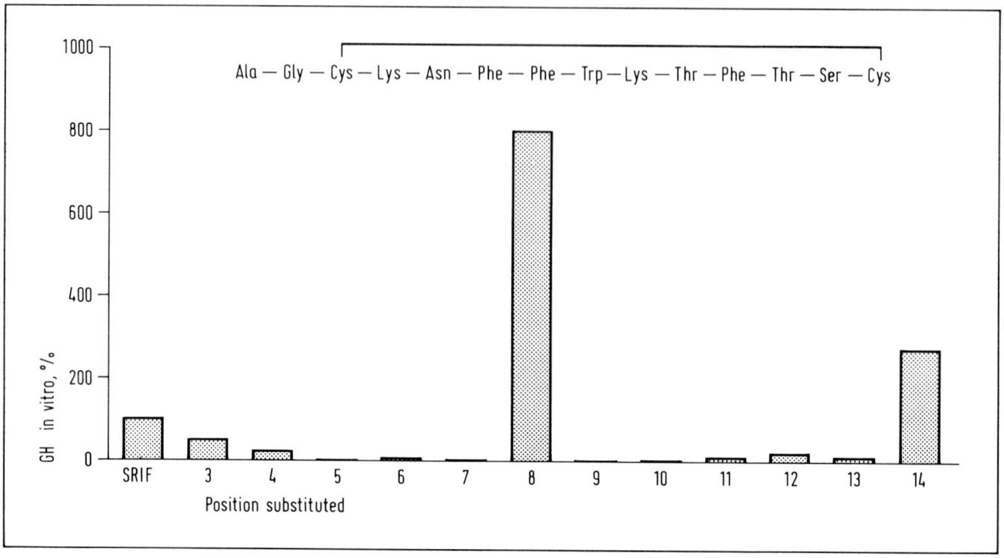

Fig. 2. Relative potencies of somatostatin analogs which are singly substituted with D-amino acids. SRIF = somatostatin = 100%; GH = growth hormone

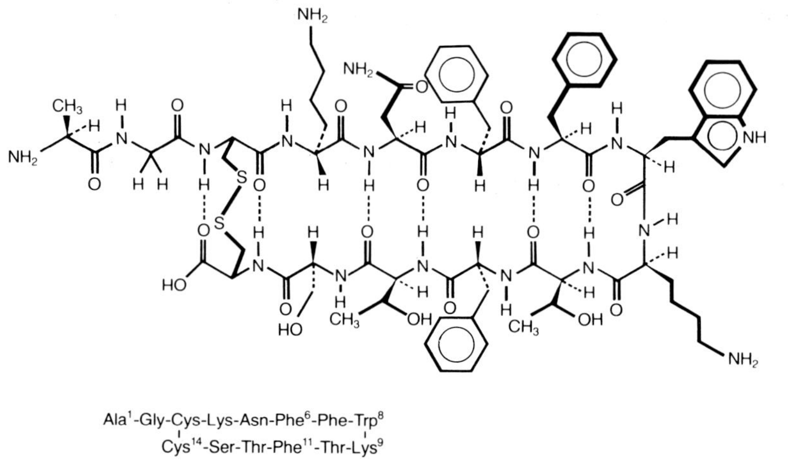

Fig. 3. A hypothetical conformation of somatostatin

available one can use the second-best physicochemical method, namely nuclear magnetic resonance studies [14]. This is a rather time-consuming procedure and needs highly specialized experts, but can still offer a quite useful structural hypothesis.

Figure 3 shows a hypothetical conformation of somatostatin, achieved at by model-building, chemical intuition, and some NMR studies. It reveals a so-called β-sheet structure which is held together by the disulfide bridge of cystine and H-bonds. In the corner we can see Trp and Lys, both 'untouchable' amino acids for biological activity, except with the already mentioned L → D-Trp change.

Further important information for the active site can be deduced by systematic replacement of all amino acids in SRIF by a neutral amino acid such as Ala. The total inactivity of analogs with Ala in positions 6, 7, 8 or 9 indicates that these residues are part of the pharmacophore. Similarly, yet more information can be gained by systematically

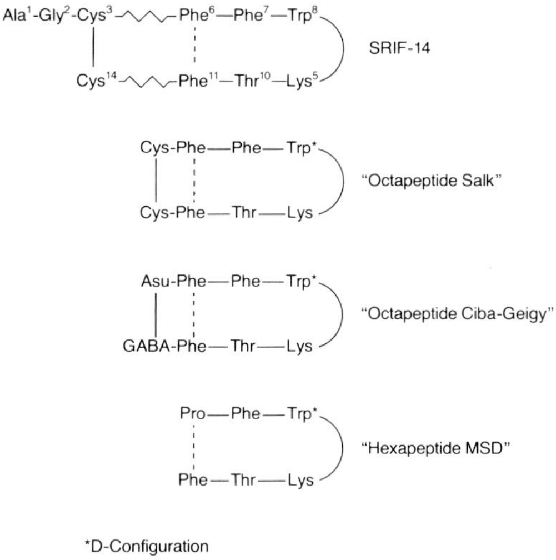

Fig. 4. A variety of somatostatin analogs of reduced size. SRIF = somatostatin

deleting single amino acids from the natural sequence. Such studies showed that the first two amino acids, Ala-Gly, are not necessary for full biological activity [12].

This body of information, accessible to everybody, prompted the synthesis of hundreds of SRIF analogs in many research centers all over the world.

Some of the most interesting structures are shown in Figure 4. Note that all of these share a common feature, namely the tetrapeptide active site Phe^7-Trp^8-Lys^9-Thr^{10} [13]. All of them are active and rather stable SRIF analogs.

Chemistry of Sandostatin

Our synthetic work also started from that very essential part of the molecule, held together by a disulfide bridge (Fig. 5). This lead proved to be almost inactive both in vitro and in vivo. However, this very weak potency could be improved dramatically by systematic addition of amino acids on both sides.

For this 'stepwise strategy' we tested each analog for GH inhibitory potency in the rat. Some of the interesting analogs are summarized in Table 1. Adding D-Phe at the N-terminus already increased potency to the level of natural SRIF but only the simultaneous prolongation with Ser and, even better, with Thr at the carboxyl end resulted in biological activity of the analogs which considerably surpassed that of natural SRIF [1].

This thorough program of chemical modification enabled us to select the most active and adequate peptide for further development. We coded it SMS 201-995 (it may also be found in the literature under the names of octreotide and Sandostatin®).

The synthesis of an octapeptide nowadays is no longer an heroic achievement and can be performed in many ways. What is more

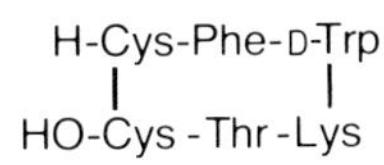

Fig. 5. The Sandoz lead compound for a program of synthetic analogs which led to Sandostatin

Table 1. Structures and biological activities of some octapeptide analogs of somatostatin. SRIF = somatostatin, SMS = Sandostatin

A-Cys-Phe-D-Trp-Lys-Thr-Cys-B

	Substituents		Potency ↓ GH (SRIF = 100)	
	A	B	in vitro	in vivo
1	H	NH_2	<0.1	1.4
2	H	D-Ser(NH_2)	<0.1	3.3
3	Asn	D-Ser(NH_2)	<0.1	3.3
4	D-Phe	OH	<0.1	ND
5	D-Phe	NH_2	4	165
6	D-Phe	D-Ser(NH_2)	12	680
7	D-Phe	D-Thr(NH_2)	47	1160
8	D-Phe	D-Thr(ol)	54	1100
SMS	D-Phe	L-Thr(ol)	300	7000

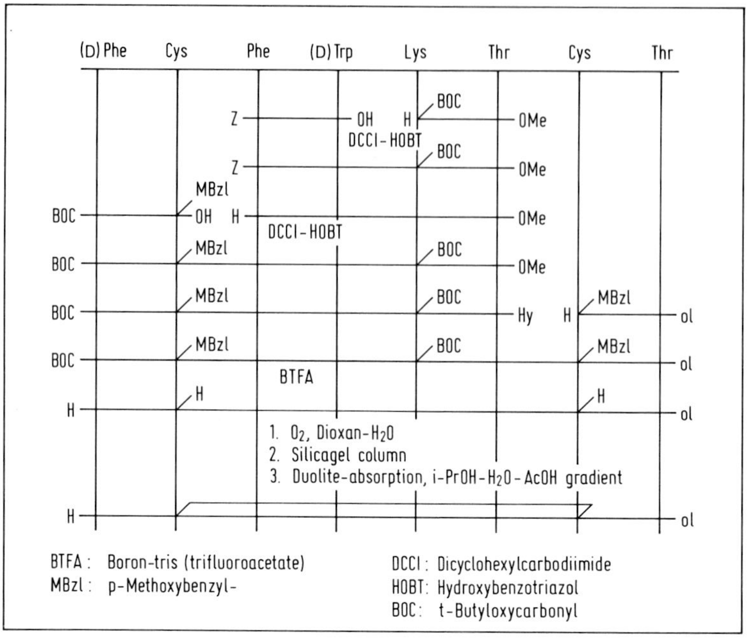

Fig. 6. Fragment-condensation synthesis of Sandostatin

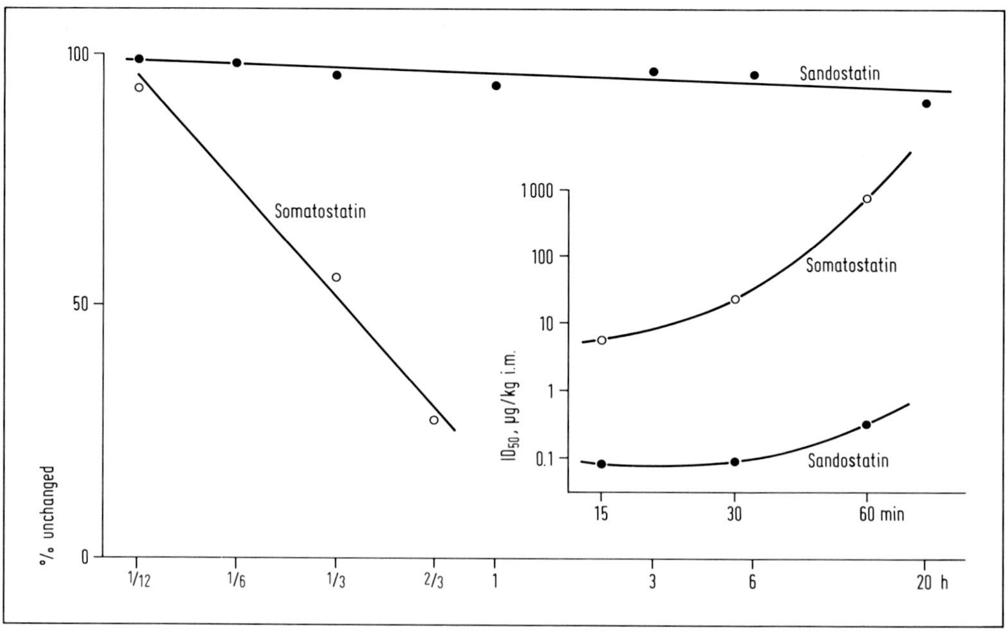

Fig. 7. Stability of Sandostatin and somatostatin at 37 °C in ultrafiltrate of rat kidney homogenate

difficult is the use of a method which is simple, economic and yields a product with at least 98% purity. This is the quality authorities demand for a peptide drug used in man. Taking into account that in this case we speak of a classical – not solid-phase – synthetic approach, with 25 distinct steps (Fig. 6) in which neither intermediates nor end product can be purified by crystallization, the quality requirements for manufacturing are enormous.

We have achieved industrial-scale production, however, which delivers a product whose purity and homogeneity are identical to that attained in the laboratory. To give you some idea of the quantities involved, we needed half a kilogram of Sandostatin alone for the long-term toxicity studies in rats and dogs.

We have invested a great deal of effort in protecting Sandostatin against enzymatic degradation. Introduction of D-Phe at the N-terminus protects against exopeptidases, as does the amino-alcohol Thr(ol) at the C-terminus. The disulfide bridge itself offers some protection, and the D-Trp protects a position which would otherwise be cleaved by a specific endopeptidase. Figure 7 shows the remarkable stability of Sandostatin in a system, kidney homogenate, known to degrade natural peptide hormones aggressively within a matter of minutes.

Similar excellent stability was observed at 37 °C in porcine gastroduodenal juice and in scrapings of rat intestinal mucosa.

Preclinical Pharmacology of Sandostatin

Sandostatin was selected in structure activity studies because of its outstanding GH inhibitory potency. The endocrinological investigations were then extended to the mode of application, duration of action and to specificity against other pancreatic peptides.

After i.m. application in the rat, good dose-response curves of Sandostatin compared with natural SRIF in the inhibition of GH, insulin and glucagon can be demonstrated (Fig. 8).

For example, fifteen minutes after administration to male rats in nembutal anaesthesia, Sandostatin is 70 times more active than SRIF. Insulin was stimulated by application of 0.5 g/kg glucose and in this model Sandostatin was only 3 times more active than SRIF in inhibiting insulin. This gives a very important and desirable selectivity in favour of GH inhibition (70:3). Finally, insulin-stimulated glucagon was also inhibited more potently (by a factor of 23) than by SRIF.

To study the role of different routes of administration (i.v., s.c., p.o.) we have developed a specific radioimmunoassay with a

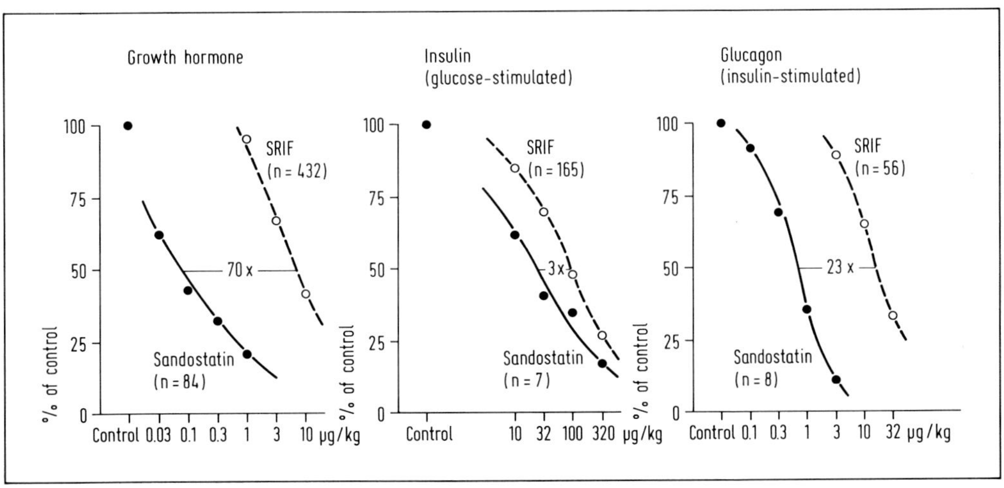

Fig. 8. Inhibiting effects of Sandostatin (SMS) and somatostatin (SRIF) on hormone secretion in the nembutal-anaesthetized rat, 15 min after i.m. injection

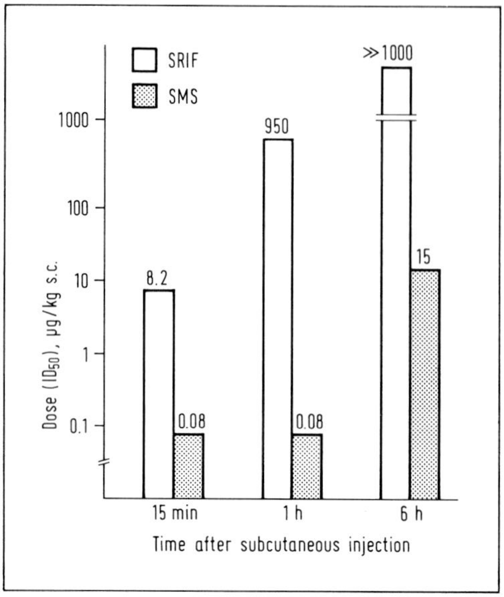

Fig. 9. GH-inhibitory potency of Sandostatin (SMS) and of somatostatin (SRIF) at various times after subcutaneous administration

sensitivity of 2 pg/tube and no cross-reactivity with natural SRIF. Studies in the rat show that after application of equal amounts of Sandostatin by all three routes, absorption is fast and bioavailability is almost quantitative, but compared with i.v. administration the elimination after s.c. and p.o. administration is much slower.

These observations are also relevant in functional tests, since natural SRIF loses more than 99% of its activity 1 h after s.c. application whereas Sandostatin is as active as SRIF after 15 min (Fig. 9).

With results similar to those in the rat, higher potency and specificity of Sandostatin could be demonstrated in the rhesus monkey (Table 2) after intravenous infusion. Sandostatin inhibited GH 45 times and insulin 1.3 times more potently than SRIF.

The advantages of s.c. application found in the rat could also be demonstrated in rhesus monkeys and it seems that the elimination in monkeys (based on plasma level) is even slower (Fig. 10). Sufficiently high levels of Sandostatin can also be measured after oral administration in the rat (Fig. 9). The same is found in the monkey, but the doses required are 50 to 100 times higher than by the s.c. route (Fig. 11).

Pharmacokinetic Studies

Metabolic studies with peptides are rather complicated and need a lot of tedious work, starting with the synthesis of a tritiated form with which the determination of biological half-life, absorption rate, distribution pattern, elmination and residue analysis are feasible.

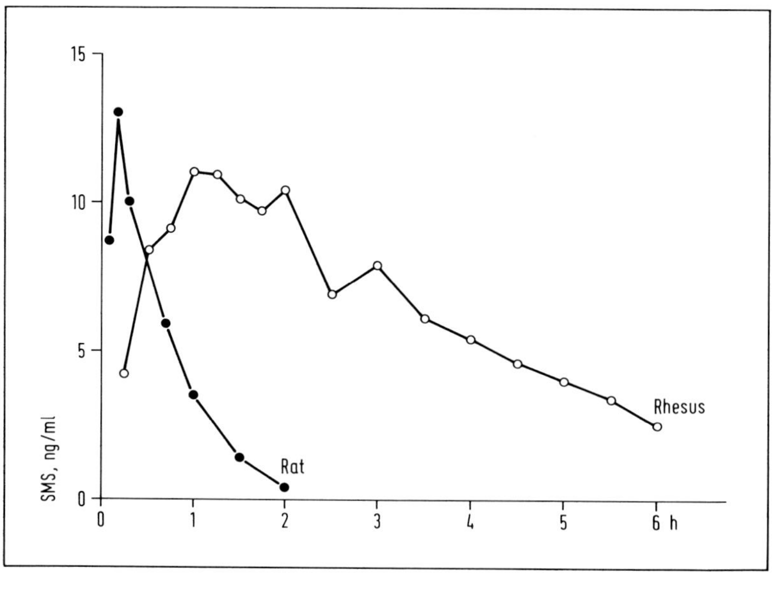

Fig. 10. Plasma levels of Sandostatin (SMS) in the rat and the rhesus monkey after subcutaneous administration of 10 µg/kg

Table 2. Comparison of the pharmacodynamic effects of Sandostatin (SMS) and somatostatin (SRIF) in the rhesus monkey. GH = growth hormone

Hormone	SMS ID_{50} µg/kg/h	SRIF ID_{50} µg/kg/h	Potency ratio SRIF = 1	Insulin/GH or glucagon/GH ratio		Selectivity factor SRIF = 1
				SMS	SRIF	
GH ↓	0.04	1.7	45			
Insulin ↓	3.8	4.9	1.3	100	3	33
Glucagon ↓	0.075	0.8	11	2	0.5	4

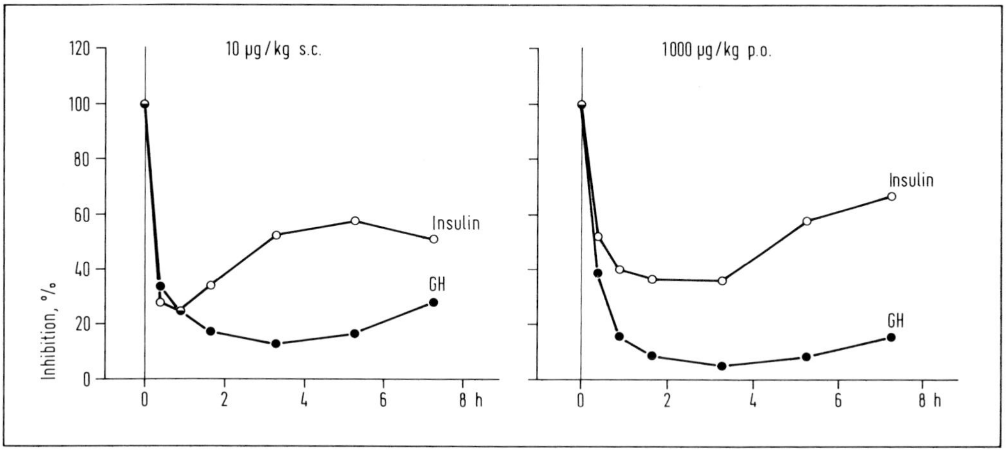

Fig. 11. Activity of Sandostatin in inhibiting growth hormone (GH) and insulin secretion in the rhesus monkey after subcutaneous and oral administration

	1/2 h	4 h
Plasma	737.0	12.0
GI-tract	525.0	14.0
Skin	547.0	48.0
Thymus	94.0	4.7
Thyroid	163.0	<32.0
Adrenals	153.0	67.0
Kidney	1182.0	235.0
Liver	523.0	17.0
Pancreas	208.0	75.0
Hypothalamus	8.3	<1.1
Pituitary	120.0	<67.0

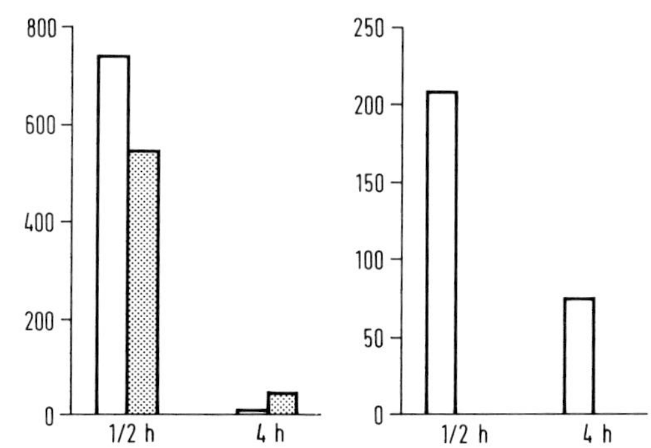

Fig. 12. Tissue distribution of Sandostatin in rats after intravenous administration of 1 mg/kg

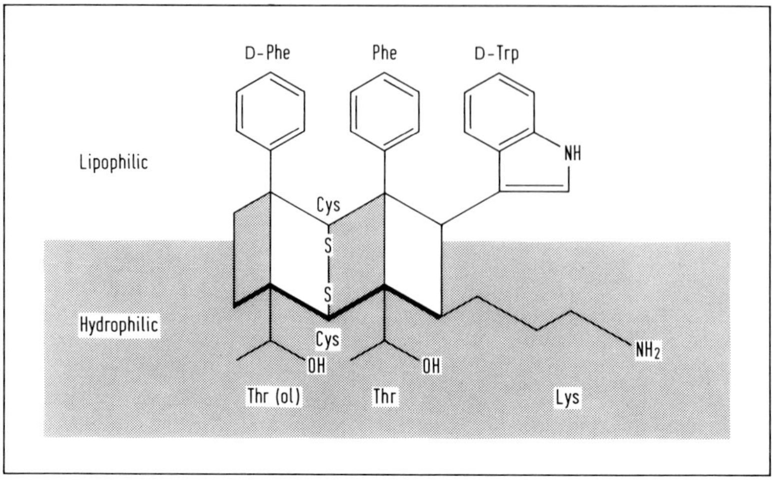

Fig. 13. The amphiphilic properties of Sandostatin

Figure 12 shows i.v. and s.c. pharmacokinetic studies in the rat. Different organs were analyzed for their Sandostatin content after acid methanol extraction procedure.

Clear differences in distribution pattern between assumed target and non-target organs can be seen. Whereas Sandostatin plasma concentration falls to less than 10% after 7 h, the peptide accumulates in the pancreas after 4 h and large amounts are still present there after 7 h. This very slow elimination from a target organ may explain the long duration of action, especially after s.c. administration.

Another important pharmacokinetic aspect is the route of elimination. After i.v. application in the rat, 25% of the Sandostatin dose was recovered unchanged from urine and none from the faeces. In the bile-duct cannulated rat, however, 73% of the drug could be found in the bile. From these results we may conclude that Sandostatin is excreted mainly via bile and cleaved by the bacterial flora during passage through the intestinal tract.

The unusual and outstanding properties of Sandostatin can also be partly explained by its unique physicochemical properties. Due to the amphiphilic character of the molecule (Fig. 13), the polar structure permits an ideal embedding of Sandostatin in biopolymers such as receptors or plasma proteins.

Receptor Studies

The polyvalent biological actions of SRIF can be explained by a wide distribution of specific *SRIF receptors* in the organ [11]. From previous studies it is known that in the rat receptors are present in the pituitary, endocrine and exocrine pancreas, in the gastrointestinal tract, the adrenals and the CNS. The measurements are carried out either by binding to homogenates in vitro or visualised with autoradiography. Various radioligands can be used, such as analogs of SRIF-14 or SRIF-28 or analogs of a stable SRIF analog namely iodinated Tyr^3-Sandostatin [7, 9]. High affinity and saturable binding sites were identified in all tissues; 3 typical binding experiments are shown in Figure 14.

Within the central nervous system there is a topographically very precise distribution of SRIF receptors, as could be demonstrated in the rat. They are mainly located in cortical areas and in the limbic system (hippocampus, amygdala and septum). In the pituitary gland of the rat, SRIF receptors are located in the anterior part, particularly on somatotrophs, but also on thyreotrophs and lactotrophs. In the pancreas, within the islets the A, B, D cells all possess SRIF receptors, a fact which is compatible with the inhibitory action of Sandostatin on insulin or glucagon.

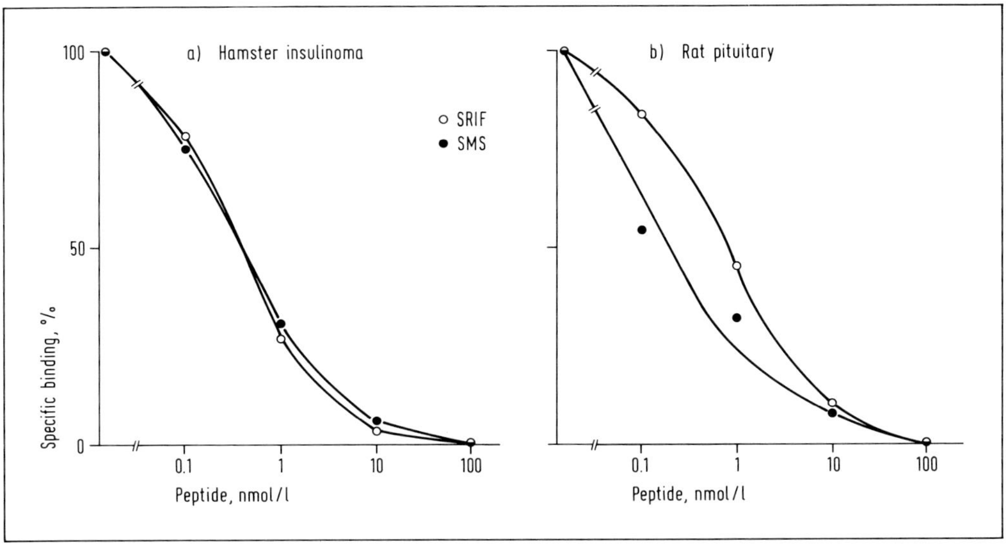

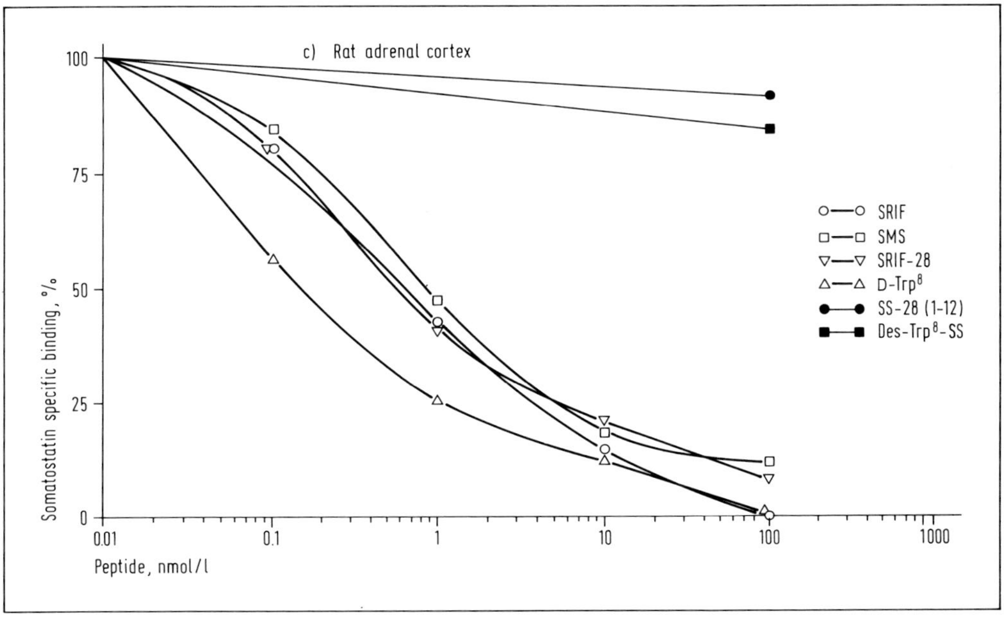

Fig. 14. Displacement of the specific binding of [^{125}I-Tyr^{11}]-somatostatin (SRIF) by Sandostatin (SMS) and SRIF in a) hamster insulinoma, b) rat pituitary, and c) rat adrenal cortex homogenates

In the GI tract of the rat the detection of SRIF receptors is more difficult. However, they could be found in the stomach mucosa. The precise role of SRIF receptors in inhibition of various GI hormones has still to be elucidated.

Interestingly, the rat adrenal medulla also contains SRIF receptors which might mediate aldosterone release [6].

A very great number of studies already published demonstrate that somatostatin receptors could also be detected in normal human tissues. Moreover the presence of SRIF receptors has been described in different human tumour tissues by Reubi, Maurer, Werder, Landolt and Lamberts, e.g. in adenomas, GRFomas, VIPomas [4].

In some of these tumours a good correlation between the presence of SRIF receptors and the in vivo responsiveness to Sandostatin could be found. Such measurement of receptors in humans might be very important for the prediction of new therapeutical applications for SRIF analogs. Table 3 shows the binding of [^{125}I-Tyr^{11}]-SRIF to 5 human GH-secreting adenomas [8].

Table 3. Dissociation constants (K_D) and receptor densities (B_{max}) of [^{125}I-Tyr^{11}]-SRIF binding sites in five human GH-secreting adenomas (1–5) compared with normal rat pituitary

Tissue	[^{125}I-Tyr^{11}]-SRIF binding sites	
	K_D (nmol/l)	B_{max} (f mol/mg protein)
1	0.57	757
2	1.48	800
3	1.04 ± 0.01	441 ± 29.0
4	0.24 ± 0.04	103 ± 56.6
5	1.04 ± 0.11	1058 ± 101.8
Normal rat pituitary	0.95	100

Mean ± S.D. of 2–3 experiments

The presence of SRIF receptors could be detected in all of 13 human meningioma samples [10]. Figure 15 shows detailed binding studies on one such sample. Pharmacologically inactive SRIF analogs such as Des-Trp^8-SRIF or LHRH do not displace the labelled SRIF analogs, thus demonstrating pharmacological specificity.

Toxicity Testing

Finally, Sandostatin had to be tested in intensive *toxicological* trials prior to clinical investigations. In a 26-week intraperitoneal study Sandostatin was administered in doses of 0.02, 0.1 and 1 mg/kg/day in the rat. The tolerance was extremely good and histological examinations revealed no changes attributable to Sandostatin treatment. The non-toxic effect level could be set at 1 mg/

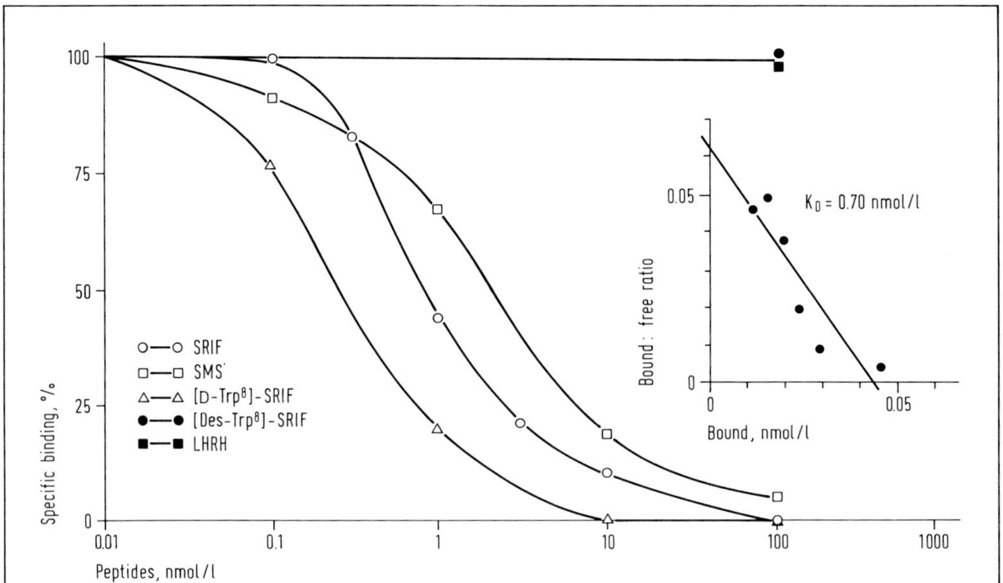

Fig. 15. Somatostatin receptors; displacement of specific binding of [^{125}I-Tyr^{11}]-somatostatin (SRIF) in a human meningioma sample. SMS = Sandostatin; LHRH = luteinizing hormone releasing hormone

kg/day, which gives a safely factor of approx. 150–1500 in relation to the average doses for various indications in humans.

Conclusion

Recollecting the goals we had in mind at the commencement of our program of SRIF analogs, we can say that from the preclinical point of view, we have been successful. Starting from a small conformationally defined fragment of the natural substance, we were able to design and synthesize Sandostatin (SMS 201-995), a very potent and stable peptide of relatively simple structure with a very attractive profile of biological activities.

In extensive pharmacological, metabolic, and toxicological studies of this compound, we have provided our clinical colleagues with a drug which enables them to investigate the therapeutic potential of somatostatin in both expected and new, unexpected indications.

Acknowledgement: The results presented here are the work of the concerted effort of the "Somatostatin Team". Thus it is a pleasure to acknowledge the dedicated efforts of Wilfried Bauer, Ulrich Briner, Wolfgang Doepfner, Roland Haller, René Huguenin, Peter Marbach and Trevor Petcher. Thanks are due also to our many colleagues in Metabolic Studies, Toxicology and Clinical Research, all of whom have helped to bring Sandostatin to the point where it can be introduced into human therapy.

References

1. W. Bauer, U. Briner, W. Doepfner, R. Haller, R. Huguenin, P. Marbach, T. J. Petcher, J. Pless: Life Sci *31*, 1133–1140 (1982)
2. P. Brazeau, W. Vale, R. Burgus, N. Ling, M. Butscher, J. Rivier, R. Guillemin: Science *179*, 77–79 (1973)
3. M. Brown, J. Rivier, W. Vale: Endocrinology *98*, 336–343 (1976)
4. S. W. J. Lamberts, J. C. Reubi, P. Uitterlinden, J. Zuidervijk, P. van den Werff, P. van Hal: Endocrinology *118* (No. 6), 2188 (1986)
5. N. Marks, F. Stern: FEBS Lett *55*, 220–224 (1975)
6. R. Maurer, J. C. Reubi: Mol Cell Endocrinol *45*, 81–90 (1986)
7. J. C. Reubi: Life Sci *36*, 1829 (1985)
8. J. C. Reubi, A. Landolt: J Clin Endocrinol Metab *59*, 1148–1151 (1984)
9. J. C. Reubi, R. Maurer: Neuroscience *15*, 1183 (1985)
10. J. C. Reubi, R. Maurer, J. G. M. Klijn, S. Z. Stefanko, J. A. Foekens, G. Blaauw, M. A. Blankenstein, S. W. J. Lamberts: J Clin Endocrinol Metab *63* (No. 2), 433 (1986)
11. C. B. Srikant, Y. C. Patel: Proc Natl Acad Sci USA *78*, 3930 (1981)
12. W. Vale, J. Rivier, N. Ling, M. Brown: Metabolism *27* [Suppl I], 1391–1401 (1978)
13. D. Veber, R. Freidinger, D. Schwenk, W. Palavede, F. Holly, R. Strachan, R. Nutt, B. Arison, C. Hamnich, W. Randall, M. Glitzer, R. Saperstein, R. Hirschmann; Nature *292*, 55–58 (1981)
14. C. Wynants, G. van Binst, H. R. Loosli: Int J Pept Protein Res *25*, 615–621 (1985)

3. Carcinoid Tumours and the Carcinoid Syndrome

H. F. Woods, N. D. S. Bax, J. A. C. Thorpe*, J. A. R. Smith*

The University Department of Pharmacology and Therapeutics, Royal Hallamshire Hospital, Sheffield, UK, and* The Northern General Hospital, Sheffield, UK

Introduction

The purpose of this paper is to describe the clinical features, pathology and treatment of carcinoid tumours and the carcinoid syndrome. The content is based upon our personal experience of the management of the disorder and the original literature.

Incidence

The gastrointestinal tract is the most frequent site of occurrence of carcinoid tumours. Thus, Godwin [8] using data collated by the National Cancer Institute in Bethesda (USA) reported that, within the gut, the appendix, rectum and ileum were most often involved, accounting for 44, 15 and 22% of tumours respectively. Tumours in the thoracic cavity accounted for about 10% of cases in the series.

Marks [16] recorded that the most common sites for carcinoid tumours in the gastrointestinal tract were the appendix, the jejuno-ileum and the rectum, these accounting for 35, 21 and 15% of gut tumours respectively. In our series (Table 1) the small bowel, the appendix and the large bowel were the most common intra-abdominal sites, accounting for 36, 13 and 9% of the tumours seen. We have estimated the incidence of carcinoid tumours in the Trent Region of the United Kingdom using statistics supplied by the Trent Region Cancer Registration Bureau (see also [31]).

Of the population of the British Isles, 8.5% live in the Trent Region (Fig. 1) and the crude incidence of intra-abdominal car-

Table 1. Carcinoid tumours – primary tumour sites, Sheffield series 1978–1987

Site	Number	%
Stomach	2	3
Small bowel	24	36
Large bowel	6	9
Appendix	9	13
Pancreas	3	5
Porta hepatis	1	1
Lung	15	22
Ovary	2	3
Breast	1	1
Unknown	4	7
Total	67	

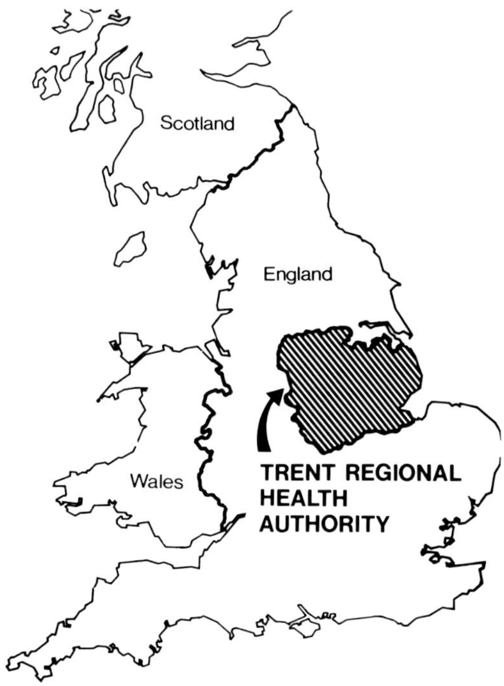

Fig. 1. The geography of the Trent Regional Health Authority

Table 2. Incidence of intra-abdominal carcinoid tumours. The data are derived from the Trent Regional Cancer Registration Bureau and do not include tumours of the appendix. The figures relating to colon cancer have been included for comparison

Year	Number of intra-abdominal carcinoid tumours	Number of colon cancer tumours	Total population of Trent Region (millions)	Crude incidence of abdominal tumours (cases per 100 000 of population per year)	
				Carcinoid	Colon cancer
1981	23	1320	4.60	0.50	28.7
1982	11	1383	4.60	0.24	30.1
1983	18	1439	4.60	0.39	31.3
1984	23	1416	4.61	0.50	30.7
1985	16	1299	4.62	0.35	28.1

cinoid tumours in that population is shown in Table 2 for the years 1981–1985. The table also shows the incidence of malignant tumours of the colon, for purposes of comparison. These figures demonstrate the rarity of the condition. In our experience abdominal carcinoid tumours are rare below the age of 40 years.

The incidence of intrathoracic carcinoid tumours is lower than that in the abdomen. In the Trent Region, the incidence in the years 1981–1985 has varied between 0.07 and 0.15 cases per 100 000 of population per year.

Abdominal Carcinoid Tumours

Small Bowel Tumours

Carcinoid tumours of the small bowel formed the largest group of abdominal carcinoid tumours in our series. Within the group there was a preponderance of male patients (M:F ratio 2:1). The ages of the patients at presentation were between 39 and 75 years, the mean being 60 years.

The symptoms and signs at presentation are listed in Table 3. In our experience it is common for patients to have had symptoms for a number of years before the diagnosis was made. Thus, 18 patients had had symptoms for at least a year before diagnosis and, of these, 9 had a history of symptoms for five years or more.

The main presentation is that of intestinal obstruction which can be acute or subacute. In some cases a right-sided abdominal mass is palpable. The typical history consists of episodic abdominal pain which is right-sided or is felt across the upper abdomen and is either constant or is colicky in nature. At first the symptoms are not specific and lead to extensive investigations. These investigations, which often include gastroscopy, cholecystograms, barium series and ultrasound and CT scanning frequently do not lead to a diagnosis. In some cases, however, barium studies are abnormal showing nonfilling of the ascending colon and caecum on barium enema, or an abnormal mucosal pattern in the terminal ileum on small bowel enema. In the latter case the mucosal pattern may resemble that seen in Crohn's disease.

Table 3. Presenting symptoms and signs in cases of small bowel carcinoid tumour (n = 24)

Symptom	No.
Diarrhoea	17
Pain	17
Flushing	12
Weight loss	7
Valvular heart disease	3
Wheezing	1
Epiphora	1
Pigmentation	1

The natural history is for the attacks of abdominal pain to become more frequent and for their intensity to increase. In some cases, the patient then presents with acute intestinal obstruction and in others there can be several episodes of subacute obstruction before laparotomy.

A few cases present with metastatic disease or the carcinoid syndrome.

There are three types of finding at laparotomy. In the first, the tumour forms the nidus of a mass in the right iliac fossa. The mass consists of loops of small bowel and the ascending colon stuck down to each other and to the tumour by dense fibrous tissue. In the second type there is a single small bowel tumour which may be the site of an intussusception, and in the third type there is no mass. In this variant the tumour or multiple tumours are palpable through the bowel wall and are visible as nodules within the bowel wall.

The diagnosis is not always clear at laparotomy and depends upon histological examination of the tumour. The majority of laparotomies reveal either local invasion through the bowel wall or the presence of distant metastases. The literature supports this experience: Marks [16] reported local invasion in 54% of cases and distant metastases in 62%; Sanders and Axtell [27] recorded distant spread in 33% of cases. The liver is often involved. The deposits may be large and occasionally single, or small and visible on the liver surface. The presence of liver secondaries may not be suspected before laparotomy because they are not detected by ultrasound or isotopic scans when they are small. In this context we have recently managed a case where serial histopathological sections revealed microscopic secondary deposits within the liver substance.

Marks [16] has suggested that the likelihood of distant spread and local invasion is related to the size of the primary tumour. Spread was rare with tumours of 1 cm in diameter at diagnosis, whereas it was almost inevitable with a tumour over 2 cm in diameter. There are rare variants of intra-abdominal tumour spread: chylous ascites can occur because of occlusion of the main lymphatics by tumour infiltration of the posterior abdominal wall, and in other cases the entire peritoneal surface is covered by a thin layer of tumour.

Large Bowel Tumours

Carcinoid tumours of the large bowel are difficult to distinguish from adenocarcinoma of the colon so far as their mode of presentation is concerned. The main features are abdominal pain, rectal bleeding and intestinal obstruction. Symptoms may be present for up to two years before the diagnosis is made and the appearances on barium enema x-ray examination are identical to those produced by adenocarcinoma of the colon.

Pathology

The cells of carcinoid tumours are derived from those of the APUD (amine precursor uptake and decarboxylation) series [25] and there are histological similarities to other neuroendocrine tumours. The cells are usually arranged in a regular pattern and are small and polygonal or round. The nuclei may contain granules and are basophilic. Tumours may have a glandular pattern with rosettes and strands of cells. There are characteristic histochemical properties of the cells, giving positive argentaffin and diazo reactions, and argyrophil granules occur frequently.

Carcinoid tumours contain and secrete 5-hydroxytryptamine and substantial amounts of its metabolite 5-hydroxyindoleacetic acid may be excreted in the urine. The ability to synthesize 5-hydroxytryptamine is not universal, and some tumours secrete dopamine and noradrenaline [9]. Others are the site of ectopic hormone production. Small bowel carcinoid tumours are often multiple. In the ileum, Moertel et al. [20–22] found that 29% had a multicentric origin and Marks [16] found that 4% of his patients had multiple jejunal or ileal tumours. The lesions may be tumour nodules within the bowel wall or discrete masses in the lumen. In our experience there can be discrete tumours at more than one site in the bowel [31].

There is an association between carcinoid tumours and primary malignant tumours at other sites. This has been described in a number of series of small bowel carcinoid tumours in particular [16, 20–22]. However, in our experience the association is rare. Large bowel carcinoid tumours are only occasionally associated with malignancy at other sites.

The Carcinoid Syndrome

The existence of a characteristic systemic illness in some patients with carcinoid tumours has been recognized for many years. The first comprehensive description of what is now known as the carcinoid syndrome was that of Cassidy [6, 7]. He described a 31-year-old male who had dilated small skin vessels over the malar regions and nose and also flushing of the face precipitated by emotional factors and eating.

In Cassidy's second paper [7] the postmortem findings of a pelvic tumour mass with hepatic secondary deposits and valvular pulmonary stenosis were described.

Similar cases were described later by Millman [19], Björck et al. [5], Isler and Hedinger [12] and Rosenbaum and colleagues [26]. The case reports were followed by a comprehensive description of the carcinoid syndrome by Thorson [29].

The main components of the syndrome are flushing, diarrhoea, cardiac valvular lesions, and wheezing. Thorson [29] listed the manifestations of the syndrome and their relative incidences (Table 4). There is great variability in terms of the relative intensity of each component of the syndrome in each patient. Thorson [29] did not mention weight loss, which can be profound and is an almost invariable feature.

Table 4. The manifestation of the carcinoid syndrome. (After [29])

General		
Total number of cases	79*	
Males	48	
Females	29	
Age at presentation (years)		
Males	18–80	
Females	33–80	
Manifestation	**No.**	**%**
Flushing	74	93.7
Intestinal hypermotility	68	86.1
Bronchial asthma	18	22.8
Oedema	52	65.8
Heart lesions	41	51.9
Pellagra-like skin lesions	5	6.3
Peptic ulcers	5	6.3
Arthralgia	6	7.6

* The sex of two patients is not stated.

Flushing

Flushing is the most common manifestation of the carcinoid syndrome. In 1968 Grahame-Smith [10] subdivided flushing into 4 types:

Type 1) A diffuse erythematous flush that involves the face, neck and upper anterior chest wall and, to a lesser extent, the skin of the abdomen, back, and palms. The flush lasts from 2 to 5 min and is often paroxysmal. The facial colour is usually normal between episodes.

Type 2) This type affects the same areas as type 1. It is longer lasting and violaceous in colour. These patients often have a permanent cyanotic flush over the nose and malar regions. There are many facial telangiectases and congested conjunctivae.

Type 3) In patients with bronchial carcinoid tumours the flush can be prolonged and intense. The flush is less red than in type 1 and is accompanied by lacrimation and conjunctival congestion. Palpitations and hypotension are occasionally present, together with facial swelling and an exaggeration of normal facial creases. This type of flushing is very distressing and may be associated with diarrhoea.

Type 4) A bright red patchy (geographical) flush consisting of red and pale areas. The patchiness is often seen at the root of the neck. This type is often associated with gastric carcinoid tumours producing histamine.

In patients with small bowel carcinoids, the flushing can be precipitated by activities such as eating, drinking, physical exercise, experiencing strong emotions, and ethanol ingestion. Some patients find that particular foods precipitate flushing and others that hot drinks do the same.

A particular pattern has been present in several of our patients: soon after they have risen and eaten the first meal of the day there is a rapid onset of facial flushing, gripping abdominal pain, and urgency of defaecation. This occurs mostly at the start of the day and is not necessarily present after other meals. This flushing can be accompanied by watering of the eyes, which is not unique to pulmonary carcinoids. These symptoms often wane as the day passes.

The pharmacology of flushing has been investigated, and a causative role for bradykinin has been demonstrated. There is evidence that 5-hydroxytryptamine may act synergistically with bradykinin in some cases, but not all patients with flushing have elevated 5-hydroxyindoleacetic acid excretion. Vasoactive amines can provoke a flush through the release of kallikrein [15].

Diarrhoea

Diarrhoea is the second most common symptom of the carcinoid syndrome. It is often accompanied by abdominal colicky pains and associated with episodes of flushing. The patient may complain of anything from a small increase in the frequency of passing stools to passing more than 20 watery or semi-solid stools per day. It its severest form, defaecation may be explosive and borborygmi very loud. In some patients, usually early in the disease, diarrhoea may be episodic, perhaps occurring for a day or two, followed by normal bowel function for days or even weeks. The diarrhoea is often worse soon after awakening. The cause of the diarrhoea may be excess 5-hydroxytryptamine, since this symptom is often treated successfully by methysergide, a 5-hydroxytryptamine antagonist.

Diarrhoea and the intestinal hypermotility seen in the carcinoid syndrome may result in malabsorption. This is, however, found in only a few patients with diarrhoea and may improve following treatment with methysergide. In our experience, malabsorption is seen only in patients who have undergone extensive small bowel resection.

Heart Lesions

Right heart failure may be found in the carcinoid syndrome. This feature can be difficult to diagnose, since the liver may be enlarged and tender due to secondary deposits, and peripheral oedema may reflect hypoalbuminaemia. The jugular venous pulse is thus of critical diagnostic importance, and on auscultation a systolic murmur may be heard. The two most common cardiac abnormalities are tricuspid incompetence and pulmonary stenosis. The left-side heart valves are rarely affected.

The heart failure usually responds to diuretic treatment, but the success of either medical or surgical treatment depends partly on the extent of any underlying coronary artery disease.

In rare cases, secondary deposits of carcinoid tumour may be found in the heart. We have a case in which a carcinoid secondary deposit was found in the left ventricle during an operation to replace an aortic valve.

Bronchial Asthma

Asthma has been reported in up to 20% of cases of the carcinoid syndrome, although Grahame-Smith [10] reports a prevalence of 10%. Wheezing may accompany flushing. Bronchial asthma was rare in our patients.

Other Clinical Features

During a carcinoid flush there is often tachycardia, a decrease in systolic blood pressure, lacrimation, and sensations of heat and sometimes anxiety. The facial flush may become permanent, leaving the patient with facial cyanosis and telangiectasia.

Nicotinic acid production is much decreased in patients with the carcinoid syndrome, since the metabolism of dietary tryptophan is diverted down the metabolic pathway that results in the formation of 5-hydroxytryptamine. Pellagra may develop and accompany the mental changes seen occasionally in the carcinoid syndrome. These changes are typically depression, excitability, and confusion.

Renal failure is a rare complication due to ureteric obstruction caused by retroperitoneal fibrosis.

Treatment

The aims of treatment are listed in Table 5.

Table 5. Treatment of carcinoid tumours – aims of therapy

- To resect the primary tumour
- To reduce tumour mass
- To inhibit the synthesis, prevent the release or block the action of pharmacologically active tumour products
- To prevent the development or the progression of the remote effects of the tumour
- To treat dietary deficiencies resulting from the presence of the tumour

Surgical Treatment

The first aim is to overcome any obstruction caused by the tumour. This means resection of the primary tumour and any loops of small bowel involved in the tumour mass. In some cases, a right hemicolectomy has to be performed.

When tumour is present outside the gut, as much tumour as possible should be removed. This includes mesenteric and para-aortic lymph nodes infiltrated with tumour and hepatic secondary deposits. The latter grow slowly and have a false 'capsule' of normal liver tissue surrounding them. The deposits can easily be removed after the liver capsule has been opened. Occasionally, the hepatic spread is in the form of large deposits which may be removed piecemeal. In cases in which multiple deposits are present, partial resection of the liver can be of benefit [32].

Surgical treatment may extend beyond the removal of the primary tumour and secondary deposits. The secondary deposits in the liver receive their blood supply from the hepatic artery. Interruption of their arterial supply results in tumour necrosis, and the 2 procedures that have been used are hepatic artery ligation and hepatic arterial embolization. These methods are possible because the liver has a dual blood supply which protects the normal tissue from ischaemic damage and infarction when the tumour arterial supply is interrupted.

Hepatic Artery Ligation

This procedure is used to treat patients with widespread hepatic tumour deposits but has largely been superseded by hepatic arterial embolization. Ligation of the hepatic artery may be preceded by cholecystectomy.

Hepatic Artery Embolization

In 1977 Allison and colleagues [1] reported an amelioration of symptoms following hepatic artery embolization in two patients with the carcinoid syndrome. In two subsequent articles this group described the use of the therapy in more detail [2, 17]. The procedure consists of the following parts: (1) the prevention of complications resulting from the release of tumour products by pretreatment with drugs that block serotonin synthesis and release; (2) the prophylactic use of antimicrobials, steroids, and aprotinin started on the day of the procedure; (3) angiography to determine the extent of hepatic tumour deposits and the patency of the portal vein; (4) if the portal vein is patent, selective catheterization of the hepatic arterial supply and selective embolization of the tumour vasculature with absorbable gelatin sponge or human dura mater. The extent of embolization is demonstrated by further angiography; (5) careful post-embolization monitoring with continuation of antimicrobials and serotonin antagonists for at least 5 days; and (6) assessment of the success of the procedure from the patient's symptoms and biochemical estimations.

Following embolization there is a fever and leucocytosis which, in the absence of infection, is most probably due to tissue necrosis. The liver enzyme activities in serum rise, as does the urinary excretion of 5-hydroxyindoleacetic acid. After a few days all these return to normal.

Embolization may be complicated by septicaemia, liver abscess, abdominal pain, pleural effusion, and encephalopathy. Maton et al. [17] concluded that it was the treatment of choice for patients with severe symptoms of carcinoid syndrome that did not respond to drug therapy. Our experience is less extensive, but we have found that it is possible to induce profound remission of symptoms using this procedure.

Surgical Treatment of Remote Effects of Tumour

Surgical treatment is occasionally helpful when the tumour has caused remote effects. For example, the fibrosis that can occur as part of the carcinoid syndrome may give rise to lesions that can be treated surgically. Fibrosis around the small bowel can cause obstruction that requires resection, and we have also managed cases in which dense retroperitoneal fibrosis has obstructed the ureters at the pelvic brim. In one case the ureters were freed by dissecting them from the fibrous tissue.

The fibrosis of the right-side heart valves can be so severe as to necessitate valve replacement. This is unusual; in our experience a limiting factor in such cases is the occurrence of extensive coronary artery disease, shown by angiography.

Drug Therapy

The drug therapy of carcinoid tumours and the carcinoid syndrome is best considered in relation to the synthesis, release, and action of pharmacologically active tumour products [10].

We have found that the symptoms of flushing alone or diarrhoea and flushing can be controlled in most patients with a combination of cyproheptadine and codeine phosphate. The dose of codeine phosphate required to control the stool frequency may be high. In cases in which the diarrhoea is difficult to control, parachlorophenylalanine in doses of up to 4 g/day can be tried. In one case however, we found this drug to block the flushing without affecting the stool frequency [4], and it can cause myalgia and depression.

Cytotoxic chemotherapy has been used in patients with widespread tumour. Some patients respond favourably, as judged by a decrease in tumour mass and liver size and a lowered 5-hydroxyindoleacetic acid excretion [14, 18, 23]. Infusion chemotherapy has been used either prior to hepatic artery ligation or as a systemic treatment [24, 30]. Our experience with this form of therapy is limited, as we have favoured hepatic artery embolization in cases in which other drug therapy has failed.

Table 6. Prognosis of carcinoid tumours. The data are taken from Godwin [8]. The figures in brackets are from Anderson and Wilson [3], Thompson et al.: [28] and Marks [16]

Primary Site	Prognosis as %, 5-year survival
Stomach	52
Small bowel	54 (47–62 with hepatic 2°)
Appendix	(99)
Colon	52
Rectum and rectosigmoid	83 (89)
Lung and bronchi	82

Harris and Smith [11] reported tumour regression in two patients treated with cyproheptadine alone. The mechanism is not clear, and the authors report that a further five patients did not show an objective response. These observations need to be extended.

The introduction of the long-acting somatostatin analogue Sandostatin® has provided a drug which offers the chance of long-term remission of symptoms in patients with the carcinoid syndrome [13]. This compound is the subject of subsequent papers in this book.

Prognosis

The prognosis in carcinoid disease is very variable and it is therefore difficult to predict for an individual patient. The rate of growth of the primary tumours and their metastases is frequently slow, and we have seen patients who survived up to 15 and 30 years from diagnosis.

Table 6 shows the prognosis for carcinoid tumours at various primary sites. The data are taken from the literature and it is important to note that long-term survival is possible in cases where there is extensive spread of tumour. Our figures for small bowel and large bowel tumours are in close agreement with those listed in Table 6.

Acknowledgements: The authors are indebted to the Trent Regional Health Authority Cancer Registration Bureau, who provided the tumour incidence data. We also thank the physicians and surgeons who referred cases. The collection and collation of data was made possible by a grant from the Willie Handley Cancer Research Fund of the University of Sheffield.

References

1. Allison, D. J. et al.: Treatment of carcinoid liver metastases by hepatic artery embolisation. Lancet *2*:1323, 1977
2. Allison, D. J. et al.: Therapeutic embolisation of the hepatic artery: A review of 75 procedures. Lancet *1*:595, 1985
3. Anderson, J. R., Wilson, B. G.: Carcinoid tumours of the appendix. Br J Surg *72*:545, 1985
4. Bax, N. D. S. et al.: Clinical and biochemical effects of parachlorophenylalanine in a patient with the carcinoid syndrome. Postgrad Med J *58*:493, 1982
5. Björck, G. et al.: Unusual cyanosis in a boy with congenital pulmonary stenosis and tricuspid insufficiency. Fatal outcome after angiocardiography. Am Heart J *44*:143, 1952
6. Cassidy, M. A.: Abdominal carcinomatosis with probable adrenal involvement. Proc R Soc Med *24*:139, 1930
7. Cassidy, M. A.: Post mortem findings in case shown on October 10th 1930 as one of abdominal carcinomatosis with probable adrenal involvement. Proc R Soc Med *24*:920, 1931
8. Godwin, D. J.: Carcinoid tumours. Cancer *36*:560, 1975
9. Goedert, M. et al.: Dopamine, norepinephrine and serotonin production by an intestinal carcinoid tumour. Cancer *45*:104, 1980
10. Grahame-Smith, D. G.: The carcinoid syndrome. Am J Cardiol *21*:376, 1968
11. Harris, A. L., Smith J. E.: Regression of carcinoid tumour with cyproheptadine. Br Med J *285*:475, 1982
12. Isler, P., Hedinger, C.: Meastasierendes Dünndarmcarcinoid mit schweren vorwiegend das rechte Herz betreffenden Klappenfehlern und Pulmonalstenosen, ein eigenartiger Symptomenkomplex. Schweiz Med Wochenschr *83*:4, 1953
13. Kvols, L. K. et al.: Treatment of the malignant carcinoid syndrome. N Engl J Med *315*:613, 1986
14. Legha, S. S. et al.: Chemotherapy for metastatic carcinoid tumours. Experience with 32 patients and a review of the literature. Cancer Treat Rep *61*:1699, 1977
15. Levine, R. J., Sjoerdsma, A.: Pressor amines and the carcinoid flush. Ann Intern Med *58*:818, 1963
16. Marks, C.: Carcinoid Tumours – A Clinicopathologic Study. Hall, Boston, 1979
17. Maton, P. L. et al.: Role of hepatic arterial embolisation in the carcinoid syndrome. Br Med J *287*:932, 1983
18. Mengel, C. E.: Therapy of the malignant carcinoid syndrome. Ann Intern Med *62*:587, 1965
19. Millman, S.: Tricuspid stenosis and pulmonary stenosis complicating carcinoma of the intestine with metastases to liver. Am Heart J *25*:391, 1943
20. Moertel, C. G. et al.: Multiple primary malignant neoplasms, part I. Cancer *14*:221, 1961
21. Moertel, C. G. et al.: Multiple primary malignant neoplasms, part II. Cancer *14*:231, 1961
22. Moertel, C. G. et al.: Multiple primary malignant neoplasms, part III. Cancer *14*:238, 1961
23. Moertel, C. G. et al.: Phase II study of streptozotocin (NSC-85998) in the treatment of advanced gastrointestinal cancer. Cancer Chemother Rep *55*:303, 1971
24. Murray-Lyon, I. M. et al.: Treatment of secondary hepatic tumours by ligation of hepatic artery and infusion of cytotoxic drugs. Lancet *2*:172, 1970
25. Pearse, A. G. E., Welbourn, R. B.: The apudomas. Br J Hosp Med *10*:617, 1973
26. Rosenbaum, F. F. et al.: Essential telangiectasia, pulmonic and tricuspid stenosis and neoplastic liver disease. A possible new clinical syndrome. J Lab Clin Med *42*:941, 1953
27. Sanders, R. J., Axtell, H. K.: Carcinoids of the gastrointestinal tract. Surg Gynecol Obstet *119*:369, 1964
28. Thompson, G. B. et al.: Carcinoid tumours of the gastrointestinal tract: Presentation, management, and prognosis. Surgery *98*: 1054, 1985
29. Thorson, A. H.: Studies on carcinoid disease. Acta Med Scand *161* [Suppl 334]:1, 1958
30. Watkins, E. Jr. et al.: Surgical basis for arterial infusion chemotherapy of disseminated carcinoma of the liver. Surg Gynecol Obstet *130*:581, 1976
31. Woods, H. F. et al.: Small bowel carcinoid tumours. World J Surg *9*:921, 1985
32. Zeegen, R. et al.: Massive hepatic resection for the carcinoid syndrome. Gut *10*:617, 1969

4. Tumors of the Gastroenteropancreatic Axis

T. S. Gaginella, T. M. O'Dorisio, H. S. Mekhjian, M. S. O'Dorisio, E. A. Woltering

The Ohio State University, College of Medicine, Columbus, Ohio, USA

VIPomas (VIP: vasoactive intestinal peptide), gastrinomas, glucagonomas, insulinomas and GRFomas (GRF: growth hormone releasing factor) comprise the tumors of the gastroenteropancreatic (GEP) system. Patients with mixed pancreatic endocrine tumors usually present with symptoms characteristic of only one peptide, for example, hypoglycemia due to insulinoma. Although controversy exists over the exact site of origin of GEP endocrine cells and the etiology of the tumors, the APUD (amine precursor uptake and decarboxylation) cell concept of Pearse [99] provides a framework for understanding how endocrine tumor cells might produce multiple peptides [91]. In cases of 'non-functional' endocrine tumors, peptides with less well-defined pathophysiologic functions (e.g. pancreatic polypeptide) may be secreted.

Endocrine tumor cells may produce peptides that are the natural products of a given cell type (e.g. gastrin by gastrinomas, insulin by insulinomas), or they may produce peptides foreign to the cells that constitute the tumor. These peptides usually originate from different cell lines within the same tumor or from one cell capable of producing several different hormones. For example, some gastrinomas are associated with elevated plasma levels of glucagon, insulin and somatostatin [92]. To avoid ambiguity, tumors of the GEP axis should be described by their most prominent secretory product, not by their most prevalent cell type.

VIPoma

Zollinger and Ellison contributed greatly to gut endocrinology with their report of two patients with gastric hypersecretion, diarrhea and jejunal ulceration [143]. Subsequently it was noted that certain patients with non-beta-cell tumors and severe diarrhea did not fit the criteria for diagnosis of gastrinoma [103, 129]. Further studies suggested an association between achlorhydria, watery diarrhea and non-beta-cell pancreatic tumors [87]. The latter syndrome, now thought to arise primarily from the excessive production and release of vasoactive intestinal peptide (VIP), was originally termed 'pancreatic cholera', and later WDHA (watery diarrhea, hypokalemia, achlorhydria) syndrome [74]. Over the last 20 years the association between pancreatic tumors and watery diarrhea has been confirmed [9, 63, 129].

Incidence

According to the register for endocrine tumors of the GEP system established in 1978 in Northern Ireland [16], VIPomas account for 2% of all GEP tumors encountered through 1983. All of the patients with VIPomas had elevated levels of VIP.

Pathophysiology

Several different endocrine tumors are associated with high tissue and/or plasma levels of VIP. These include neuroblastoma, ganglioneuroma, bronchogenic carcinoma and phenochromocytoma (Table 1). Some islet- and non-islet-cell tumors may secrete additional peptides that contribute to the watery diarrhea, but VIP is the primary candidate for mediating the clinically observed manifestations of the syndrome [60, 85, 90]. Indeed, VIP infusion can reproduce the signs

Table 1. Tumors associated with elevated VIP levels. (Modified from [36])

Tumor type
Ovarian-uterine adnexa
Islet cell adenoma or hyperplasia
Neuroblastoma
Ganglioneuroma
Pheochromocytoma
Medullary thyroid carcinoma
Bronchogenic carcinoma
Mastocytoma

and symptoms of the watery diarrhea syndrome (WDS) (Table 2).

The precise cell type and origin of VIPomas, which are predominantly located in the pancreas, is not known. Special silver-staining suggests that the cells producing the VIP are derived from APUD stem cells [121]. VIP-staining nerve endings and APUD cells are found in VIP-secreting pheochromocytomas, ganglioneuroblastomas and neuroblastomas [121].

Ingestion of fat, glucose or amino acids does not release VIP into the circulation. Portal vein concentrations of VIP increase, however, after vagal stimulation in pigs [117]. Neural stimulation evokes VIP release from the enteric nerves of the rabbit small intestine [39] and the vagal branches to the rat stomach [100]. In addition, VIP is released from brain synaptosomes by membrane depolarization with potassium [43]. Although VIP may serve physiologically as a neuromodulator, it is unknown whether such an action is of significance in the pathophysiology of VIP-induced electrolyte secretion.

Although questions had been raised regarding whether or not VIP is the causative agent of WDS or merely a marker of the disorder [42], part of the confusion revolved around incomplete knowledge regarding the duration of action of VIP and the plasma levels necessary to evoke the watery diarrhea. Indeed, exogenous VIP administration for two hours in pigs did not mimic the pathophysiology characteristic of patients with WDS. However, when VIP was infused chronically (up to 10 h) in pigs [85], and man [60], VIP levels within the range of those reported in patients with VIP-secreting tumors were achieved and watery diarrhea with flushing was observed. In the normal subjects, as in patients with WDS, there were significant increases in sodium and bicarbonate loss in the feces and no evidence of carbohydrate or fat malabsorption [60]. VIPomas are thought to secrete VIP episodically and, in contrast to gastrinoma (in which gastrin release can be induced by stimuli such as secretin), provocative release of VIP from a tumor has not been reported.

Whether or not VIP plays a role physiologically as a modulator of intestinal water and electrolyte transport or serves only as a pathophysiologic humoral mediator is still not precisely understood. The association of VIP with neural elements in the mucosa and submucosa [36, 38, 121] and the presence of VIP receptors on epithelial cells [1, 36] suggests that it may indeed be physiologically relevant. A number of in vitro and in vivo studies have demonstrated that VIP can induce active serosal-to-mucosal chloride secretion. Intravenous infusion of VIP (13 mg/min) for 15 min induced net secretion in the dog jejunum and ileum [3]. Intraarterial infusion (0.08 μg/kg/min) of VIP also promptly reverses net water and electrolyte absorption to secretion in the canine jejunum [64]. In this model the effects of VIP were readily reversible upon removal of the peptide from the circulation. Mailman [72] demonstrated that VIP induced sodium and water secretion into the canine ileum after intravenous infusion at a rate of 10.5 μg/kg/h. Interestingly, he found that atropine blocked the effect of VIP, suggesting that VIP may release acetylcholine, itself a secre-

Table 2. Effects of VIP consistent with signs and symptoms of watery diarrhea syndrome. (Modified from [36])

Symptom	Comment
Secretory diarrhea	Alkaline isotonic; > 500 ml/day
Hypokalemia	K^+ loss in stool
Hypochlorhydria (rarely achlorhydria)	Inhibition of gastric secretion
Hyperglycemia	Glycogenolysis
Flushing	Vasodilation
Atonic gall bladder	Muscle relaxation

tagogue [15, 52]. We found that intravenous infusion of 14.3 μg/kg/h of VIP reversed rat colonic absorption to secretion and reduced ileal absorption by 73%: the effect was reversible upon cessation of VIP infusion [141]. These effects of VIP can be antagonized by angiotensin II and norepinephrine [106].

The mechanism of VIP action on electrolyte transport has been studied to some extent in vitro. The peptide causes colonic electrolyte secretion in the rat and rabbit [18, 104, 118, 133]. In the rabbit ileum, the response to VIP (6×10^{-7} mole) was immediate and associated with increases in intracellular 3′,5′-cyclic adenosine monophosphate (cAMP) production. Human ileal tissue responded in a manner similar to that of the rabbit [118]. Whether the effect of cAMP is due to inhibition of the entry of sodium chloride into mucosal cells or to chloride secretion from crypt cells to the lumen has not been clearly established. In either case, chloride, sodium and water accumulate on the lumenal side of the mucosa and would lead to diarrhea. Thus the fluid accumulation may result from excessive secretion in the small intestine, producing fluid in volume greater than the absorptive capacity (approximately 6 l) of the colon [22]. An effect of VIP directly on the colon would also lead to net secretion and excess water in the stool.

Somatostatin inhibits the action of VIP in vitro [18, 24] and in vivo [25]. This effect is thought to be due to inhibition of adenylate cyclase or the action of cAMP at the epithelial cell level [94].

Finally, although it was initially thought that intestinal motility was not increased in WDS, experimental studies have now demonstrated that intra-arterial or intralumenal administration of VIP can alter intestinal motor function [120]. One can only speculate that this effect may contribute to the diarrhea observed in patients with VIPoma and WDS.

Signs and Symptoms

Perhaps the most consistent clinical observation in VIPomas is severe watery diarrhea and hypokalemia. As the tumor grows, the diarrhea becomes more continuous, whereas in the early stages it tends to be episodic and intermittent. The profound hypokalemia is due to loss of potassium in the stool, partly the result of active secretion by the colon [34]; this can amount to as much as 300 mol/l of potassium loss in the stool daily [90]. The potassium loss is further aggravated by secondary hyperaldosteronism resulting from hypovolemia [68]. VIP also stimulates renin secretion by a direct mechanism, contributing to the hypokalemia by stimulating the release of aldosterone [102].

Flushing is seen in roughly 20% of the patients with WDS [11, 90, 129], presumably mediated by VIP [26]. The most pronounced flushing occurs in the head and trunk region and is characterized by erythematous, patchy and sometimes urticarial lesions. Tachyphylaxis occurs to the flushing effect produced by VIP [26, 85], possibly explaining the low (20%) incidence of this symptom in patients with WDS.

Hypochlorhydria, but rarely achlorhydria, is observed in about 80% of patients with WDS [91]. VIP is a relatively weak inhibitor of pentagastrin-stimulated gastric secretion in man [50]. However, essentially all of the peptides which have been measured in elevated levels in the plasma of patients with WDS are also inhibitors of gastric acid secretion. Hypercalcemia is observed in some patients with VIPomas and may be due to enhanced osteolytic activity of VIP [8], or it may be related to factors secondary to the diarrhea. The incidence of hypercalcemia is reported to be from 25 to 75% in patients with WDS [90]. Tetany is also sometimes associated with the syndrome and may be due to hypomagnesemia secondary to the diarrhea. Some patients (20–50%) develop hyperglycemia. This may be due to hepatic glycogenolytic activity of VIP [44]. The hyperglycemia is probably enhanced by hypokalemia, which blunts insulin release.

Laboratory Tests and Diagnosis

A powerful tool in making the diagnosis of VIPoma is a sensitive and specific VIP radioimmunoassay. Normal plasma VIP concentrations are between 0 and 190 pg/ml [8, 113]. In our laboratory the range of normal VIP levels in fasting plasma samples is 0 to 170 pg/ml [88]. Although it is important to obtain measurements of VIP levels in individuals suspected of having WDS, a single plasma VIP level is of very limited usefulness. It is possible that, between episodes of watery diarrhea, the VIPoma may not be secreting VIP, thus creating a false impression of the potential role of VIP. Since the clinician is faced with the difficult decision whether or not to have the patient explored surgically, the diagnosis should be based on the measurement of plasma samples obtained at various times, especially those during which the patient may be experiencing the severest symptoms. In a group of 2900 samples we screened for plasma VIP, 88% fell below our limit of detection (50 pg/ml of plasma). In our series, 29 patients were found to have elevated levels of VIP in their plasma and they were later documented at surgery to have VIPomas [90]. Their mean VIP value was 956 $\pm$ 285 pg/ml; the lowest level was 225 pg/ml. Four of the patients had VIPomas without metastases at the time of surgery; 16 had gross metastases, most frequently to the liver. We noted 8 VIP-secreting ganglioneuroblastomas-pheochromocytomas with watery diarrhea in our series; six of these were children less than five years old with ganglioneuroma or ganglioneuroblastoma.

The main clinical criteria for the diagnosis of VIPoma are the establishment of secretory diarrhea, identification of VIP as the secretagogue and localization of the tumor. Secretory diarrhea is defined as fecal water loss usually greater than one 1 l/day; the stool is isotonic with plasma. The osmolality of the stool can be calculated as the sum of stool sodium and potassium concentrations multiplied by two. The diarrhea in WDS is often nocturnal and, as in cholera, it persists after fasting up to 72 h. After a diagnosis of chronic secretory diarrhea is established, a variety of causes, including chronic laxative abuse and pseudopancreatic cholera must be excluded [8, 107, 108].

Differentiation of Zollinger-Ellison syndrome from VIPoma may sometimes be difficult to make on clinical grounds alone. The measurement of gastric acid secretion is then crucial in providing diagnostic clues, since gastric acid hypersecretion is virtually always present with Zollinger-Ellison syndrome; in VIPoma, acid secretion is inhibited and gastric volume will usually be normal. Abdominal pain is a prominent feature of Zollinger-Ellison syndrome, but is an infrequent initial presenting complaint in WDS. Metabolic acidosis is not seen in Zollinger-Ellison syndrome, but is frequently associated with WDS. In addition, plasma levels of gastrin are elevated in gastrinoma, whereas VIP is generally elevated in patients with WDS.

A variety of diagnostic procedures such as abdominal ultrasonography [119], computerized tomography [86], and angiography [46] are sometimes useful in identifying the size of pancreatic tumors. WDS is occasionally associated with pancreatic hyperplasia that can escape detection by these diagnostic procedures [90].

Management and Treatment

It is essential that the first line of treatment be directed at correcting the severe fluid and electrolyte imbalance and the metabolic acidosis. It may be necessary to support the patient with intravenous fluids and, when possible, to supplement them with an oral glucose-electrolyte solution. Such solutions tend to reduce the net fluid and electrolyte loss from the intestine by stimulating jejunal water absorption. Obviously the route of administration and the magnitude of replacement required will depend on the condition of the individual patient. A number of different drugs have been used in an attempt to inhibit or reverse the secretion [90]. Prednisone, 60–80 mg (or equivalent dose of another glucocorticoid) sometimes controls initial episodes of diarrhea in VIPoma [67]. The mechanism of this effect is not understood, but it may involve a direct enhancement of sodium absorption in the small or large intestine. This is speculation based upon experimental work demonstrating that methylprednisolone induced Na/K-ATPase and reversed cholera toxin-induced intestinal secretion [19]. It may also be that steroids inhibit the release of VIP from the tumor [93].

Other pharmacologic agents that reduce experimentally induced intestinal secretion include alpha-2 adrenergic agonists (e.g. clonidine), indomethacin, lithium carbonate, somatostatin, phenylthiazines and propranolol [90, 101]. Of these agents, indomethacin [54], lithium carbonate [97] and trifluoroperazine [27] have been demonstrated to be beneficial in treating WDS. Somatostatin is potent in experimental systems but is difficult to use in man because of its short half-life. Recently, however, an analog of somatostatin, octreotide (Sandostatin®) has shown great promise as therapy for VIPoma. Subcutaneous injection of this drug produces a long-lasting inhibition of the diarrhea associated with this and other GEP tumors and diarrheas of other etiologies [37, 116]. At this writing Sandostatin® is available on a compassionate need basis. However, it will undoubtedly become a first-line weapon in the treatment of WDS.

The most effective and definitive means of treating VIPoma is surgery. After a diagnosis has been established, patients should be surgically explored. In most cases the tumor will be found to be present in the distal two-thirds of the pancreas. In approximately 80% of the patients discrete tumors are reported. Because it is believed that approximately 50% of VIPomas are benign, they are potentially resectable. Removal of ganglioneuroblastomas is curative in about 70% of children subjected to surgery for VIP-secreting tumors [69]. More studies are required before total pancreatic resection in suspected VIPoma can be recommended. On the basis of current data it is our opinion that blind total pancreatectomy is not justifiable. Chemotherapy, after surgical debulking, is recommended. Streptozotocin and 5-FU and chlorozotocin are reported to produce a 60 to 70% response rate, associated with normalization of plasma VIP levels and disappearance of diarrhea [58].

Gastrinoma (Zollinger-Ellison Syndrome)

A syndrome of excessive gastric acid secretion, diarrhea and primary jejunal ulceration was described in 1955 by Zollinger and Ellison [143]. This classic report stimulated a new awareness in endocrinologists and gastroenterologists of the role and relevance of peptides in gastrointestinal diseases. Although the mediator of the pathophysiology was not identified in the first two patients described, the authors were aware that this non-beta cell tumor elaborated a potent ulcerogenic factor. Within about 12 years biochemical studies demonstrated that gastrin was produced in large quantities by these tumors and was probably responsible for the gastric hypersecretion and ulceration [47]. Bioassay for quantification of gastrin was replaced by radioimmunoassay for determining plasma and tissue levels of gastrin [81]. RIA is much more specific and sensitive for detecting gastrin, and has been used to establish unequivocally elevated gastrin levels in the sera of patients with Zollinger-Ellison syndrome (ZES). Although for many years the primary approach to ZES was total gastrectomy, the recognition of different patient subgroups in ZES and the advent of newer potent gastric antisecretory drugs has resulted in a more specific therapeutic approach to the disease.

Incidence

Patients from 7 to 90 years of age have been reported with gastrinomas. Most often, however, a diagnosis is made between 30 and 50 years of age [53, 56]. More cases are reported in males [56], although there does not appear to be a clear sex predominance. Abdominal pain is reported in up to 95% of patients with ZES [53, 31] and about 75% are symptomatic for ulcer disease.

In the Belfast study [16] the annual incidence of gastrinomas per 100000 population from 1980 to 1985 was 0.04. Gastrinomas represented 9% of GEP tumors; thus gastrinomas, although much rarer than carcinoids (which represented 55% of the tumors), are still four times more common than VIPomas.

Pathophysiology

Gastrin is produced by the G cells, which are found in highest concentration in the pyloric and antral area of the gastric mucosa and to some extent in the upper small intestine [80]. The hormone exists in several forms, principally G-17, which accounts for about 95%

of gastrin immunoreactivity, and G-34. The primary stimulus for gastrin release is feeding and protein dietary stimulants. Antral distension and vagal stimulation also raise plasma levels of gastrin [134, review], while acidification of the antrum inhibits secretion [136]. Gastrin secretion from gastrinomas can be provoked by the intravenous administration of secretin (a paradoxic phenomenon) or calcium [57].

Most of the immunoreactive gastrin released in response to a test meal in man is G-34, although G-17 is much more potent (approximately 5-fold) than G-34 as a gastric acid secretagogue [137]. Other gastrins, named big gastrin and mini gastrin (gastrin-14) have been characterized but their significance relative to G-17 and G-34 in ZES is unknown. Gastrin also increases the contractility of the gastric antrum and has trophic effects on the gastric mucosa, so that an excess of the hormone in ZES may be associated with gastric hypermotility and mucosal hypertrophy or hyperplasia. This last fact may be potentially important in non-endocrine gut tumor growth (e.g. colonic carcinoma).

Gastric hypersecretion is thought to be the cause of abdominal pain reported in up to 60% of the patients [53, 56]. The excessive amounts of gastric acid in the duodenum can inactivate pancreatic enzymes, leading to steatorrhea, and direct damage to the small bowel mucosa can decrease the absorption of nutrients. Bile salts are precipitated by low intralumenal pH, so that part of the malabsorption of dietary fats is thought to be due to inadequate micelle formation [45]. Diarrhea observed in ZES (6 to 15 stools/day) is due to a combination of the large volume of gastric fluid entering the small intestine, the mucosal damage (which allows solute to accumulate in the lumen), and possibly the formation of hydroxylated fatty acids by the action of colonic bacteria on excess dietary fat. The hydroxy fatty acids can induce fluid secretion by the colon [6, 101].

Signs and Symptoms

As already noted, the most prominent clinical signs and symptoms of ZES upon initial presentation are often those of uncomplicated peptic ulcer disease. Thus, abdominal pain is reported in the majority of cases and approximately 18% of the patients have diarrhea as an initial symptom [91]. During the course of the disease diarrhea occurs in up to 60% of the patients [53, 56]. The actual prevelance of steatorrhea is uncertain but it is a relatively common finding.

Laboratory Tests and Diagnosis

The most valuable laboratory test in ZES is the measurement of plasma gastrin levels by RIA. Serum gastrin levels are generally greater than 200 pg/ml in ZES patients; occasionally they are normal as the result of a day-to-day variation [135] which may be the result of quality control in the laboratory or perhaps of the cyclic nature of gastrin secretion by the tumor. In cases that are, for other reasons, thought to be ZES it is best to sample at different times and on different days. Hypergastrinemia can also occur in renal failure, short-bowel syndrome, hyperparathyroidism, gastric outlet obstruction and antral G-cell hyperplasia [91]. Disorders characterized by hypergastrinemia and normal or low gastric acid secretion include atrophic gastritis, gastric cancer, pernicious anemia, post-vagotomy syndrome and pheochromocytoma; basal gastrin levels also increase with age [82, 91].

Another important laboratory test is the measurement of basal and maximal acid output. It is usually accepted that basal acid output in excess of 15 mmol/l/h in patients without prior acid-reducing gastric surgery is diagnostic for gastrinoma. An overnight (12-h) gastric acid secretion exceeding 1 l occurs in 85% of patients with gastrinoma. Other patients may secrete more than 100 mmol/l free acid during this period [31]. Some patients with ordinary peptic ulcer disease secrete at this rate and 25% of gastrinoma patients do not meet this criterion. A good diagnostic criterion is the ratio of basal to maximal or peak acid output. A ratio greater than 0.6 is suggestive of gastrinoma [111]. This is because basal secretory levels do not increase significantly after the administration of a stimulant of acid secretion since there is already maximal parietal cell activity due to high circulating levels of the tumor gastrin. Care must be exercised with this criterion, since there is substantial overlap of ZES and duodenal ulcer patients in this ratio.

Physical findings in ZES are usually absent, apart from non-specific signs of weight loss, epigastric tenderness, diarrhea and some dehydration. Abdominal palpation is usually not helpful, since the gastrinoma is generally small and difficult to identify even at surgery. Endoscopy is particularly useful for documenting the extent of ulcer disease. The stomach is usually unremarkable in ZES, although gastric ulcer and mucosal erosions sometimes occur. Duodenitis and ulcers of the duodenal bulb and the immediate parabulbar area are observed in approximately 75% of cases [56, 109], and jejunal ulcers are also sometimes observed. Peptic ulcer associated with hyperparathyroidism or multiple endocrine neoplasia, as well as a family history of ulcer disease, should arouse suspicion of a gastrinoma. It is sometimes useful to use glucagon (1 mg i.v.) to reduce hypermotility of the proximal duodenum so that focal abnormalities can be biopsied. A side view endoscope is also helpful in some instances. Although usually localized to the pancreas, the primary tumor may also occur in the gastric mucosa or in the duodenal wall [31, 56, 77, 91].

Provocative tests are also useful in making a diagnosis of ZES. These tests utilize secretin, calcium, bombesin and test meals as stimulants of gastrin release and hypersecretion [23, 65, 83]. Normal subjects and patients with uncomplicated peptic ulcer disease show no change, a slight decrease or slight increase in gastrin responses to secretin [83]. However, those with gastrinoma display a paradoxical increase in serum gastrin after intravenous secretin [83]. It is relevant to note that differences in response can be obtained, depending upon the source of the secretin; highly purified Secretin-Kabi (2 U/kg body weight) should be given i.v. A rise in plasma gastrin of 200 pg/ml or 50% increase above basal gastrin levels within minutes of secretin infusion should be considered a positive response [65, 83]. Although false negative responses are sometimes seen, more than 90% of gastrinoma patients will exhibit an absolute rise in gastrin in the region of 200 pg/ml.

Calcium infusion (15 mg/kg body weight of elemental calcium i.v. over 4 h) induces a 2- to 3-fold rise in serum gastrin and strongly suggests gastrinoma [23]. This test should not be used in patients with primary hyperparathyroidism or those with multiple endocrine neoplasia syndrome. It is less diagnostic than secretin and is frequently associated with false positive and false negative responses as well as adverse reactions [83].

The tetradecapeptide bombesin is a potent stimulant of gastrin secretion [33]. In combination with the calcium test, infusion of bombesin is sometimes helpful in differentiating ZES patients with pancreatic gastrinoma from those with duodenal tumors [4]. This method is, however, not a standard one and results should be interpreted with caution until more cases have verified its reliability.

Responses to a standard meal also differ in ZES as compared with antral G-cell hyperplasia. Individuals with ZES generally exhibit less than a 50% rise in serum gastrin above basal in response to the meal, whereas those with G-cell hyperplasia usually show a greater increase [20, 83, 53].

In summary, diagnosis of ZES should be approached by measuring basal and maximal pentagastrin-stimulated acid secretion, in conjunction with determination by specific RIA of basal as well as stimulated plasma levels of gastrin. These tests should be done in the absence of anticholinergic or H_2-receptor antagonists.

Management

Since the advent of potent H_2-receptor antagonists the clinician has at his disposal not only acute but also long-term management of patients with ZES. Surgical management is not routinely recommended because medical therapy is highly effective and the surgical cure rate is low (approximately 5%) [56, 91]. Certainly, the H_2-receptor antagonists such as cimetidine, ranitidine and famotidine have dramatically improved the medical management of ZES patients. Cimetidine has been used acutely, by intravenous infusion, to reduce the massive gastric secretion and stabilize the patient prior to surgery or other treatment. Up to 15 g/day of cimetidine or 6 g/day of ranitidine, sometimes together with anticholinergic drugs, may be required to control hypersecretion in patients presenting with acute symptoms of ZES [77]. Close monitoring of the patient should be instituted and plasma levels of chloride greater than 100 mmol/l, with plasma pH less than 7.45, should be achieved. Removal of the gastric secretions via nasogastric suction is important to avoid complications of further ulceration and severe esophageal inflammation due to reflux. If more potent gastric antisecretory agents (e.g. proton pump inhibitors such as omeprazole) become available, they may find worthy application in the acute and, possibly the long-term, management of ZES. Another likely candidate for the medical management of gastrinoma is Sandostatin, which acutely lowers serum gastrin levels and gastric acid secretion in patients with proven gastrinoma [32].

Long-term management of ZES involves the maintenance of symptomatic control and the healing of ulcers with pharmacotherapy. Since different individuals will present with different disease patterns, a single management strategy will not always be adequate. However, if patients are titrated with an appropriate dose of H_2-receptor antagonist, with or without anticholinergic therapy, marked or complete symptomatic improvement can occur in up to 90% of the patients [56]. Currently, ranitidine is preferred to cimetidine in the treatment of the hypersecretion associated with gastrinoma, although the only difference between these agents is quantitative, in terms of their potency. Earlier studies utilizing high doses of cimetidine were associated with anti-androgenic side effects (eg. gynecomasty in males), which does not appear to occur with ranitidine, at equipotent doses [35]. Occasionally patients become tolerant or resistant to the antisecretory effects of the H_2-receptor antagonists [77]. Although the reason for this is not understood patients who require a high dose of cimetidine initially usually also require a correspondingly high dose of ranitidine.

The future of the medical control of gastric hypersecretion in gastrinoma is being forged by the development of new drugs with mechanisms of action different from those of the H_2-receptor antagonist. Omeprazole, a benzimidazole analog, irreversibly inhibits the H^+/K^+-ATPase (proton pump) of the gastric parietal cells. This drug has an extremely long duration of action (a single oral dose of 80 mg reduced the basal acid output by 83% for 24 h after the dose [77]). Although this drug shows great promise in the medical therapy of gastrinoma, long-term (two years), high-dose toxicity studies in rats have demonstrated that the animals develop sustained hypergastrinemia (over 2000 pg/ml) associated with gastric carcinoid tumor formation [77]. On the basis of clinical data, omeprazole appears to have little effect on serum gastrin levels in gastrinoma. Another promising therapeutic agent is Sandostatin®. A subcutaneous injection of 200 μg of this drug dramatically inhibited basal acid output to 0.3 mmol/h and reduced serum gastrin levels to 42 pg/ml [12]. The basal acid output returned to normal but serum gastrin was still at the treatment level 12 h after the single injection. The drug did not alter parietal cell mass. The mechanism for the antisecretory effect is not completely understood but probably involves inhibition of parietal cell histamine-stimulated adenylate cyclase and cAMP-dependent protein kinase.

There are a number of situations where surgical intervention in gastrinoma is warranted. These include total gastrectomy to relieve acid peptic disease, excision of a well-defined gastrinoma to effect a 'cure', debulking surgery as palliation and, in highly selected cases, vagotomy as a means of enhancing pharmacotherapy [77]. Most of the surgery for gastrinoma was done before the appearance of the H_2-receptor antagonists and routine RIA of gastrin. It is reasonable to carry out surgical exploration in all patients with ZES who do not have documented metastatic disease, assuming that there are no serious medical contraindications to surgery [56]. Zollinger has followed throughout their lives 40 patients in whom he has performed surgery for gastrinoma, Cushing's syndrome or bacteremia [91].

Glucagonoma

The existence of tumors involving glucagon has been suspected since 1942, and they received increased attention after the identification in 1966 of diabetes associated with a pancreatic tumor and the production of glucagon [79]. Glucagonoma is associated with a characteristic skin rash and necrolytic migratory erythema [122, 139]. Anemia, weight loss, glossitis, venous thrombosis and psychiatric disturbances (depression) are often noted in the syndrome [91, 131].

Pathophysiology

Glucagon shares amino acid homologies with secretin, VIP, gastric inhibitory peptide, phosphohexoseisomerase and growth hormone releasing factor, with which it also shares biological actions. It is produced by the pancreatic alpha cells and its secretion is stimulated by hypoglycemia and certain amino acids. In some cases hyperglucagonemia may result in stimulation by glucagon of intestinal fluid and electrolyte secretion [91]. Although one would expect glucose intolerance, a more definite feature of the syndrome is hypoaminoacidemia. Plasma levels of amino acids are low and may contribute to the pathogenesis of the skin rash [51]. Indeed, glucagon counteracts the effects of insulin on glucose and amino acids and its effects are particularly pronounced on glycogenic amino acids. Many patients with glucagonoma have normal blood glucose values in spite of increased glucagon levels; there is no direct relationship between the degree of diabetes and glucagon levels in these patients.

Psychiatric disturbances such as depression are probably not due to a neurological defect, although neuropathy of the lower extremities, optic atrophy and ataxia have been reported in glucagonoma patients who subsequently return to normal upon successful treatment of the glucagonoma [51]. The weight loss and anemia may be related to increased ureagenesis at the expense of the free amino acid pool and inhibition by glucagon of erythropoiesis.

Signs, Symptoms and Diagnosis

The most striking finding in glucagonoma syndrome is the necrolytic skin rash, which is distributed over the perioral and perigenital regions, the fingers, feet and legs. This rash occurs in about 80% of the patients, while diabetes has a prevalence of 80%, anemia 60%, and glossitis 60% [91]. Angular stomatitis, cheilosis and pitting of the nails with onycholysis are also associated with the syndrome. Hypoaminoacidemia is often a feature of the disease and to such an extent that it can be a diagnostic factor. Hyperglucagonemia of up to 1500 pg/ml in the presence of the characteristic rash (with or without hypoaminoacidemia) is usually diagnostic for glucagonoma syndrome. This level of hyperglucagonemia is much higher than that usually observed in patients with diabetes mellitus, acute trauma, cirrhosis, brain injuries, renal failure, Cushing's syndrome or bacteremia [132].

The body and tail of the pancreas are the site of about 70% of glucagonomas, of which 90% are malignant and over 60% have metastases to the liver [91]. Since these tumors are usually more than 2 cm in diameter, selective pancreatic angiograms and CT scanning are useful in confirming their presence. Both sexes appear to be affected with equal frequency.

Treatment

The severity of the dermatosis is reduced upon removal of the glucagonoma. If a diagnosis can be made while the tumor is still localized, surgical resection can be curative [49, 127, 130], but surgical debulking and chemotherapy are often necessary to prolong survival [62, 75] because of the prevalence of metastases [92]. Interestingly, Kahn et al. [59] reported that infusion of somatostatin and related analogs in a patient with glucagonoma produced a depression in glucagon levels, without affecting blood glucose. More recently, Anderson and Bloom [2] used Sandostatin to manage three patients with metastatic glucagonoma. Administration of the drug (50 μg s.c. twice daily) produced symptomatic relief. There was an initial suppression of plasma glucagon and over a one-month period the rash disappeared.

Insulinoma

Insulinomas, when malignant, represent about 10% of all beta-cell tumors of the pancreas [13]. The incidence of benign and neoplastic insulinoma is estimated to be about 1 in 1 000 000/year [14]. In a European evaluation, the annual incidence of insulinomas per 100 000 population (from 1980 to 1985) was 0.09; the percentage of insulinomas encountered up to 1983 was 17% [16]. Patients are usually symptomatic when the tumor exceeds 0.5 g in mass, without metastases. Sixty per cent of insulinomas are found in women and the average age at the time of diagnosis is 45 years; about 1500 cases of insulinoma have been described since 1980 [78].

Pathophysiology

Insulinoma is associated with the abnormal physiology one would expect from an excess of circulating insulin. Thus, hypoglycemia and insulin shock are prominent features. The hypoglycemia has a pronounced effect on the nervous system, leading to neurological changes including confusion, dizziness, visual changes and epilepsy; fainting can occur episodically in 90% or more of the patients [78]. The hypoglycemic episodes in insulinoma usually occur in the fasting state when plasma levels of insulin are elevated above 25 IU/ml.

Signs, Symptoms and Diagnosis

Patients with insulinoma often live for years with subclinical disease and no overt symptoms. As already noted, the signs and symptoms are those of pronounced hypoglycemia, including disorientation, seizures, unconsciousness or coma, and personality changes. Diagnosis is made upon demonstration of fasting hypoglycemia with glucose levels usually below 40 mg/dl and insulin levels above 25 IU/ml. Obesity is present in 15 to 48% of the patients [78] and acutely they may present with sweating, palpitations, tremors and hunger.

Ultrasound and computerized tomography are not very useful in making the diagnosis of insulinoma because 60% of the solitary tumors are less than 2 mm in diameter. A 29 to 90% success rate has been reported with selective arteriographic techniques for pre-operative localization of the tumors [78].

Management and Treatment

Surgical resection is the definitive treatment for insulinoma. However, because of widespread metastases, it is often necessary to combine a surgical approach with chemotherapy such as streptozotocin, 5-FU or dacarbazine. Pre-operative administration of diazoxide may be helpful in controlling the symptoms of hypoglycemia. A trial use of diazoxide prior to surgery may be useful in determining whether the patient will respond to this therapy post-operatively, for it may be necessary to use this or other drugs even after surgery for palliation of the insulinoma. Side effects from the diazoxide, however, include erratic changes in plasma glucose and pedal edema. Parenteral glucagon may also be helpful in acute episodes of hypoglycemia.

The somatostatin analog Sandostatin has been demonstrated to be effective as therapy in pancreatic neoplasia [70, 71, 95]. Significant improvements in peripheral edema, serum electrolytes and ascites were noted in a 61-year-old woman who had been diagnosed ten years earlier as having inoperable insulinoma metastatic to the liver [71]. Hypoglycemic episodes were reduced and CT scans indicated stabilization of the pancreatic and metastatic disease. In another case, involving a 79-year-old woman, subcutaneous injection of 50 µg of Sandostatin twice daily reduced serum insulin levels by about 50%, but serum glucose remained elevated. One dose remained effective for 30 min to 6 h after administration [95]. This new drug shows great promise for palliation of malignant insulinoma.

GRFoma

Pancreatic islet cell tumors are reported to produce growth hormone releasing factor

(GRF) associated with clinical symptoms of excessive growth hormone secretion and acromegaly [5, 17, 126]. These tumors are thought to be as rare as one in 40 000 000 per year.

Signs and Symptoms

The signs and symptoms are those expected from excess growth hormone secretion. Growth hormone levels in excess of 1 to 3 ng/ml, especially if persistent in multiple blood samples and combined with elevated GRF binding are diagnostic. Acromegalics often exhibit a paradoxical increase in serum growth hormone following oral glucose. The most obvious signs are enlargement of the feet and hands and facial changes which include enlargement of the mandible, widening gaps between the teeth, enlargement of the lips and thickening of the skin of the forehead [73]. Peripheral neuropathy and sensory changes in the hands are not uncommon features. Other endocrine abnormalities in GRFoma are galactorrhea, amenorrhea and hypopituitarism.

Management and Treatment

Removal of the source of the GRF will stop the progression of the acromegaly and other manifestations of the syndrome. Surgical excision of the tumor, when identifiable at surgery, is thought to be curative. The changes in bone growth that occurred under stimulation of growth hormone are not reversible. Evidence of the patient's normal status can be obtained by evaluating glucose tolerance and insulin secretion as well as by establishing the absence of other endocrine abnormalities.

Four patients with symptoms thought to be due to GRFoma were evaluated for their response to Sandostatin over a period of up to 18 months. Mean daily dosage was 350 μg, ranging from 200 to 600 μg. Three out of the four patients improved symptomatically and the improvement was associated with a decrease in circulating levels of growth hormone [28].

References

1. Amiranaff B, Laburthe M, Rosselin G: Characterization of specific binding sites for vasoactive intestinal peptide in rat intestinal epithelial cell membrane. Biochem Biophys Acta *627*:215–224, 1980
2. Anderson JV, Bloom SR: Neuroendocrine tumors of the gut: Long-term therapy with the somatostatin analogue SMS 201-995. Scand J Gastroenterol *21*:115–128, 1986
3. Barbezat GO, Grossman M: Intestinal secretion: stimulation by peptides. Science *1874*:422–424, 1971
4. Basso N, Lezche E, Materia A, et al.: Studies with bombesin in the Zollinger-Ellison syndrome. Br J Surg *68*:97–100, 1981
5. Berger G, Trouillas J, Bloch B, et al.: Multihormonal carcinoid tumor of the pancreas, secreting growth hormone-releasing factor as a cause of acromegaly. Cancer *54*:2097–2108, 1984
6. Binder HJ: Fecal fatty acids – mediators of diarrhea? Gastroenterology *65*:847–850, 1973
7. Bloom SR: VIP and watery diarrhea. VI. In: Bloom SR (ed) Gut hormones. Churchill-Livingstone, Edinburgh, pp 583–588, 1978
8. Bloom SR, Polak JM: VIP measurement in distinguishing Verner-Morrison syndrome and pseudo-Verner-Morrison syndrome. Clin Endocrinol *5*:223s–228s, 1976
9. Bloom SR, Polak JM: Vipomas. In: Said SI (ed) Vasoactive intestinal peptides. Raven Press, New York, p 457, 1982
10. Bloom SR, Polak JM, Pearse AGE: Vasoactive intestinal peptide and watery-diarrhea syndrome. Lancet *2*:14–16, 1973
11. Bloom SR, Long RG, Bryant MG, Mitchell SJ, Polak JM: Clinical, biochemical and pathological studies on 62 VIPomas. Gastroenterology *78*:1143, 1980
12. Bonfils S, Ruszniewski P, Costil V, Laucournet H, Vatier J, Rene E, Mignon M: Prolonged treatment of Zollinger-Ellison syndrome by long-acting somatostatin. Lancet March: 554–555, 1986
13. Broder LE, Carter SK: Pancreatic islet cell carcinoma. II. Results of streptozotocin treatment in 52 patients. Ann Intern Med *79:* 108–114, 1973
14. Broughtan TA, Leslie JD, Soto JM, Hermann RE: Pancreatic islet cell tumors. Surgery *90*:671–678, 1986
15. Browning JG, Hardcastle J, Hardcastle PT, Sanford PA: The role of acetylcholine in the regulation of ion transport by rat colon mucosa. J Physiol *272*:737–754, 1977
16. Buchanan KD, Johnston CF, O'Hare M, Ardill J, Shaw C, Collins J, Watson R,

Atkinson A, Hadden DR, Kennedy TL, Sloan JM: Neuroendocrine tumors: A European view. Am J Med *81*:14–27, 1986
17. Caplan RH, Kobb L, Abellera RM, et al.: Cure of acromegaly by operative removal of an islet cell tumor of the pancreas. Am J Med *65*:874–882, 1978
18. Carter RF, Bitar KN, Zfass AM, Makhlouf GM: Inhibition of VIP-stimulated intestinal secretion and cyclic AMP production by somatostatin in the rat. Gastroenterology *73*:726–730, 1978
19. Charney AN, Donowitz M: Prevention and reversal of cholera enterotoxin-induced intestinal secretion by methylprednisolone induction of Na^+-K^+-ATPase. J Clin Invest *57*:1590–1599, 1976
20. Creutzfeldt W, Arnold R, Creutzfeldt C, Track NS: Pathomorphological, biochemical, and diagnostic aspects of gastrinoma (Zollinger-Ellison syndrome). Hum Pathol *6*:47–76, 1975
21. Damgaard-Petersen K, Stage JG: CT scanning in patients with Zollinger-Ellison syndrome and carcinoid syndrome. Scand J Gastroenterol *14*:117–122, 1979
22. Debongnie JC, Phillips SF: Capacity of the human colon to absorb fluid. Gastroenterology *74*:698–703, 1978
23. Deveney CW, Deveney KS, Jaffe BM, et al.: Use of calcium and secretin in the diagnosis of gastrinoma (Zollinger-Ellison syndrome). Ann Intern Med *87*:680–686, 1977
24. Dharmsathaphorn K, Binder JJ, Dobbins JW: Somatostatin stimulates sodium and chloride absorption in the rabbit ileum. Gastroenterology *78*:1559–1565, 1980
25. Dharmsathaphorn K, Sherwin RS, Dobbins JW: Somatostatin inhibits fluid secretion in the rat jejunum. Gastroenterology *78*:1554–1558, 1980
26. Domschke S, Domschke W, Bloom SR, et al.: Vasoactive intestinal peptide in man: Pharmacokinetics, metabolic and circulatory effects. Gut *19*:1409–1453, 1978
27. Donowitz M, Elta G, Bloom SR, et al.: Trifluoroperazine reversal of secretory diarrhea in pancreatic cholera. Ann Intern Med *93*:284–285, 1980
28. Dunne MJ, Elton R, Fletcher T, Hofker P, Shui J: Sandostatin and gastroenteropancreatic endocrine tumors. Therapeutic characteristics. (This volume) 1989
29. Dunnick NR, Doppman JL, Mills SR, McCarthy DM: Computed tomograph detection of non-beta pancreatic islet cell tumors. Radiology *135*:117–120, 1980
30. Ebeid AM, Murray PD, Fische JE: Vasoactive intestinal peptide and the watery diarrhea syndrome. Ann Surg *187*:411–416, 1978
31. Ellison EH, Wilson SD: The Zollinger-Ellison syndrome: Reappraisal and evaluation of 260 registered cases. Ann Surg *160*:512–528, 1964
32. Ellison EC, O'Dorisio TM, Woltering EA, Sparks J, Mekhjian HS, Fromkes JJ, Carey LC: Suppression of gastrin and gastric acid secretion in the Zollinger-Ellison syndrome by long-acting somatostatin (SMS 201-995). Scand J Gastroenterol *21*:206–211, 1986
33. Erspamer V, Melchiorri P: Active polypeptides of the amphibian skin and their synthetic analogue. Pure Appl Chem *35*:463–494, 1973
34. Foster ES, Sandle GI, Hayslett JP, Binder HJ: Cyclic adenosine monophosphate stimulates active potassium secretion in the rat colon. Gastroenterology *84*:324–330, 1983
35. Gaginella TS, Bauman JH: Ranitidine hydrochloride. Drug Intell Clin Pharm *17*: 873–885, 1983
36. Gaginella TS, O'Dorisio TM: Vasoactive intestinal polypeptide. In: Binder HJ (ed) Neuromodulator of intestinal secretion on mechanisms of intestinal secretion. Liss, New York, pp 231–247, 1979
37. Gaginella TS, O'Dorisio TM: Octreotide: Entering the new era of peptidomimetic therapy. Drug Intell Clin Pharm *22*:154–155, 1988
38. Gaginella TS, Mekhjian HS, O'Dorisio TM: Vasoactive intestinal peptide: Quantification by radioimmunoassay in isolated cells, mucosa, and muscle of the hamster intestine. Gastroenterology *74*:718–721, 1978
39. Gaginella TS, O'Dorisio TM, Hubel KH: Release of vasoactive intestinal polypeptide by electrical field stimulation of rabbit ileum. Regul Pept *2*:165–174, 1981
40. Gaginella TS, Hubel KA, O'Dorisio TM: Effects of vasoactive intestinal peptide on intestinal chloride secretion. Ibid ref. 9, pp 211–221, 1982
41. Gaginella TS, Hubel KA, O'Dorisio TM: Vasoactive intestinal polypeptide and intestinal chloride secretion. In: Said I (ed) Vasoactive intestinal peptide. Raven Press, New York, pp 211–222, 1982 (Advances in peptide hormone research series; vol 1)
42. Gardner JD, McCarthy DM: VIP and watery diarrhea I – arguments against VIP being the cause of the watery diarrhea syndrome. In: Bloom SR (ed) Gut hormones. Churchill-Livingstone, Edinburgh, pp 570–573, 1978
43. Giachetti H, Said SI, Reynolds RC, et al.: Vasoactive intestinal polypeptide in brain:

Localization in, and release from isolated nerve terminals. Proc Natl Acad Sci USA *74*:3424–3428, 1977
44. Go VLW, Korinek JK: Effect of vasoactive intestinal polypeptide in man: Pharmacokinetics, metabolic and circulatory effects. Gut *19*:1409–1453, 1982
45. Go VLW, Polez JR, Hofmann AF, et al.: Disturbances in fat digestion induced by acidic jejunal pH due to gastric hypersecretion in man. Gastroenterology *58*:638–646, 1970
46. Gold RP, Black TJ, Rotterdan H, Casarella WJ: Radiologic and pathologic characteristics of the WDHA syndrome. Am J Roentgenol *127*:397–401, 1976
47. Gregory RA, Tracy HJ, French JM, Sircus W: Extraction of a gastrin-like substance from a pancreatic tumor in a case of Zollinger-Ellison syndrome. Lancet *1*:1045–1048, 1960
48. Gregory RA, Grossman MI, Tracy HJ, Bentley PH: Nature of the gastric secretagogue in Zollinger-Ellison tumors. Lancet *2*:543–544, 1967
49. Higgins GA, Recont L, Fischman AB: The glucagonoma syndrome: Surgically curable diabetes. Am J Surg *137*:145–148, 1979
50. Holm-Bentzen M, Schultz A, Fahrenkrug J, et al.: Effects of VIP (vasoactive intestinal polypeptide) on gastric acid secretion in man. Hepatogastroenterology *27*:126, 1980
51. Holst JJ: Glucagon-producing tumors. In: Cohen S, Soloway RD (eds) Contemporary issues in gastroenterology. Churchill-Livingstone, New York, pp 57–84, 1985
52. Isaacs PET, Corbett CL, Riley AK, Hawker PC, Turnberg LA: In vitro behavior of human intestinal mucosa. The influence of acetylcholine on ion transport. J Clin Invest *58*:535–542, 1976
53. Isenberg JI, Walsh JH, Grossman MI: Zollinger-Ellison syndrome. Gastroenterology *65*:140–165, 1973
54. Jaffe BM, Kapen DF, DeSchryver-Kecskemeti K, et al.: Indomethacin-responsive pancreatic cholera. N Engl J Med *297*:817–821, 1977
55. Jansen-Goemont A, Engelhault J: Intractable diarrhea in a boy with vasoactive intestinal peptide-producing ganglioneuroblastoma. Pediatrics *59*:710–716, 1977
56. Jensen RT, et al.: Zollinger-Ellison syndrome: Current concepts and management. Ann Intern Med *98*:59–75, 1983
57. Johnson LR: New aspects of the trophic action of gastrointestinal hormones. Gastroenterology *772*:788–792, 1977
58. Kahn CR, Levy AG, Gardner JD, et al.: Pancreatic Cholera: Beneficial effects of treatment with streptozotocin. N Engl J Med *292*:941–945, 1975
59. Kahn D, Bhatena SJ, Recaset L, Rivier J: Use of somatostatin analogs in a patient with glucagonoma. J Clin Endocrinol Metab *53*:543–560, 1981
60. Kane MG, O'Dorisio TM, Krejs GJ: Production of secretory diarrhea by intravenous infusion of vasoactive intestinal polypeptide. N Engl J Med *390*:1482–1485, 1983
61. Katz MD, Erstad BL, Rose C: Treatment of severe cryptosporidium-related diarrhea with octreotide in a patient with AIDS. Drug Intell Clin Pharm *22*:134–136, 1988
62. Knandekor JD, Oyer D, Miller HJ, et al.: Neurologic involvement in glucagonoma syndrome. Response to combination chemotherapy with 5-fluorouracil and streptozotocin. Cancer *44*:2014–2016, 1979
63. Kraft AR, Tompkins RK, Zollinger R: Recognition and management of the diarrheal syndrome caused by non-beta cell tumors of the pancreas. Am J Surg *119*:163–170, 1970
64. Krejs GJ, Barkley RM, Read NW, Fordtran JS: Intestinal secretion induced by vasoactive intestinal polypeptide. A comparison with cholera toxin in the canine jejunum in vivo. J Clin Invest *61*:1337–1345, 1978
65. Lamers CBH, Van Tongeren JHM: Comparative study of the value of calcium, secretin, and meal stimulated increase in serum gastrin to the diagnosis of the Zollinger-Ellison syndrome. Gut *18*:128–135, 1979
66. Larsson LI: Localization of vasoactive intestinal polypeptide: A critical appraisal. In: Said SE (ed) Vasoactive intestinal peptide. Raven Press, New York, pp 51–63, 1982
67. Lennon JR, Sircus W, Bloom SR, et al.: Investigation and treatment of a recurrent VIPoma. Gut *16*:821–822, 1975
68. Levitan R, Ingelfinger FJ: Effect of d-aldosterone on salt and water absorption from the intact human colon. J Clin Invest *44*: 801–808, 1965
69. Long RG, Bryant MG, Mitchell SJ, et al.: Clinicopathological study of pancreatic and ganglioneuroblastoma tumors secreting vasoactive intestinal polypeptide (Vipomas). Br Med J *282*:1767–1771, 1981
70. Longnecker SM: Somatostatin and octreotide: Literature review and description of therapeutic activity in pancreatic neoplasia. Drug Intell Clin Pharm *22*:99–106, 1988
71. Longnecker SM: Remission of symptoms of chemotherapy-refractory metastatic insulinoma using octreotide. Drug Intell Clin Pharm *22*:136–138, 1988

72. Mailman D: Effects of vasoactive intestinal polypeptide on intestinal absorption and blood flow. J Physiol *279*:121–132, 1978
73. Malarkey WB: The pituitary and hypothalamus. In: Mazzaferri EL (ed) Textbook of endocrinology, 3rd edn. Medical Examination Publishing, New York, pp 25–88, 1985
74. Marks IN, Bank S, Louw JH: Islet cell tumor of the pancreas with reversible watery diarrhea and achlorhydria. Gastroenterology *52*:695–708, 1967
75. Marynick SP, Fagadau WR, Duncan LA: Malignant glucagonoma syndrome: Response to chemotherapy. Ann Intern Med *93*:453–454, 1980
76. Maton PN, O'Dorisio TM, Howe BA, McArthur KE, Howard JM, Cherner JA, Malarkey TB, Collen MJ, Gardner JD, Jensen RT: Effect of long-acting somatostatin analogue (SMS 201-995) in a patient with pancreatic cholera. Med Intell *312*:17–21, 1985
77. McCarthy DM, Jensen RT: Zollinger-Ellison syndrome – current issues. In: Cohen S, Soloway RD (eds) Contemporary issues in gastroenterology, vol 5. Churchill-Livingstone, New York, pp 25–55, 1985
78. McFadden D, Jaffe BM: Surgical approaches to endocrine-producing tumors of the gastrointestinal tract. In: Cohen S, Soloway RD (eds) Contemporary issues in gastroenterology. Churchill-Livingstone, New York, pp 139–157, 1985
79. McGavran MH, Unger RH, Recant L, et al.: A glucagon-secreting alpha-cell carcinoma of the pancreas. N Engl J Med *274*:1408–1413, 1966
80. McGuigan JE: Gastrin mucosal intracellular localization of gastrin by immunofluorescence. Gastroenterology *55*:315–327, 1969
81. McGuigan JE, Trudeau WL: Immunological measurement of elevated levels of gastrin in the serum of patients with pancreatic tumors of the Zollinger-Ellison variety. N Engl J Med *278*:1308–1313, 1968
82. McGuigan JE, Trudeau WL: Serum gastrin concentrations in pernicious anemia. N Engl J Med *282*:358–361, 1970
83. McGuigan JE, Wolfe MM: Secretin injection test in the diagnosis of gastrinoma. Gastroenterology *79*:1324–1331, 1980
84. Mitchell CH, Sinatra FR, Crest FW, Griffin R, Sunshine P: Intractable watery diarrhea, ganglioneuroblastoma, and vasoactive intestinal peptide. J Pediatr *89*:593–595, 1976
85. Modlin IM, Bloom SR, Mitchell SJ: Experimental evidence for vasoactive intestinal peptide as the cause of the watery diarrhea syndrome. Gastroenterology *75*:1051–1054, 1978
86. Moss AA: Computed axial tomographic scanning. In: Slesinger MH, Fordtran JS (eds) Gastrointestinal disease. Pathophysiology, diagnosis, management, 3rd edn. Saunders, Philadelphia, pp 1707–1726, 1983
87. Murray JS, Paton RR, Pope CE II: Pancreatic tumor associated with flushing and diarrhea. Report of a case. N Engl J Med *264*:436–439, 1961
88. O'Dorisio TM: Pathophysiology of VIP. II. In: Bloom SR (ed) Gut hormones. Churchill-Livingstone, Edinburgh, pp 484–487, 1978
89. O'Dorisio TM: VIP and watery diarrhea. In: Bloom SR (ed) Gut hormones. Churchill-Livingstone, Edinburgh, pp 581–585, 1978
90. O'Dorisio TM, Mekhjian HS: VIPoma syndrome. In: Cohen S, Soloway RD (eds) Contemporary issues in gastroenterology. Churchill-Livingstone, Edinburgh, pp 101–116, 1984
91. O'Dorsio TM, O'Dorisio MS: Endocrine tumors of the gastroenteropancreatic (GEP) axis. In: Mazzaferri E (ed) Endocrinology. Medical Examination Publishing, New York, pp 76–81, 1985
92. O'Dorisio TM, Vinik AI: Pancreatic polypeptide and mixed hormone producing tumors of the gastrointestinal tract. In: Cohen S, Soloway RD (eds) Contemporary issues in gastroenterology. Churchill-Livingstone, Edinburgh, pp 117–128, 1984
93. O'Dorisio TM, Woltering EA, Ellison EC, et al.: Suppression of vasoactive intestinal peptide release from a dispersed islet cell tumor by hydrocortisone. Regul Pept *6*:319, 1983
94. O'Dorisio TM, Gaginella TS, Mekhjian HS, Rao B, O'Dorisio MS: Somatostatin and analogs in the treatment of VIPomas. Proc NY Acad Sci *527*:528–535, 1988
95. Osei K, O'Dorisio TM: Malignant insulinoma: Effects of somatostatin analog (Compound 201-995) on serum glucose, growth, and gastro-entero-pancreatic hormones. Ann Intern Med *103*:223–225, 1985
96. Pais SD: Angiographic demonstration of a vasoactive intestinal polypeptide-secreting pheochromocytoma in a patient with WDHA syndrome. Am J Roentgenol *130*: 172–174, 1978
97. Pandol SJ, Korman LY, McCarthy OM, Gardner JD: Beneficial effect of oral lithium carbonate in the treatment of pancreatic cholera syndrome. N Engl J Med *302*:1403–1404, 1980

98. Pearse AGE: Common cytochemical properties of cells producing polypeptide-hormone secretion, with particular reference to calcitonin and the thyroid C-cells. Vet Rec *79*:587–590, 1966
99. Pearse AGE: The APUD concept and hormone production. In: Abe K (ed) Clinics in endocrinology. Saunders, Philadelphia, pp 211–222, 1980
100. Penderson R, O'Dorisio T, Howe B, et al.: Vagal release of IR-VIP and IR-gastrin from the isolated perfused rat stomach. Mol Cell Endocrinol *23*:225–231, 1981
101. Phillips SF, Gaginella TS: Intestinal secretion as a mechanism in diarrheal disease. In: Jerzy GB (ed) Progress in gastroenterology, vol 3. Grune & Stratton, New York, pp 481–504, 1977
102. Porter JP, Ganong WF: Relation of vasoactive intestinal polypeptide to renin secretion. In: Said SI (ed) Vasoactive intestinal peptide. Raven Press, New York, pp 285–297, 1982
103. Priest WM, Alexander MK: Islet-cell tumor of the pancreas with peptic ulceration, diarrhea and hypokalemia. Lancet *2*:1145–1147, 1957
104. Racusen LC, Binder HJ: Alteration of large intestinal electrolyte transport by vasoactive intestinal polypeptide in the rat. Gastroenterology *73*:790–796, 1977
105. Rambaud JC, Modigliani R, Matuchansky C, Bloom S, Said SI, Pessayre D, Bernier JJ: Pancreatic cholera. Gastroenterology *69*:110–122, 1975
106. Rao MB, O'Dorisio TM, George JM, Gaginella TS: Angiotensin II and norepinephrine antagonize the effect of vasoactive intestinal peptide on rat ileum and colon. Peptides *5*:291–294, 1984
107. Read NW, Krejs G, Read MG, et al.: Chronic diarrhea of unknown origin. Gastroenterology *78*:264–271, 1980
108. Read NW, Read MG, Krejs GJ, et al.: A report of five patients with large volume secretory diarrhea but no evidence of endocrine tumor or laxative abuse. Dig Dis Sci *78*:264–271, 1982
109. Regan PT, Malagelada JR: A reappraisal of clinical, roentgenographic, and endoscopic features of the Zollinger-Ellison syndrome. Mayo Clin Proc *53*:19–23, 1978
110. Richter G, Stockmann F, Lembcke B, Conlon JM, Creutzfeldt W: Short-term administration of the somatostatin analogue SMS 201-995 in patients with carcinoid tumors. Scand J Gastroenterol *21*:193–198, 1986
111. Ruppert RD, Greenberger NJ, Beman FM: Gastric secretion in ulcerogenic tumors of the pancreas. Ann Intern Med *67*:808–815, 1967
112. Said SI: Evidence for secretion of vasoactive intestinal peptide by tumors of pancreas, adrenal medulla, thyroid and lung: Support for the unifying APUD concept. Clin Endocrinol *5*:201 s–204 s, 1976
113. Said SI, Faloona GR: Elevated plasma and tissue levels of vasoactive intestinal polypeptide in a watery-diarrhea syndrome due to pancreatic, bronchogenic and other tumors. N Engl J Med *293*:155–160, 1975
114. Said SI, Mutt V: Isolation from porcine intestinal wall of a vasoactive octacosapeptide related to secretin and to glucagon. Eur J Biochem *29*:199–204, 1972
115. Santangelo WC, O'Dorisio TM, Kim JG, Severino G, Krejs GJ: Pancreatic cholera syndrome: effect of a synthetic somatostatin analog on intestinal water and ion transport. Ann Intern Med *103*:363–367, 1985
116. Santangelo WC, O'Dorisio TM, Kim JG, Severino G, Krejs G: VIPoma syndrome: effect of a synthetic somatostatin analogue. Scand J Gastroenterol *21*:187–190, 1986
117. Schaffalitzky de Muckadell OB, Fahrenkrug J, Holst JJ: Release of vasoactive intestinal polypeptide (VIP) by electric stimulation of the vagal nerves. Gastroenterology *72*:373–375, 1977
118. Schwartz CJ, Kimberg DV, Sheerin HE, Field M, Said SI: Vasoactive intestinal peptide stimulation of adenylate cyclase and active electrolyte secretion in intestinal mucosa. J Clin Invest *54*:536–544, 1974
119. Shawker TH, Doppman JL, Dunnick NR, et al.: Ultrasonic investigation of pancreatic islet cell tumors. J Ultrasound Med *1*:193, 1982
120. Snisky CA, Wolfe MM, Martin JL, et al.: Myoelectric effects of vasoactive intestinal peptide on rabbit small intestine. Am J Physiol *244*:G 46–G 51, 1983
121. Solcia E, Capella C, Buffa R, et al.: Histology, histochemistry and ultrastructure of diarrheogenic VIP-secreting tumors (VIPomas). In: Said SI (ed) Vasoactive intestinal peptide. Raven Press, New York, pp 495–602, 1982
122. Sweet RD: A dermatosis specifically associated with a tumor of pancreatic alpha cells. Br J Dermatol *19*:301–308, 1974
123. Swift PGF, Bloom SR, Harris F: Watery diarrhea and ganglioneuroma with secretion of vasoactive intestinal peptide. Arch Dis Child *50*:896–899, 1975
124. Taylor AR, Chulajata D, Jones DH, Withwam JG: Adrenal tumor secreting vasoactive intestinal peptide and noradrenaline. Anesthesia *32*:1012–1016, 1977

125. Thompson JC, Reeder DD, Villar HV, Fender HR: Natural history and experience with diagnosis and treatment of the Zollinger-Ellison syndrome. Surg Gynecol Obstet *140*:721–739, 1975
126. Thorner MO, Perryman RL, Chonin MJ, et al.: Somatotrophic hyperplasia. Successful treatment of acromegaly by removal of a pancreatic islet tumor secreting a growth hormone-releasing factor. J Clin Invest *70*: 965–977, 1982
127. Unger RH, Orci L: Glucagon and the A cell. Physiology and pathophysiology. N Engl J Med *304*:1518–1524, 1981
128. Verner JV, Morrison AB: Islet cell tumor and a syndrome of refractory watery diarrhea and hypokalemia. Am J Med *25*: 374–380, 1958
129. Verner JV, Morrison AB: Endocrine pancreatic islet disease with diarrhea: Report of a case due to diffuse hyperplasia of non beta islet tissue with a review of 54 additional cases. Arch Intern Med *133*:492–500, 1974
130. Villar HV, Johnson DG, Lynch PJ, et al.: Pattern of immunoreactive glucagon in portal, arterial and peripheral plasma before and after removal of glucagonoma. Am J Surg *141*:148–152, 1981
131. Vinik AI, Strodel WE, Lloyd RV, Thompson HW: Unusual gastroenteropancreatic (GEP) tumors and their hormones. In: Thompson NW, Vinik AI (eds) Endocrine surgery update. Grune & Stratton, New York, pp 293–320, 1983
132. Vinik AI, Strodel WE, O'Dorisio TM: Endocrine tumors of the gastroenteropancreatic axis. In: Santern A (ed) Endocrine related tumors. Martinus-Nijhoff, Amsterdam, pp 305–345, 1984
133. Waldman DB, Gardner JD, Zfass AM, Makhlouf GM: Effects of vasoactive intestinal peptide on rat colonic transport and adenylate cyclase activity. Gastroenterology *73*:518–523, 1977
134. Walsh JH: Gastrin. In: Bloom SR, Polak JM (eds) Gut hormones. Churchill-Livingstone, Edinburgh, pp 163–170, 1981
135. Walsh JH, Grossman MI: Gastrin. N Engl J Med *292*:1324–1334, 1975
136. Walsh JH, Richardson CT, Fordtran JS: pH dependence of acid secretion and gastrin release in normal and ulcer subjects. J Clin Invest *55*:462–468, 1975
137. Walsh JH, Isenberg JI, Ansfield J, et al.: Clearance and acid-stimulating action of human big and little gastrins in duodenal ulcer subjects. J Clin Invest *57*:1125–1131, 1976
138. Wesley RR, Vinik AI, O'Dorisio TM, et al.: A new syndrome of symptomatic cutaneous mastocytoma producing vasoactive intestinal polypeptide (VIP). Gastroenterology *82*:963–967, 1982
139. Wilkinson DS: Necrolytic migratory erythemia with carcinoma of the pancreas. Trans St Johns Hosp Dermatol Soc *59*:244–247, 1973
140. Wilson SD, Mathison JA, Schulte WJ, et al.: The role of bioassay in the diagnosis of ulcerogenic tumors. Arch Surg *97*:437–441, 1968
141. Wu ZC, O'Dorisio TM, Cataland S, et al.: Effects of pancreatic polypeptide and vasoactive intestinal polypeptide on rat ileal and colonic water and electrolyte transport in vivo. Dig Dis Sci *24*:625–630, 1979
142. Yalow RS, Berson SA: Radioimmunoassay of gastrin. Gastroenterology *58*:1–14, 1970
143. Zollinger RM, Ellison EH: Primary peptic ulcerations of the jejunum associated with islet cell tumors of the pancreas. Ann Surg *142*:709–723, 1955
144. Zollinger RM, Ellison EL, O'Dorisio TM, Sparks J: Thirty years experience with gastrinoma. World J Surg *8*:552–560, 1984

5. The Use of Sandostatin® in Insulinomas. The Relation Between In Vivo Responses, the Presence of Somatostatin Receptors and the Development of Tachyphylaxis

S. W. J. Lamberts, J.-C. Reubi

Department of Medicine, Erasmus University, Rotterdam, The Netherlands, and Sandoz Research Institute, Berne, Switzerland

Introduction

Patients with insulin-secreting islet cell tumors are at risk for severe, protracted hypoglycemia. Surgical removal of the tumor is the treatment of choice. During the diagnostic work up, medical treatment for hypoglycemia is often mandatory, while adequate protection against hypoglycemia during operation is sometimes difficult to achieve. In cases of malignant (metastatic) insulinomas, curative surgery is, in most instances, not possible, necessitating additional (medical) therapy to protect these patients from damage caused by hypoglycemic attacks.

After it had been shown that natural somatostatin suppresses normal insulin secretion [1], conflicting reports have appeared in the literature on the effect of somatostatin on insulin secretion in patients with insulinomas [3, 7]. Given the short half-life of natural somatostatin, the hormone has to be administered by continuous intravenous infusion in order to control hypoglycemia effectively, while post-infusion rebound hypersecretion of insulin and the ensuing hypoglycemia is a major risk.

We investigated a) the acute effects of a single 50 µg dose and of repeated administration of Sandostatin® (octreotide) in insulinoma patients, b) the role of the presence and the type of somatostatin receptors on endocrine pancreatic tumors, and c) the possible mechanism of escape from therapy. Part of these results have been reported previously [6, 10, 11].

The Acute Effects of Sandostatin®

In our first two insulinoma patients, a single subcutaneously administered dose of 50 µg Sandostatin suppressed circulating insulin levels by more than 50% and increased plasma glucose levels for 6–8 h after the injection [see also 11]. No undesirable effects after administration were observed. As opposed to insulin suppression obtained with native somatostatin, no rebound increase in insulin levels was observed after administration of the analogue. In a third patient, no inhibitory effect of the analogue on insulin secretion could be measured, but glucose levels increased significantly between 2 and 4 h after drug administration, compared with the levels on a control day.

Two of these patients were treated for up to 5 days with two or three daily subcutaneous injections of Sandostatin (daily dose ranging from 100 to 300 µg). During this time glucose concentrations were slightly increased over pretreatment levels, while no hypoglycemic attacks occurred.

In a fourth patient with a metastatic insulinoma 50 µg Sandostatin induced an acute hypoglycemic attack after 60 min (glucose 1.6 mmol/l), which was treated with intravenous glucose.

Somatostatin Receptors on Endocrine Pancreatic Tumors

Thirteen hormone-producing tumors from the human gastrointestinal tract were tested for their content of specific somatostatin receptors, using receptor autoradiography and in vitro binding assay with tumor homogenates [see 10].

All 4 gastrinomas tested had high numbers of somatostatin receptors, as did 4 of 5 vasoactive intestinal peptide (VIP)-producing tumors. Somatostatin receptors were, however, found on only 2 out of 5 insulinomas.

Apart from a lower incidence of somatostatin receptors in insulinomas, the two somatostatin-positive insulinomas were also more strongly labeled with a somatostatin-28 radioligand than with a somatostatin-14 and a Sandostatin radioligand. In one of these two tumors (the one removed from the patient who responded *in vivo* with an acute hypoglycemia after a single dose of 50 µg Sandostatin; see above), it was possible to carry out further biochemical studies with the tumor homogenate. This showed high-affinity binding sites for somatostatin-28 (K_D 0.49 nM with a B_{max} of the receptors of 1280 fmoles per mg protein), while the affinity and the number of binding sites for somatostatin-14 and for Sandostatin were between 10 and 80 times lower.

The Possible Mechanism(s) of 'Escape' from Sandostatin Therapy

Escape from Sandostatin therapy in patients with metastatic endocrine pancreatic tumors is infrequent [6]. However, we followed two patients with metastatic endocrine pancreatic tumors who responded initially well to Sandostatin therapy but had symptom breakthrough after several weeks. In the first patient, who had a malignant insulinoma, both the number of hypoglycemic attacks and the increased insulin levels decreased initially, but returned to pretreatment intensity and concentrations within 10 days of the start of therapy with 200 µg Sandostatin daily. After a short interruption of therapy, no effect was observed on re-institution of therapy with 400 µg Sandostatin daily. In the other patient, with a metastatic vipoma, diarrhea, hypokalemia, and plasma VIP levels decreased initially in response to 300 µg Sandostatin per day, but returned to pretreatment severity and values after two weeks of therapy. An increase in the dose to 600 µg/day produced transient improvement, but finally both the volume of diarrhea and VIP levels were worse than before Sandostatin therapy. During Sandostatin treatment no change in tumor size was detected. The plasma Sandostatin concentration at the end of therapy was in the 'therapeutic' range.

Because we were unable to study Sandostatin's mechanism of action relative to the breakthrough of symptoms in these two patients, we studied the effect of Sandostatin treatment, specifically on the number and characteristics of somatostatin receptors, in Syrian hamsters with transplanted insulinomas. We had previously shown that these transplantable insulinomas contain large numbers of specific somatostatin receptors [9].

Four groups of five hamsters with this tumor were treated twice daily for 3 days with subcutaneous injections of either saline or Sandostatin in various doses (10 µg/kg/day, 100 µg/kg/day or 1000 µg/kg/day in two injections). Twenty hours following the last injection (a period long enough to dissociate Sandostatin from its receptors), the individual tumors were removed, and binding assays for somatostatin were performed using ^{125}I-[Tyr^{11}]-somatostatin. The density of the somatostatin receptors in insulinomas from Sandostatin-pretreated hamsters was significantly reduced, i.e., 37% and 41% of controls using the 100 and 1000 µg/kg/day doses, respectively ($p < 0.005$ vs. control in both dose schedules). Scatchard analysis of saturation binding data, however, did not show significant changes in the affinity of the receptor for somatostatin.

In another experiment, hamsters with insulinoma tumors were treated for four days with various daily doses of Sandostatin (0.1 µg/kg, 10 µg/kg, 1 mg/kg and 100 mg/kg) divided into twice-daily subcutaneous injections. The tumors were surgically removed 3 h after the last injection and studied via autoradiography. The density of somatostatin receptors decreased with increasing doses of Sandostatin.

Discussion

In most patients, chronic therapy with Sandostatin has been shown to control effectively the clinical signs and symptoms caused by hypersecretion of the endocrine tumor peptides. However, in patients with insulinomas, caution is needed.

In the present study, human insulinomas, in contrast to gut endocrine tumors, did not always contain somatostatin receptors [10]. In addition, some of the insulinomas contained mainly somatostatin-28 receptors, while the number and affinity of somatostatin-14 and/or Sandostatin receptors was between 10 and 100 times lower. In one of these patients with a malignant insulinoma containing mainly somatostatin-28 receptors, the acute subcutaneous administration of 50 μg Sandostatin caused a prompt hypoglycemia: tumorous hypersecretion of insulin was not affected, but the release of the counter-regulatory hormones glucagon and growth hormone was suppressed, and there was a delay in gut transit-time and in glucose absorption. It therefore seems advisable to select insulinoma patients for Sandostatin therapy only after a well-controlled trial in which the first dose of the drug is administered in the hospital, where rapid intravenous infusion of glucose can be given if necessary.

In the present study, we followed two patients in whom an 'escape' from Sandostatin therapy occurred within 14 days after the start. The mechanism involved the inhibition of both insulin (insulinoma patient) and VIP (VIPoma patient), and their respective clinical effects (reappearance of hypoglycemic attacks and watery diarrhea with potassium loss). Increasing the Sandostatin dose was not effective in the first patient, and only temporarily effective in the second.

Several possibilities might explain the occurrence of this escape from therapy. First, an accelerated enzymatic breakdown of Sandostatin might occur in some patients. This can be excluded, however, in our second patient who, 3 h after the subcutaneous administration of 200 μg of the analogue, had circulating SMS 201-995 levels which can be considered to be in the 'therapeutic' range. Second, a rapid growth of the primary tumor, or its metastases, might explain the secondary 'escape' from Sandostatin therapy. However, this was probably not the case in our two patients. Echography studies of the tumor in the second patient did not point to this possibility. A third possibility is the development of antibodies to Sandostatin in these patients. However, in the second patient, the hyperglycemia that developed during therapy normalized immediately after stopping the drug. This implies that Sandostatin remained active in its inhibitory effect on insulin secretion in this patient even when hormone secretion by the VIPoma had become insensitive to Sandostatin therapy. The fourth, and most likely explanation, is down-regulation of somatostatin receptors on these endocrine pancreatic tumors during chronic Sandostatin therapy.

In the present study, we documented that somatostatin receptors on an insulinoma (in this case a transplantable hamster insulinoma) can be down-regulated by pretreatment with high doses of Sandostatin. It is unclear, however, to what extent such a down-regulation will affect the functional processes which are begun by Sandostatin activation of these receptors. Repeated administration of high doses of Sandostatin induces desensitization or tachyphylaxis of its inhibitory effect on normal GH secretion in the rat, and on its inhibitory effect on the growth of transplantable PRL-secreting pituitary tumors [4].

The 40% diminution in somatostatin receptors on hamster insulinomas pretreated with very high doses of Sandostatin might be insufficient to affect the functional response of these tumor cells to Sandostatin. On the other hand, no down-regulation was observed after pretreatment in vivo with 10 μg/kg of Sandostatin per day. We have shown in hamsters bearing transplantable insulinomas that 200 μg/kg Sandostatin given subcutaneously once a day for 33 days (5 days/week) significantly inhibited tumor growth by 50% [8]. Intermittent, once-daily administration of the analogue may prevent the loss or permit the regeneration of receptors on this type of endocrine pancreatic tumor.

Currently, the mechanism of this desensitization phenomenon or tachyphylaxis to Sandostatin in endocrine pancreatic tumors is not known. In acromegalic patients, both tumorous GH from the pituitary, and insulin secretion by normal beta-cells remain highly sensitive to the analogue during long-term therapy, while the beneficial clinical effects persists [5]. In addition, continuous infusion of Sandostatin for 30 days in a newborn with nesidioblastosis was highly effective in suppressing insulin secretion without signs or symptoms of resistance to therapy [2].

In the two patients described in the present study an 'escape' from Sandostatin therapy resulted in the recurrence of hypoglycemia in one patient, and of diarrhea and hypokalemia in the other. In patients with (malignant) insulinomas, this symptom breakthrough can be especially dangerous. Close clinical monitoring with careful instruction should therefore be given to insulinoma patients during Sandostatin treatment. However, the results from studies on the effects of chronic Sandostatin therapy in other patients with endocrine pancreatic tumors and carcinoids fortunately show that the 'escape' phenomenon observed in our two patients rarely occurs.

References

1. Alberti K. G. M. M., Christensen N. J., Christensen S. E., Prange-Hanse J., Iversen J., Lundbaek K., Syer-Hansen K., Ørskov H.: Inhibition of insulin secretion by somatostatin. Lancet 1973; *ii*:1299–1301
2. Bruining G. J., Bosschaart A. N., Aarsen R. S. R., Lamberts S. W. J., Sauer P. J. J., del Pozo E.: Normalization of glucose homeostasis by a long-acting somatostatin analogue SMS 201-995 in a newborn with nesidioblastosis. Acta Endocrinol 1986; *113*:334–340
3. Christensen S. E., Hansen A. P., Lundbaek K., Ørskov H., Syer-Hansen K.: Somatostatin and insulinomas. Lancet 1975; *i*:1426
4. Lamberts S. W. J., Reubi J. C., Uitterlinden P., Zuiderwijk J., van den Werff P., van Hal P.: Studies on the mechanism of action of the inhibitory effect of the somatostatin analogue SMS 201-995 on the growth of the prolactin/adrenocorticotropin-secreting pituitary tumor 7315a. Endocrinology 1986; *118*:2188–2194
5. Lamberts S. W. J., Uitterlinden P., Verschoor L., van Dongen K. J., del Pozo E.: Long-term treatment of acromegaly with the somatostatin analogue SMS 201-995. N Engl J Med 1986; *313*:1576–1580
6. Lamberts S. W. J., Pieters G. F. F. M., Metselaar H. J., Ong G. L., Tan H. S., Reubi J. C.: Patients with metastatic endocrine pancreatic tumors seldom escape from therapy with a long-acting somatostatin analogue. Acta Endocrinol (Copenh) 1988; in press
7. Lorenzi M., Gerich J. E., Karam J. H., Forsham P. H.: Failure of somatostatin to inhibit tolbutamide-induced insulin secretion in patients with insulinomas: a possible diagnostic tool. J Clin Endocrinol Metab 1975; *40*:1121–1124
8. Reubi J. C.: A somatostatin analogue inhibits chondrosarcoma and insulinoma tumor growth. Acta Endocrinol 1985; *109*:108–114
9. Reubi J. C., Rivier J., Perrin M., Brown M., Vale W.: Specific high affinity binding sites for somatostatin-28 on pancreatic β-cells: Differences with brain somatostatin receptors. Endocrinology 1982; *110*:1049–1051
10. Reubi J. C., Häcki W., Lamberts S. W. J.: Hormone-producing gastrointestinal tumors contain high density of somatostatin receptors: diagnostical and therapeutic implications. J Clin Endocrinol Metab 1987; *65*: 1127–1135
11. Verschoor L., Uitterlinden P., Lamberts S. W. J., del Pozo E.: On the use of a new somatostatin analogue in the treatment of hypoglycaemia in patients with insulinoma. Clin Endocrinol 1986; *25*:555–560

6. Sandostatin®: Assay and Efficacy in VIPoma and Insulinoma

T. M. O'Dorisio, T. S. Gaginella, M. S. O'Dorisio, R. W. Meleca, D. A. Wray, K. Osei

The Ohio State University, College of Medicine, Columbus, Ohio, USA

This communication is divided into three sections. The first deals with the clinical application of gut peptide radioimmunoassay (RIA) and a description of the Sandostatin® RIA performed at The Ohio State University. The second section briefly addresses the utility of peptide RIA in endocrine tumors of the gastroenteropancreatic (GEP) system and a rationale for Sandostatin therapy specifically as it pertains to VIPoma/watery diarrhea syndrome (WDS). The final section discusses observations regarding chronic Sandostatin therapy of our patient with malignant insulinoma.

Since the discovery of the peptide hormone 'secretin' by Bayliss and Starling in 1902, more than 35 different peptides have been identified in the GEP system [7]. The vast majority of the gut peptides were discovered between 1950 and 1970 and paralleled the development of sophisticated gel filtration and purification methodologies. These early years served as a fertile milieu for the discovery and description of the RIA by Yalow and Berson in 1959 [13]. The discovery of RIA spawned the development of immunocytochemistry, in which specific peptide-releasing endocrine cells and nerve fibers could be visually localized. Although many superb RIAs and immunocytochemical laboratories have been established both in Europe and in the United States, recognition for securing the importance of RIA and immunocytochemistry in gut endocrinology should be given to Drs S. R. Bloom and J. M. Pollack of the Royal Postgraduate Medical School in London. Their studies have led to the localization of several peptides in the GI tract and to the identification of peptides as major secretagogues in neuroendocrine tumors of the GEP system.

Gastrointestinal regulating peptides may travel via the circulation (as classical hormones) to their target organ (endocrine action); they may be released from endocrine cells to exert an action on adjacent target cells (paracrine action); or they may be released from a peptidergic neuron and diffuse across a neuronal gap to reach their target cell (neurocrine action). Regardless of the physiologic action as hormone, paracrine or neurocrine peptide, when secreted in excessive amounts, these peptides may all act in a pathophysiologic manner. One example of this pathohumoral effect is operative in VIPoma, from which vasoactive intestinal peptide (VIP)-secreting tumor cells release VIP into the bloodstream, translocating it to target tissues as a peptide hormone.

The RIA and the subsequent development of immunocytochemistry has allowed us to understand normal regulatory function through the study of states of peptide excess. These states of peptide excess (endocrine tumors) have been described in previous chapters. Since 1973, several sensitive and specific RIAs for many of the gut peptides have been developed at The Ohio State University [8]. Our assays employ heterologous antiserum raised to highly pure or synthetic peptides of the GEP system. These include VIP, gastrin, pancreatic peptide (PP), somatostatin, calcitonin, calcitonin gene related peptide (CGRP), insulin, glucagon, substance-P, neurotensin, gastrin releasing peptide (GRP, bombesin), glucose-dependent insulinotropic peptide (GIP) and atrial natriuretic peptide (ANF). With the exception of somatostatin, which is acetone-extracted from plasma prior to assay, all RIAs done in our laboratory use freshly collected fasting EDTA-plasma. The assays have been effective in screening large numbers of plasma samples from patients with suspected GEP tumors [8]. Approximate range values in normal unaffected subjects have been utilized to determine upper limits in normal subjects. Peptide measurements at our institution quantify peptides in both normal and tumor tissue. Tissue is prepared with an acetic acid/alcohol solution, lyophilized, reconstituted in 50 mmol/l acetic acid and assayed directly at several dilutions. We have been able to confirm the co-occurrence of peptides in many of the major GEP endocrine tumors and have formed a working hypothesis that co-occurring peptide release may modify the otherwise classic clinical expression of many endocrine tumors [8]. We have been able to discern that co-occurring production of somatostatin is inversely correlated with the clinical expressiveness of otherwise major GEP tumors [8].

The novel long-acting somatostatin analog, octreotide (Sandostatin®) has helped define the pivotal role played by somatostatin in both normal and abnormal intestinal physiology. The effectiveness of this unique peptidomimetic agent serves as the major theme of this communication. Thus far, published reports have shown Sandostatin to be effective in the management of major symptoms and syndromes associated with several of the major endocrine tumors including VIPomas, malignant carcinoid tumors, malignant insulinoma, glucagonomas, PPomas, and growth hormone secreting tumors as well as growth hormone releasing factor tumors (cf bibliographic citations). Because Sandostatin has been so effective in the treatment of symptomatic neuroendocrine tumors, few clinical dose-response studies have been done. Further, the initial dose of Sandostatin in symptomatic tumors is, at present, empiric. We have modified the Sandostatin assay of Bauer and colleagues [1] and have utilized this assay for both clinical and research investigation. The Sandostatin antibody RBA (courtesy of Dr Peter Marbach, Sandoz, Basle) was used in the assay. Tyrosinated Sandostatin (courtesy of Sandoz, Basle) was used for labelling. The iodination of the tyrosinated (T) Sandostatin is done by the chloramine-T method. Two micrograms of T-Sandostatin is used with 1 mCi ^{125}I. Chloramine T (12.5 µg) is added in the reaction carried for 25 s. Sodium metabisulfite (120 µg) stops the reaction. The solution is placed over a ten-centimeter column packed with dry Whatman CF-1 fibrocellulose. The column is washed with 20 ml of 50 mmol/l sodium phosphate, pH and then 1 ml frac-

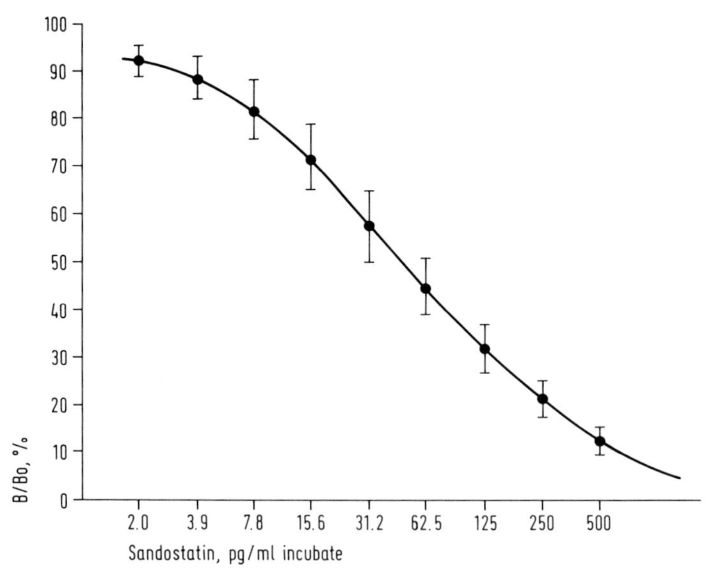

Fig. 1. Standard Sandostatin® RIA curve (mean ± 2SD) performed at The Ohio State University. The standard curves utilize charcoal-stripped plasma or, if tissue Sandostatin is measured, 0.05 N acetic acid. Second antibody precipitation is used for both plasma and tissue Sandostatin measurement. Intra- and inter-assay coefficients of variation are 4% and 17% respectively, for both plasma and tissue measurements

tions are eluted utilizing 200 mmol/l acetic acid/10% charcoal-stripped human plasma. The first eluted fraction contains free iodine followed by a peak of radiolabelled peptide; this second fraction has been found to have excellent binding with little or no apparent radiation damage.

Figure 1 shows a composite Sandostatin standard RIA curve (mean ± 2 SD) generated at The Ohio State University. This assay has a sensitivity of 39 pg/ml of plasma. No cross-reactivity is observed with any of 15 gut peptides normally tested to date nor with somatostatin 1–14 at concentrations up to 10 ng/ml of incubate. Our assay appears to be helpful in determining both plasma half-life and tissue levels of Sandostatin in several clinical studies using Sandostatin therapy for various symptomatic neuroendocrine tumors. Further, utilizing this tyrosinated Sandostatin label, we have developed methodology for determination of Sandostatin antibodies. Briefly, this modified antibody assay involves treatment of plasma with 0.12 N HCl, dextran charcoal vortexing, neutralizing with 0.12 N sodium chloride, incubation with $I^{125}T$ Sandostatin, precipitation with 25% polyethylene glycol (10% human serum) und counting. Thus far, we have tested 100 patients treated for various periods of time with Sandostatin. The period of treatment of these patients ranged from 6–18 months. No significant antibody titer (that is, more than 10% nonspecific binding, normal upper limit) has been detected. One infant treated with the analog for secretory diarrhea had a partial response to Sandostatin (60% in reduction of diarrhea) and a transient rise of Sandostatin detectable antibody (15%). However, repeated testing of this patient during administration of the analog failed to reproduce a titer of more than 10% [3]. Thus, it does not appear that Sandostatin is immunogenic.

As we have learned from the chapter 2 of J. Pless, Sandostatin is a long-acting analog of the naturally occurring somatostatin. The rationale for both the development and the clinical use of a Sandostatin analog is best demonstrated in the management of the VIPoma/WDS [5]. Since somatostatin's discovery in 1972, much has been learned regarding its regulatory role. As it modulates inhibition of growth hormone via the hypothalamic-pituitary portal circulation, it is considered a true endocrine or hormone substance. Because of its unique location in both the pancreatic islet cell and in peptidergic nerve fibers, somatostatin is suggested to have an important role in the gut as both a paracrine and a neurocrine substance [11]. Native somatostatin inhibits the release or action of several gut peptides including insulin, glucagon, secretin, CCK, GIP, PP, neurotensin and motilin. Both endocrine and neurocrine effects of somatostatin have been recently reviewed [11, 12].

It is now accepted that VIP is the primary secretagogue in tumors associated with WDS. The definite causal association between VIP and intestinal secretion in humans was demonstrated by Kane and associates in 1983 [4]. These investigators found that, in normal subjects, chronic VIP infu-

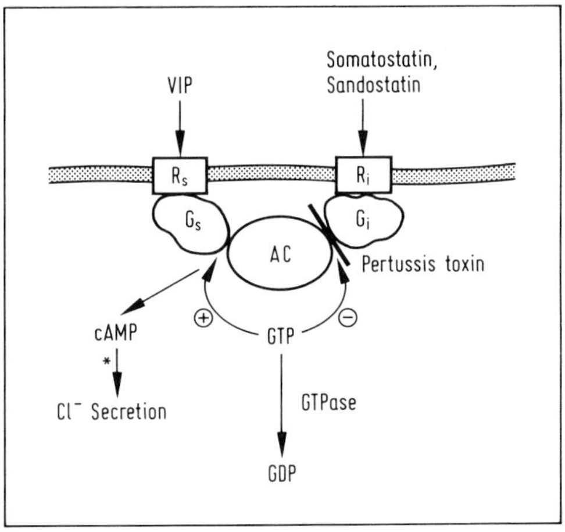

Fig. 2. Two mechanisms whereby Sandostatin® (*) blocks vasoactive intestinal peptide (VIP)-induced intestinal secretion. One mechanism involves receptor-linked activation of the inhibitory subunit (G_i) of adenylate cyclase (AC), preventing cAMP generation. The subsequent effects of cAMP on protein kinase activation are also blocked by somatostatin and Sandostatin. Pertussis toxin uncouples the inhibitory effect of somatostatin at the adenylate cyclase level. GTP and GDP are guanosine triphosphate and guanosine diphosphate respectively. G_s is the protein coupling stimulatory receptors (Rs) to adenylate cyclase, and R_i the recognition site of receptors coupled to the inhibitory (G_i) protein component of the cyclase system

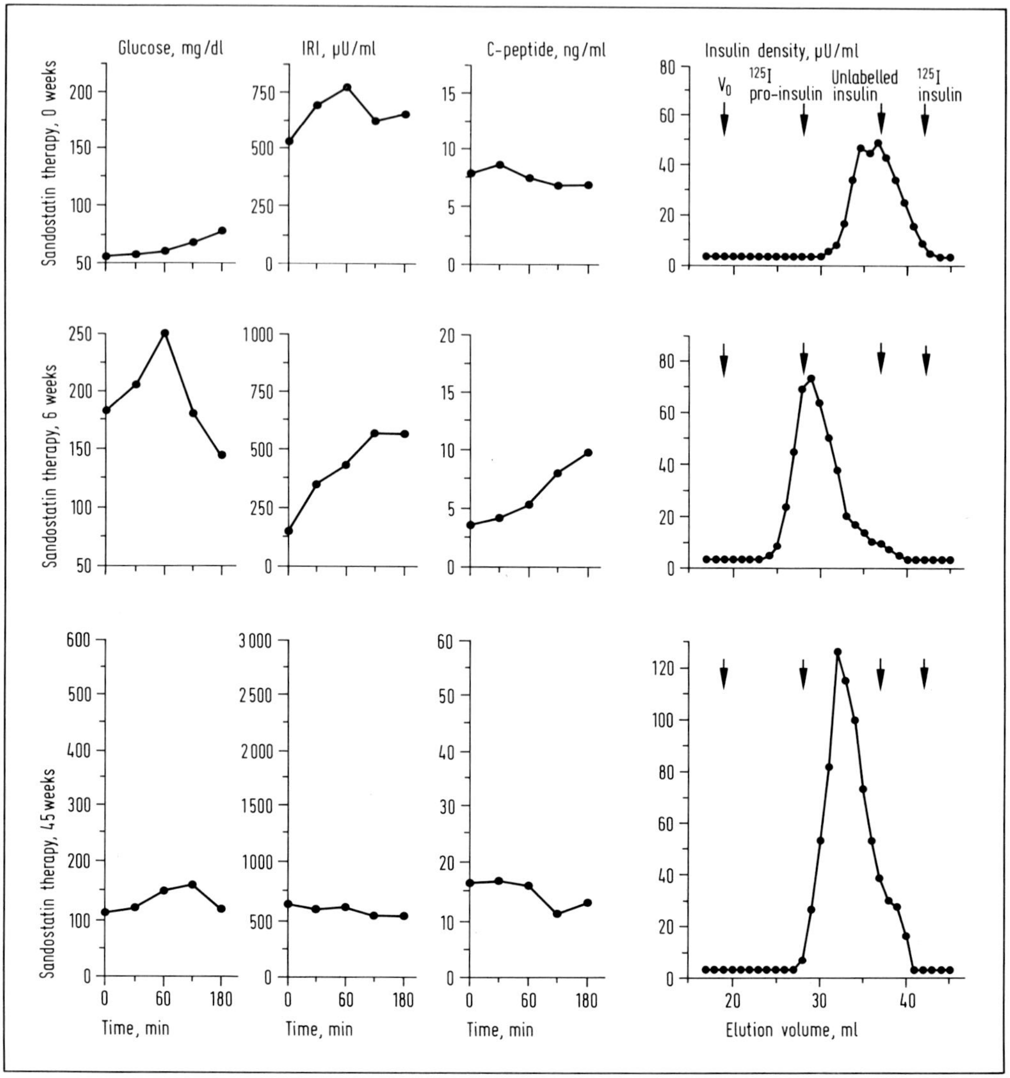

Fig. 3. Plasma glucose, immunoreactive insulin (IRI) and C-peptide levels, baseline and following a meal, in a patient with malignant insulinoma before and during (at 6 and 45 weeks) Sandostatin® therapy. Shown on the right is the corresponding elution profile of the patient's fasting plasma pre-analog and at 6 and 45 weeks of therapy. The untreated plasma was eluted on a G-50 Sephadex column using 0.05 N acetic acid with 0.05% BSA and 0.02% NaN_3, pH 3.6. Porcine insulin antibody (#12610-A) was used to measure both plasma insulin and the column eluates of the plasma. Markers included Blue Dextran (V_0) I^{125} pro-insulin (MW approx. 9000 Daltons) and both labelled and unlabelled insulin (MW approx. 6000 Daltons)

sion mimicking levels observed in patients with VIPoma/WDS resulted in a secretory diarrheal state. Native somatostatin inhibits the effect of a number of hormones, as we have already observed. However, the precise role of somatostatin as an antagonist of normal or pathologic action of VIP is less well delineated. We can consider Sandostatin to have the same properties as native somatostatin in terms of the mechanisms by which it inhibits VIP-mediated intestinal secretion. Whether or not the beneficial effects of the native somatostatin or Sandostatin in patients with VIPoma/WDS are due solely to inhibition of release of VIP from its tumor site and/or inhibition of the action of VIP on its target cell (intestinal epithelial cell) is unknown at the present time. However, several studies including those of Maton and colleagues [5] point to a direct common action of Sandostatin on inhibition of VIP-induced intestinal secretion. We have recently reported that native somatostatin antagonizes the secretory effect of VIP in rat ileal and colonic perfusion experiments [9]. These experiments demonstrated functional antagonism by somatostatin on VIP-stimulated intestinal secretion. VIP induces intestinal secretion through the adenylate cyclase-cAMP pathway. Further, somatostatin and, presumably, Sandostatin appear to antagonize intestinal secretion directly via inhibition of adenylate cyclase [6]. Figure 2 offers a schema which illustrates the possible modes of action of somatostatin on VIP-induced epithelial target cells. As can be noted, there are at least two sites where Sandostatin may antagonize VIP action.

The final comments of this communication address our observations on a patient with malignant insulinoma, treated with Sandostatin [13]. Gel chromatography (G-50 Sephadex) was employed, using the patient's fasting plasma pre-Sandostatin therapy and at 6 and 45 weeks of Sandostatin therapy. The plasma eluates were measured using an insulin RIA porcine antibody #12610-A, which appears to recognize not only insulin but also larger forms of insulin. Figure 3 demonstrates both fasting and meal-stimulated glucose immunoreactivity insulin (IRI) and C-peptide-like immunoreactivity, as well as the Sephadex elution profiles of our patient with the malignant insulinoma. Pre-analog blood sugars were quite low in spite of intravenous 10% glucose. A large amount of insulin-like immunoreactivity was present in the plasma, probably corresponding also to pro-insulin. The excess insulin correlated with elevated C-peptide levels prior to analog therapy.

Chromatography of pre-analog plasma demonstrated a large peak which eluted in or around the unlabelled insulin marker. At six weeks, when the patient was asymptomatic and on Sandostatin, both basal and stimulated glucose levels were in a high-normal range. Further, plasma IRI was much lower, as were C-peptide levels compared with pre-analog measurements. Column chromatography at six weeks revealed a larger IRI moiety with only a very small number of elution peaks corresponding to the unlabelled insulin marker. At 45 weeks the patient was relatively symptomatic with more frequent 'break-through' episodes of hypoglycemia. The lower panel of Figure 3 demonstrates the elution profile at 45 weeks. Fasting and meal-stimulated glucose, although not grossly abnormal, were much lower than they were during the asymptomatic period but higher than during the symptomatic period (pre-analog). Insulin-like immunoreactivity was now closer to pre-analog therapy levels as were C-peptide levels. Of great interest was a shift in the column of plasma eluates showing a peak larger than the insulin peak, with a 'shelf-like' appearance of fractions corresponding to the unlabelled insulin marker.

The precise mechanism whereby Sandostatin modified the various molecular moieties in this patient could not be discerned from this study. It may well be that Sandostatin preferentially inhibited the post-transcriptional processing of pre-pro-insulin or insulin release. Whether or not Sandostatin actually modified the peptide processing within the tumor cell is a fascinating question, but opinions can be no more than speculative at this point.

References

1. Bauer W, Briner, U, Doepfner W, et al.: A very potent and selective octapeptide analogue of somatostatin with prolonged action. Life Sci 1982; *31*:133–135
2. Bloom SR, Polak JM (eds): Gut hormones, 2nd edn. Churchill-Livingstone, Edinburgh, 1981, pp 11–560
3. Jaros W, Biller J, Greer S, O'Dorisio T, Grand R: Successful treatment of idiopathic secretory diarrhea of infancy with the somatostatin analogue SMS 201-995. Gastroenterology 1988; *94*:189–193
4. Kane MG, O'Dorisio TM, Krejs GJ: Production of secretory diarrhea by intravenous infusion of vasoactive intestinal polypeptide. N Engl J Med 1983; *309*:1482–1485

5. Maton PH, O'Dorisio TM, Howe BA, et al.: Effect of a long-acting somatostatin analogue (201-995) in a patient with pancreatic cholera. N Engl J Med 1985; *312*:17–21
6. O'Dorisio MS: Neuropeptides and gastrointestinal immunity. Am J Med 1986; *81* [Suppl 6 B]:74–82
7. O'Dorisio TM: Gut endocrinology: clinical and therapeutic impact. Am J Med 1986; *81* [Suppl 6 B]:1–7
8. O'Dorisio TM, Mekhjian HS, Ellison EC, et al.: Role of peptide radioimmunoassay in understanding peptide interactions and clinical expression of gastroenteropancreatic endocrine tumors. Am J Med 1987; *82* [Suppl 5 B]:60–67
9. O'Dorisio TM, Gaginella TS, Mekhjian HS, Rao B, O'Dorisio MS: Somatostatin and analogues in the treatment of Vipoma. NY Acad Sci 1988
10. Osei K, O'Dorisio TM: Malignant insulinoma: effects of a somatostatin analog (compound 201-995) on serum glucose, growth and gastroenteropancreatic hormones. Ann Intern Med 1985; *103*:223–225
11. Reichlin S: Somatostatin: historical aspects. Scand J Gastroenterol 1986; *21*:1–10
12. Schusdziarra V, Schmid R: Physiological and pathophysiological aspects of somatostatin. Scand J Gastroenterol 1986; *21*:29–41
13. Yalow RS, Berson SA: Assay of plasma insulin in human subjects by immunologic methods. Nature 1959; *184*:1648–1649

7. Sandostatin® in Digestive Endocrine Tumors

J. A. Chayvialle, J. C. Souquet, G. Sassolas, C. Partensky

Inserm U 45, Hôpital Edouard-Herriot, Lyon, France

Some years ago, several authors reported that the tetradecapeptide somatostatin could be of value for the temporary control of inappropriate secretions from endocrine tumors of the digestive tract [2, 3, 5]. However, this therapeutic benefit was hampered by the short half-life of the peptide [6], thus requiring continuous intravenous infusion with the risk of critical rebound effects upon discontinuation. The slower catabolism of Sandostatin® (octreotide, SMS 201-995), along with its relative target specificity and administration via the subcutaneous route, prompted its trial in patients with various types of digestive endocrine tumors. We here report the results of studies conducted in the Lyon area from November 1984 to early 1987.

Methods

The study group included 26 patients, aged 25–82 years, who gave informed consent. Cytologic or histologic proof of the endocrine tumors and/or of their secondaries was available in all but 2 patients. These two presented with typical Zollinger-Ellison syndromes (high basal acid secretion rates, high plasma gastrin levels, positive secretin tests).

The tumors comprised 9 gastrinomas, 1 insulinoma, 1 glucagonoma, 1 pancreatic tumor secreting a substance-P-like component, and 14 metastatic carcinoids. All patients in the last subgroup displayed the features of moderate to severe carcinoid syndrome, both clinically (3 or more bowel movements per day, 3 or more flushing episodes per day or permanent flush) and biologically (5-HIAA urinary output: median 480 μmol per 24 h, range 116–2200, normal <45). Plasma substance-P-like immunoreactivity was elevated in 6 (range 157–2377 pg/ml, normal <50).

Hormonal profiles were performed before and after Sandostatin therapy by measuring plasma concentrations of immunoreactive gastrin, somatostatin, vasoactive intestinal peptide, substance P, pancreatic polypeptide, calcitonin, parathormone, adrenocorticotropin, glucagon, insulin, the blood serotonin level and the 24-h urinary output of 5-HIAA. These parameters and the patients's symptoms were initially monitored for 2–3 days. Sandostatin was then administered for 3 days at a dose of 50 or 100 μg b.i.d. subcutaneously. The clinical and biological criteria were measured on day 3 of therapy together with standard biological parameters: blood cell count, blood glucose, serum electrolytes, azotemia, serum creatinine, liver function tests and urine analysis. All patients were maintained on their current therapy, including H 2-blockers in gastrinoma patients. Following this short-term evaluation, Sandostatin was continued if symptomatic relief and/or biological improvement was observed.

Gut hormones were measured with previously reported radioimmunoassays [1, 4], blood samples were taken at 8:00 am, 12 h after the last Sandostatin injection. In some gastrinoma patients the gastric contents was sampled for 1 h, starting 3 h after the morning dose of H 2-blocker with or without Sandostatin.

Part of these results was recently reported [7].

Results

Eight of the 9 gastrinoma patients showed a 33–99% reduction in basal plasma gastrin, the mean reduction in the total group of 9 subjects being 62.3 ± 10.3%, SEM ($p < 0.01$, paired t test). In one patient who had a highly malignant gastrinoma with an associated ectopic secretion of adrenocorticotropin, Sandostatin failed to alter plasma gastrin cortisol and adrenocorticotropin levels. Basal acid secretion rates were measured before and during Sandostatin treatment in 6 patients with intact or partially resected stomachs. As compared with H2-blockers alone, Sandostatin plus the patient's regular dose of H2-blocker strongly inhibited the gastric acid secretion, especially in 2 patients in whom the morning dose of 300 mg ranitidine clearly failed to control the acid secretion adequately (Table 1). Sandostatin was continued in several patients for periods up to 20 months. One had multiple endocrine neoplasia including a pancreatic gastrinoma, a residual alpha-subunit secreting pituitary tumor and parathyroid hyperplasia. She had been operated on for a grade V melanoma. Plasma gastrin remained normal while on Sandostatin. She died as a result of melanoma metastases. Another patient, in whom an antral gastrinoma had been removed, was found by ultrasound and CT scan to have three 15 mm-diameter liver secondaries one year after surgery. Acid secretion was well controlled with 300 mg ranitidine at night. Sandostatin was given continuously, resulting in plasma gastrin levels consistently lower than 50 pg/ml. The three liver secondaries were no longer detectable by either ultrasound or CT scan 6 months after starting Sandostatin therapy.

The effects of Sandostatin on the other cases of pancreatic tumor varied from patient to patient. No improvement occurred in the subject with a benign insulinoma. The patient with a pancreatic glucagonoma (metastasized to the liver) showed incomplete reduction in plasma glucagon but dramatic clearance of skin lesions. One patient had a pseudo-carcinoid syndrome and a malignant pancreatic tumor with multiple liver, bone and lung metastases, and inappropriate secretion of a substance-P-like component (blood serotonin and urinary 5-HIAA being consistently within the normal range). Sandostatin partially controlled the flushing and dyspneic attacks, especially during the first 3 h after each injection. The short-term rebound episodes were prevented by continuously infusing a larger dose (1200 mg per day with a minipump), until death occurred from metastasis.

In patients with moderate to severe carcinoid syndrome, Sandostatin resulted in a dramatic, though incomplete, improvement in biological and clinical abnormalities (Table 2). One patient had an acute intestinal obstruction four days after initiation of Sandostatin. Because the carcinoid symptoms were at their most severe at the time of admission, x-ray evaluation of the small bowel had been delayed until the diarrhea and flushing could be reduced. At laparotomy the small bowel was perforated proximal to a large, obstructing, carcinoid tumor with fibrotic mesenteritis. The patient died in the early post-operative period. Nine other patients have been treated for up to 28 months. Six patients have been stable with moderate

Table 1. Basal acid output (mmol/h) 3 h after the current dose of H2-blocker, alone or associated with 0.1 mg Sandostatin (SMS) in 6 gastrinoma patients with intact or partially resected stomachs

	Without Sandostatin	With Sandostatin
Ranitidine 150	1.5	0.5
Cimetidine 400	5.4	0.05
Ranitidine 300	12.0	0
Ranitidine 150	2.6	0
Ranitidine 300	23.8	0
Ranitidine 300	2.1	3.9

Table 2. Biological and clinical short-term evaluation of Sandostatin (0.1 mg b.i.d.) in patients with carcinoid syndrome

5-HIAA/24 h:	mean reduction: 47 ± 6.6% (SE)* (range 0–90%, n = 14)
Substance P:	mean reduction: 43.3 ± 12.6% (SE)** (range 9–99%, n = 6)
Diarrhea:	definite improvement: 9/14
Flushes:	definite improvement: 7/14

* = $p < 0.01$
** = $p > 0.05$

doses (100 µg b.i.d.), while three have required progressive increases up to 1000 µg per day. So far no antitumoral effect has been recorded in this group.

In the total study group no serious side effects were reported with Sandostatin therapy. Standard laboratory evaluations remained unchanged compared with baseline during therapy. Several patients complained of burning at the site of injection, alleviated in part by slowing the injection rate and prewarming the solution. Only one patient reported regular abdominal cramping, which was severe enough to necessitate withdrawal from the study.

Discussion

Sandostatin was effective in both the gastrinoma and carcinoid tumor patients. The efficacy of therapy for metastatic gastrinomas has greatly improved during the last few years. Adequate control of acid secretion is obtained for a time in most patients with H2-blockers. With the recently developed proton pump inhibitor, omeprazole, greater reduction of acid hypersecretion has been achieved. Sandostatin could be an alternative antisecretory agent in this clinical group. Moderate doses of Sandostatin dramatically improved the control of acid hypersecretion in two patients with high residual basal rates while on large doses of ranitidine.

An important point is that Sandostatin normalized plasma gastrin concentrations in 4 of the 9 patients. Persistently high gastrin levels are thought to trigger hyperplasia of enterochromaffin(EC)-like cells of the fundic mucosa, which could theoretically result in malignant fundic carcinoid tumors [8]. Sandostatin may be especially valuable in such responsive (malignant) gastrinoma patients, since chronic potent inhibition of gastrin release might prevent or delay fundic EC-cell hyperplasia. This, however, remains to be established.

Not all patients with the carcinoid syndrome responded to Sandostatin therapy, clinical and biological responses being incomplete. The control of advanced carcinoid syndrome is a therapeutic challenge, so any treatment that may result in some degree of secretory inhibition may be beneficial. Partial, and most often temporary, improvement may be attained through hepatic artery ligation or embolization, chemotherapy or symptomatic medications, or combinations of these approaches. The significant reduction in urinary 5-HIAA in our study is encouraging and suggests that larger doses of Sandostatin could result in even greater inhibition. No serious side effects occurred except in the one patient with an obstructing, intestinal carcinoid tumor. Since somatostatin has been reported to delay intestinal transit, Sandostatin therapy should be postponed until the possibility of a large obstructing carcinoid has been ruled out.

Overall, Sandostatin was a safe, effective and well-tolerated therapeutic alternative for the symptomatic treatment of a large number of patients with advanced, non-resectable, gut endocrine tumors. When Sandostatin can be used with other therapeutic modalities it will prove to be a major advance in the management of clinically symptomatic endocrine tumors. Although not yet established, long-term inhibition of secretory tumor activity may be extremely valuable in conditions where secondary consequences of inappropriate tumor secretions may worsen the prognosis, e.g. cardiac valvular involvement and nutritional status in carcinoid syndrome, and possibly EC-cell hyperplasia in gastrinoma.

Acknowledgements: The authors thank R. Brette, L. Descos, R. Levrat, R. Lombard-Platet, J. Pasquier and J. Thivolet for giving access to records.

References

1. Chayvialle J. A., Miyata M., Rayford P. L., Thompson J. C.: Immunoreactive somatostatin and vasoactive intestinal peptide in the digestive tract of cats. Gastroenterology, 1980, *79*:837–843
2. Curnow R. T., Carey R. M., Taylor A., Johanson A, Murad F.: Somatostatin inhibition of insulin and gastrin hypersecretion in pancreatic islet-cell carcinoma. N Engl J Med, 1975, *292*:1385–1386
3. Dharmsathaphorn K., Sherwing R. S., Cataland S., Jaffe B., Dobbins J.: Somatostatin inhibits diarrhea in carcinoid syndrome. Ann Intern Med, 1980, *92*:68–69

4. Miazza B., Palma R., Lachance J. R., Chayvialle J. A., Jonard P. P., Modigliani R.: Jejunal secretory effect of intraduodenal food in humans: a comparison of mixed nutrients, proteins, lipids, and carbohydrates. Gastroenterology, 1985, *88*:1215–1222
5. Ruskone A., Rene E., Chayvialle J. A., Bonin N., Pignal F., Kremer M., et al.: Effect of somatostatin on diarrhea and on small intestinal water and electrolyte transport in a patient with pancreatic cholera. Dig Dis Sci, 1982, *27*: 459–466
6. Sheppard M., Shapiro B., Pimstone B., Kronheim M. B., Gregory M.: The metabolic clearance and plasma half disappearance time of exogenous somatostatin in man. J Clin Endocrinol Metab, 1979, *49*:50–53
7. Souquet J. C., Sassolas G., Frichon J., Champetier P., Partensky C. H., Chayvialle J. A.: Clinical and hormonal effects of a long-acting somatostatin analogue in pancreatic endocrine tumors and in carcinoid syndrome. Cancer, 1987, *59*:1654–1660
8. Sundler F., Hakanson R., Carlsson E., Larsson H., Mattson H.: Hypergastrinemia after blockade in acid secretion in the rat: trophic effects. Digestion, 1986, *35* (1):59–69

8. VIPoma, Gastrinoma and Glucagonoma

G. J. Krejs

Department of Medicine, Karl Franzens University, Graz, Austria

The incidence of gut hormone-producing tumors is estimated to be one per 200 000 population per year. Gastrinomas are found in one person per 2 million per year, VIPomas are found in one person per 10 million per year, and glucagonomas are found in one person per 20 million per year. Somatostatinomas and GRFomas (growth hormone releasing factor) may be as rare as one case per 40 million population per year. (Data based on Tumor Registery of Belfast, Northern Ireland [2]).

Table 1 lists the clinical and biochemical features of the three gastrointestinal endocrine tumor syndromes discussed in this chapter.

Gastrinoma

In 1955, Zollinger and Ellison [17] first described a syndrome characterized by severe peptic ulcer disease that recurred after several surgical procedures, gastric hypersecretion, and the presence of a pancreatic tumor. Later, the tumors were found to produce and release the hormone gastrin into the circulation. Today the availability of a radioimmunoassay for gastrin makes the diagnosis relatively easy, and cases are often recognized early. A basal serum gastrin level above 200 pg/ml requires further assessment because gastrin levels may be elevated in other conditions.

Table 1. Clinical features of three gut hormone-producing tumor syndromes

Tumor syndrome	Clinical features	Diagnostic features
VIPoma	Watery diarrhea, hypokalemia, metabolic acidosis, hypochlorhydria	Fecal pH as high as 8.0 (colonic bicarbonate secretion), concomitant elevation of PHM (peptide histidine methionine) and calcitonin. Tumor may contain helodermin
Gastrinoma	Severe peptic ulcer disease, secretory diarrhea, in 25% part of MEN I	Serum gastrin rise after intravenous secretion, high basal and peak acid secretion, secretory diarrhea stops with omeprazole or H_2-blocker treatment
Glucagonoma	Necrolytic migratory erythema, mild diabetes, psychiatric disturbances, venous thrombosis	Excessive glucagon release after intravenous tolbutamide

Gastric acid secretion rates are high in patients with gastrinoma but may overlap with those in patients with common duodenal ulcer disease or even some healthy controls. About half the patients have a basal acid secretion rate of more than 15 mmol/h. A basal acid output equal to or greater than 60% of the peak acid output (after pentagastrin) is highly suggestive of gastrinoma. However, about half of all gastrinoma patients fail to show this pattern [5].

If serum gastrin elevation is minor (200 to less than 1000 pg/ml), a provocative test should be performed. The best provocation is provided by intravenous secretin injection (2 U/kg). In patients with gastrinoma the serum gastrin level increases promptly (within 5 or 10 min), usually by more than 200 pg/ml [5].

Clinical features other than peptic ulcer include diarrhea and steatorrhea. Diarrhea is present in one-third of the patients and may precede peptic ulcer symptoms in up to one-sixth of affected patients. The major cause of the diarrhea is the large amount of acidic fluid entering the jejunum. In one such patient we measured a pH of 1.1 in the proximal jejunum and from perfusion studies calculated the entry of 15 l of fluid per day into the small bowel in the fasting state. Suppression of gastric acid secretion with H_2-receptor antagonists abolished the diarrhea. High circulating concentrations of gastrin may play a minor role in causing diarrhea by reducing intestinal water and ion absorption. Mild steatorrhea may result from the inactivation of lipase at low pH in the intestinal lumen.

The incidence of MEN I (multiple endocrine neoplasia syndrome, type I) in gastrinoma patients is about 25%. These patients should be considered a separate group because they tend to show a better survival rate than patients with sporadic gastrinoma [18]. This is contrary to what might be expected, since gastrinomas tend to be multiple throughout the pancreas. When gastrinomas are part of MEN I, most patients also have parathyroid hyperplasia. Multiple parathyroid gland removal is often necessary.

The traditional treatment for gastrinoma has been total gastrectomy. However, studies by Richardson and colleagues [8] suggest that the treatment of choice is exploratory laparotomy, tumor resection if technically possible, and proximal gastric vagotomy. Vagotomy allows more effective treatment of acid hypersecretion with H_2-receptor antagonists even when the tumor cannot be removed. In a small number of patients curative tumor resection is possible. H_2-receptor antagonists can control hypersecretion without vagotomy, but large doses are necessary and discontinuation of medication may create a life-threatening exacerbation. Omeprazole, an inhibitor of H^+/K^+-ATPase activity in gastric mucosa, is capable of suppressing acid secretion with a single daily dose. This agent has now become the drug of choice for medical treatment of patients with gastrinomas. When tumor mass is the problem, treatment with streptozotocin and 5-fluorouracil may be successful [6].

VIPoma

In 1957 Priest and Alexander [7] described a patient with islet cell tumor, severe watery diarrhea and hypokalemia, and in 1958 Verner and Morrison [14] called attention to the syndrome of watery diarrhea, hypokalemia and death from renal failure in association with islet cell tumor. Synonyms for VIPoma include the Verner-Morrison syndrome, the watery diarrhea, hypokalemia, hypochlorhydria (WDHH) syndrome, and the pancreatic cholera syndrome.

In the pancreatic cholera syndrome, the diarrhea, as in Asiatic cholera, results from intestinal fluid secretion; some tumors, however, are outside the pancreas (neuroblastoma and ganglioneuroma in children). Bloom, Polak, and Pearse recognized that patients with this syndrome have elevated plasma levels and a high tumor content of vasoactive intestinal polypeptide (VIP) [1].

Our understanding of the physiologic role of VIP has changed considerably in the past 20 years. VIP was initially identified by Said as a vasoactive substance [10]; we now recognize its major role as a neurotransmitter or neuromodulator. Among many biological actions VIP induces intestinal electrolyte secretion. A controversy existed for many years over whether VIP was a true mediator of intestinal secretion and diarrhea in pancreatic cholera syndrome rather than a marker of the disease, since not all patients with islet cell tumors and diarrhea had elevated plasma VIP levels and elevated levels can be found in some healthy controls and in persons abusing laxatives.

VIP is the major mediator of the WDHH syndrome; many of the symptoms can be explained by its biological actions. In patients in whom tumors have been removed, diarrhea disappears when plasma VIP levels return to normal. Prolonged intravenous VIP infusion (10 h) in healthy subjects produces secretory diarrhea (mean 2.4 l/10 h) and causes metabolic acidosis, thus mimicking the clinical syndrome [3].

The major clinical manifestation of the syndrome is large-volume secretory diarrhea. Since the diarrhea is secretory, stool water is isotonic to plasma, and stool electrolytes account for all the osmolality. Diarrhea persists on fasting. In 8 patients with VIPomas we measured a mean daily stool weight of 4460 g while eating and 1977 g while fasting. For practical purposes, a stool volume of less than 700 g per day excludes the syndrome. Large amounts of potassium and bicarbonate are lost in the diarrheal stool, resulting in hypokalemia, acidosis, and volume depletion. In the few patients who have been studied carefully, secretion of water and ions by the small intestine has been demonstrated.

Achlorhydria or hypochlorhydria is often present. Of 43 patients reviewed by Verner and Morrison [15], only 14 had histamine-fast achlorhydria while another 16 had hypochlorhydria. It is likely that the tumor releases a gastric inhibitor, but it is not known whether VIP affects meal-stimulated acid secretion in humans.

Hypercalcemia occurs in half the cases [15], but the mechanism is not clear. There appears to be a negative calcium balance with increased bone resorption. Tetany is thought to be due to hypomagnesemia and may occur in the presence of hypercalcemia. Flushing is occasionally observed. Some patients have circulatory disturbances with hypotension due to peripheral vasodilation, and rebound hypertension may follow tumor removal. These symptoms can be expected from the known cardiovascular effects of VIP. Glucose intolerance is seen in about 50% of the patients with the VIPoma syndrome and is thought to be due to VIP's glycogenolytic and glucogenetic effects on the liver.

The duration of symptoms prior to diagnosis may vary from months to years, the average being three years. Metastases (liver, lymph nodes) are present in half the patients at the time of diagnosis. Death results from the complications of water and salt depletion and acidosis.

With the better understanding of the pathophysiology of VIPoma syndrome and new treatment modalities, both survival and the quality of life have been improved.

The most effective method of treating a VIPoma is total tumor excision. Unfortunately, this is often not possible because of metastases or tumor growth involving vital structures. Approximately half of the pancreatic tumors are resectable. Debulking of the tumor may be beneficial, as is hepatic arterial embolization in the case of liver metastases. Hepatic artery ligation is usually unsuccessful because of collateralization. Embolization therapy appears to destroy tumor metastases without impairing normal liver function.

VIPomas may respond to streptozocin (streptozotocin) alone or in combination with 5-fluorouracil; the remission rate may be as high as 90 per cent [6].

Several agents including indomethacin, lithium carbonate, trifluoperazine, phosphate buffer, clonidine, metoclopramide, loperamide, and steroids have been used for symptomatic relief of the often fulminant secretory diarrhea. Unfortunately, none have produced sustained improvement.

Interestingly, native somatostatin has been shown to inhibit intestinal electrolyte secretion. Ruskone et al. were the first to show a beneficial effect of native somatostatin in a patient with VIPoma syndrome [9]. The somatostatin analogue (Sandostatin® – SMS 201-995) has recently been shown to be a highly effective treatment for the fulminant diarrhea of end stage VIPoma/WDHH; in some cases there appeared to be tumor mass regression. Because its antimotility effect, Sandostatin may be beneficial in pseudopancreatic cholera syndrome, whenever the intestinal secretion is not due to tumor or high concentrations of a circulating secretagogue.

Glucagonoma

Glucagonoma is diagnosed by its characteristic skin rash, necrolytic migratory erythema, which is a figurate erythema having histologic features of toxic epidermal necrolysis [13]. The lesions are found on the buttocks, groin, perineum and thighs, beginning as red patches and progressing to bullae which break down, become encrusted, and heal with pigmentation. The lesions tend to coalesce, often with extensive skin involvement and secondary infection [13]. The lesions are less likely due to the elevated plasma glucagon levels than to the low amino acids and zinc levels which result from hyperglucagonemia. The rash disappears following complete tumor resection and subsequent normalization of glucagon levels.

Other manifestations include anorexia, glossitis, angular cheilitis, venous thrombosis, weight loss, anemia, and psychiatric disturbances such as depression [13]. Diarrhea is prominent in occasional patients and is thought to result from the secretory effects of glucagon on the small bowel mucosa (reduction of absorption or enhancement of net secretion of water and electrolytes).

Like most islet cell tumors, glucagonomas are slow growing. Patients are usually middle-aged and have a long history of symptoms related to glucagon excess. The diagnosis is confirmed by documenting elevated plasma glucagon levels in the presence of a pancreatic mass. Intravenous doses of tolbutamide cause release of tumor glucagon, but this test is usually not necessary. Moreover, it has become difficult to obtain tolbutamide for intravenous use. High glucagon levels may also occur with diabetes mellitus, pancreatitis, trauma, burns and myocardial infarction. Diagnosis therefore requires the presence of a tumor mass and the exclusion of other conditions known to elevate the plasma glucagon concentration.

Dramatic improvement of the disabling rash in this syndrome has been reported with the use of native somatostatin or the somatostatin analogue (Sandostatin®, SMS 201-995) [11, 12, 16]. Plasma glucagon did not correlate with the improvement in skin rash, suggesting that Sandostatin may have multiple mechanisms.

References

1. Bloom SR, Polak JM, Pearse AGE: Vasoactive intestinal peptide and watery-diarrhea syndrome. Lancet *2*:14–16, 1973
2. Buchanan KD, Johnston CF, O'Hare MT: Neuroendocrine tumors. A European view. Am J Med *81* [Suppl 6B]:14–22, 1986
3. Kane MG, O'Dorisio TM, Krejs GJ: Production of secretory diarrhea by intravenous infusion of vasoactive intestinal polypeptide. N Engl J Med *309*:1482–1485, 1983
4. Krejs GJ: VIPoma Syndrome. Am J Med *82* [Suppl. 5B]: 37–48, 1987
5. McGuigan JE: The Zollinger-Ellison syndrome. In: Sleisenger MH, Fordtran JS (eds) Gastrointestinal disease, 4th edn. Saunders, Philadelphia, 1989, pp 909–925
6. Moertel CG, Hanley JA, Johnson LA: Streptozocin alone compared with streptozocin plus fluorouracil in the treatment of advanced islet-cell carcinoma. N Engl J Med *303*:1189–1194, 1980
7. Priest WM, Alexander MK: Islet-cell tumor of the pancreas with peptic ulceration, diarrhea, and hypokalaemia. Lancet *2*:1145, 1957
8. Richardson CT, Peters MN, Feldman M, et al.: Treatment of Zollinger-Ellison syndrome with vagotomy, exploratory laparotomy, and H_2-receptor antagonists. A prospective study. Gastroenterology *89*:357–367, 1985
9. Ruskone A, Rene E, Chayvialle JA, et al.: Effect of somatostatin on diarrhea and small intestinal water and electrolyte transport in a patient with pancreatic cholera. Dig Dis Sci *27*:459–466, 1982
10. Said SI, Mutt V: Potent peripheral and splanchnic vasodilator peptide from normal gut. Nature *225*:863–864, 1970
11. Santangelo WC, Unger RH, Orci L, Dueno MI, Popma JJ, Krejs GJ: Somatostatin analog-induced remission of necrolytic migratory erythema without changes in plasma glucagon concentration. Pancreas *1*:464–469, 1986
12. Sohier J, Jeanmougin M, Lombrail P, Passa P: Rapid improvement of skin lesions in glucagonomas with intravenous somatostatin infusion. Lancet *1*:40, 1980
13. Stacpoole PW: The glucagonoma syndrome: clinical features, diagnosis and treatment. Endocr Rev *2*:347–363, 1981

14. Verner JV, Morrison AB: Islet cell tumor and a syndrome of refractory watery diarrhea and hypokalemia. Am J Med *25*:374–380, 1958
15. Verner JV, Morrison AB: Endocrine pancreatic islet disease with diarrhea: report of a case due to diffuse hyperplasia of nonbeta islet tissue with a review of 54 additional cases. Arch Intern Med *133*:492–500, 1974
16. Wood S, Polak JM, Bloom SR: Glucagonoma syndrome. In: Lefebvre PJ (ed) Glucagon. Handbook of experimental pharmacology, vol 66/2. Springer, Berlin Heidelberg New York Tokyo, 1983, pp 411–430
17. Zollinger RM, Ellison EC: Primary peptic ulcerations of the jejunum associated with islet cell tumors of the pancreas. Ann Surg *142*:709–728, 1955
18. Zollinger RM, Ellison EC, Fabri PJ, et al.: Primary peptic ulcerations of the jejunum associated with islet cell tumors. Twenty-five year appraisal. Ann Surg *192*:422–430, 1980

9. Rebound Effect and Escape of Diarrhea Inhibition Using Sandostatin® in VIPoma Patients

K. Gyr, A. Koelz, M. Kraenzlin, C. Beglinger, V. Meier, S. R. Bloom

Department of Internal Medicine, Kantonsspital Liestal, University of Basle, Liestal, Switzerland, and Department of Endocrinology, Hammersmith Hospital, London, UK

Introduction

We report here on two patients treated with Sandostatin® (octreotide) for pancreatic cholera due to metastatic VIPoma. After good initial responses, the inhibitory effect of Sandostatin (SMS) on diarrhea and VIP release disappeared and a significant rebound state developed while the treatment continued.

Case Reports

Patient No. 1: This 54-year-old male patient had suffered from intermittent profuse watery diarrhea since February 1978. After the diagnosis of a VIPoma of the pancreas had been established (VIP: 85 pmol/l; N < 15 pmol/l), in April 1980 the patient underwent hemipancreatectomy, splenectomy and partial resection of the omentum for a multiloculated nodular pancreatic tumor. This was an islet cell tumor which stained positive for chorionic gonadotropin (CG), alpha-hCG and VIP.

Following surgery, the patient remained symptom-free until late 1982, when watery diarrhea recurred and reached approximately 30 bowel movements a day and a volume of about 1600 ml/24 h in 1983. Liver metastases and a retrogastric tumor mass were found (VIP: 32.5 pmol/l). The patient underwent 5 courses of combined chemotherapy with streptozotocin and 5-fluorouracil between March 1983 and December 1984, with only temporary symptomatic improvement. In December 1984 the patient was re-admitted to the hospital with severe watery diarrhea, dehydration and acidosis (blood pH: 7.2). Stool output varied between 1500 and 5080 ml per 24 h. Additional growth of the liver metastases was confirmed by computer tomography. Trials with loperamide, nifedipine and prednisone failed to improve the symptoms. Sandostatin 50 µg twice daily was therefore started on December 24. A dramatic remission of the diarrhea occurred, with the patient having only 1 to 2 formed stools per day. Ten days later, the patient again developed profuse watery diarrhea while on Sandostatin treatment, and was re-admitted because of weight loss and dehydration. Increasing the dose of Sandostatin to 600 µg per day subcutaneously reduced the diarrhea markedly, but for only a short time. In a further attempt to control the situation, the drug was given intravenously at a rate of 50 µg per hour without success. To rule out tachyphylaxis to the analogue, native somatostatin was tried, but without success. Diarrhea then increased to 16 l per day and the fluid balance could barely be maintained in the intensive care unit. Plasma VIP levels had increased to 350 pmol/l. Sandostatin was stopped and VIP rose to 425 pmol/l. The patient was taken to emergency surgery and tumors were removed from the pancreas, liver and peritoneum. Diarrhea ceased on the day of operation and VIP levels fell to a minimum of 15 pmol/l on the 8th post-operative day. The patient was well for several months, but then diarrhea resumed which, however, responded to chemotherapy. Autoradiographic examination of resected tumor tissue revealed high densities of somatostatin receptors.

Patient No. 2: A 48-year-old Egyptian woman had been operated for a symptomatic pancreatic tumor in 1980 and for recurrence and metastases in 1981. Following surgery, the pre-existing diarrhea resolved and VIP plasma levels that were elevated before operation fell to less than 5 pmol/l. Until 1983 the patient had been treated several times with combined chemotherapy (streptozotocin and 5-fluorouracil), surgery or hepatic artery embolization for recurrences. In 1983 a further recurrence occurred with VIP plasma levels up to 300 pmol/l. It was then decided to start the patient on Sandostatin (2 × 50 µg s.c.). This resulted in a marked improvement of her diarrhea. The VIP levels fell to 100 pmol/l. However, 4 days after starting Sandostatin the diarrhea recurred and the VIP levels rose to 760 pmol/l. The analogue was discontinued for 2 days. With severe challenge, the patient responded dramatically for a few days. Hepatic artery embolization was then performed, but failed to control the symptoms. A third trial of Sandostatin was started, which again reduced diarrhea and VIP levels for 11 days. Then again, diarrhea increased dramatically and the VIP levels rose to 700 pmol/l. The patient was then started on prednisolone which controlled the diarrhea for up to 18 months.

Discussion

The escape of diarrhea control and VIP secretion inhibition, seen in these two patients treated with Sandostatin is similar to the phenomena observed with regard to gastric acid secretion in the rat [1]. There are several possible explanations for the escape and rebound phenomena with Sandostatin treatment: accelerated enzymatic breakdown of somatostatin, ligand-induced changes of somatostatin receptors on the target cell, or gradual adaptation of the target cells to intracellular effects of somatostatin. One way to overcome this problem of desensitization to somatostatin might be the intermittent administration of somatostatin [2].

The two cases reported here indicate that an escape of control or even a rebound effect with a dangerous exacerbation of symptoms may occur during treatment with somatostatin and its analogues in VIPoma patients. Treatment with Sandostatin should therefore be conducted under close medical supervision.

References

1. Ekelund M., Ekman R., Hakanson R., Sundler F.: Continuous infusion of somatostatin evokes escape of gastric acid inhibition in the rat. Gastroenterology 1984, *86*:861–865
2. Koelz A., Kraenzlin M., Gyr K., Meier V., Bloom St. R., Heitz Ph., Stalder H.: Escape of the response to a long-acting somatostatin analogue (SMS 201-995) in patients with vipoma. Gastroenterology 1987, *92*:527–531

10. Long-Term Treatment of VIPoma and Glucagonoma with Sandostatin®

G. Williams [1], S. R. Bloom [2]

[1] Department of Medicine, University of Liverpool, Liverpool, UK, and [2] Department of Medicine, Royal Postgraduate Medical School, Hammersmith Hospital, London, UK

Gut-associated neuroendocrine tumors grow slowly. Throughout most of their natural history, their ill-effects are due to secretion of biologically-active products rather than to tumor burden alone [4, 7]. Specific therapy to reduce tumor peptide secretion therefore has considerable theoretical appeal as an adjunct to tumor mass reduction by surgical debulking, embolization or cytotoxic drugs. The recent introduction of somatostatin analogues for clinical use has translated this theoretical hope into reality [1, 3].

We report our experience over the last four years with the somatostatin analogue, Sandostatin® (octreotide), also known as SMS 201-995, in the treatment of seven gastroenteropancreatic (GEP) tumors, specifically four VIPomas (vasoactive intestinal peptide), one mixed gastrinoma/glucagonoma and two glucagonomas.

VIPoma

The clinical features of the four VIPoma patients are shown in Table 1. When first seen at the Hammersmith Hospital, symptoms of profuse watery diarrhea and intermittent profound hypokalemia (plasma potassium concentration as low as 1 mmol/l) had been present for 6 months to 6 years.

The diagnosis was confirmed by the finding of persistently elevated plasma VIP levels, defined as >30 pmol/l.

The primary tumor was found in the pancreas in three patients and in the jejunal wall in the fourth; all patients had multiple hepatic metastases. In two patients, primary and metastastic tissues stained heavily for VIP.

As shown in Table 1, all patients had previously undergone intensive treatment. The primary tumor had been removed in two of them. All patients had received either systemic or local infusions of either streptozotocin alone or in combination with 5-fluorouracil. Three patients had undergone hepatic artery embolization [2]. Although these treatments were initially effective, symptoms recurred within a few weeks. When the patients were treated with Sandostatin, they were severely ill (intractable diarrhea, dehydration and hypokalemia) and further surgery, embolization and chemotherapy were either contraindicated or considered inappropriate.

After starting subcutaneous Sandostatin injections (initially 50–100 μg twice daily), all four patients showed at least a 50% fall in mean 24-h plasma VIP concentration. In one patient (No. 3), levels were suppressed to the normal range. Coincident with this, watery diarrhea improved: stool frequency fell from 4–8 per day to 1–2 per day, with dramatic relief of urgency of defecation and incontinence. Stool volumes fell from 1–8 l/day (mean: 4300 ml/day) to 500 ml/day or less (mean: 300 ml/day). Intravenous fluids and parenteral potassium supplements were gradually withdrawn over several days.

The improvement in quality of life, particularly alleviation of the immense personal and social handicap of debilitating and unpredictable diarrhea, which each patient reported after starting Sandostatin treatment cannot be overstated. One patient (No. 4) had been treated symptomatically with high dosages of prednisolone, which could not be withdrawn without a diarrheal relapse. She had developed severe iatrogenic Cushing's syndrome with avascular necrosis of both femoral heads. While on Sandostatin, the

Table 1. Clinical features of GEP tumor patients treated with long-term Sandostatin

Tumor type	Patient No.	Age and sex	Duration of symptoms	Primary tumor site	Previous treatment [1] Surgery	Chemo	Embolism	Duration (months) of Sandostatin treatment [2]
VIPoma	1	M, 40	6 years	Pancreas	+	+	+	48
	2	M, 55	6 months	Pancreas	–	+	+	27 [3]
	3	M, 47	1 year	Pancreas	–	+	–	18 [3]
	4	F, 47	3.5 years	Jejunum	+	+	+	30
Gastrin-glucagonoma	5	M, 66	5 years	Pancreas	+	+	–	30 [3]
Glucagonoma	6	M, 70	3 years	Pancreas	–	–	–	31
	7	F, 58	2 years	Pancreas	–	–	–	27

Notes:

[1] Treatment: Chemo = chemotherapy (mostly streptozocin ± 5-fluorouracil); Embolism = embolization

[2] Duration of symptoms = at start of Sandostatin treatment

[3] Patients who have subsequently died

prednisolone dosage was reduced from 20 mg/day to 2.5 mg/day with no increase in stool frequency or volume.

During long-term (24–48 months) therapy, the initially observed biochemical and clinical improvement was sustained in each patient for at least 6–12 weeks. In one patient (No. 3), this continued for several months. In the other three patients (Nos. 1, 2 and 4), however, mean plasma VIP concentrations rose to 300–600 pmol/l, followed 6–18 months later by a progressive return of watery diarrhea. All patients eventually suffered several acute exacerbations with symptomatic dehydration and hypokalemia despite the increase of Sandostatin dosages to 500–1500 µg/day. One patient (No. 2) died during an acute exacerbation and another (No. 3) died after over a year of symptomatic remission. In the latter patient, rapid growth of hepatic metastases occurred throughout Sandostatin therapy, despite decreases in plasma VIP levels and improvement of diarrhea. One patient (No. 1) had a further course of streptozotocin and arterial embolization of the primary pancreatic tumor, and was maintained on dexamethasone, 2–5 mg/day. The other patient (No. 4) was given increasing doses of prednisolone, with temporary symptomatic improvement.

We have performed serial CT scans of the hepatic metastases during these trials to assess the effect of Sandostatin on tumor growth. This is difficult to investigate because: a) tumor bulk is difficult to measure, even with CT scanning; b) the natural growth curve of these tumors, as well as the possible long-term effects of previous treatment, are unknown; and c) spontaneous infarction (which is well documented in prolactinomas and other pituitary tumors) may occur, giving the appearance of either a natural cure or a dramatic response to treatment. Although an early report on patient No. 1 described possible shrinkage of VIPoma hepatic metastases after several months of Sandostatin therapy [5], re-assessment after longer follow-up suggests that the hepatic metastases apparently increased in size. Modest tumor growth was noted in patients 1, 2 and 4 but was very pronounced in No. 3. It is of interest that, despite advancing tumor growth, biochemical and chemical remission for several months was noted in patient 3.

The reported gastrointestinal side effects of Sandostatin treatment (colic, bloating, urgency and occasionally paralytic ileus, diarrhea and steatorrhea) were relatively unimportant when compared with the dramatic reduction in watery diarrhea and bowel movement frequency. Mild glucose intolerance was noted in each patient. However, none developed symptoms of diabetes or required antidiabetic treatment. Anterior pituitary function remained normal.

Discussion

Sandostatin acts in part by suppressing VIP secretion. An additional anti-diarrheal effect at the gut mucosal level is suggested by two points. First, diarrhea improved dramatically with initiation of therapy, even though VIP levels (albeit reduced below pretreatment levels) remained substantially above normal (up to 200 pmol/l) in three patients. Secondly, clinical remission continued for some months following 'escape' of plasma VIP due, perhaps, to either down-regulation of the tumor's somatostatin receptors or increased tumor mass or activity. The discrepancy between clinical improvement and persistently high circulating immunoreactive VIP levels may be due in part to Sandostatin's selective suppression of a smaller, more biologically-active molecular form of VIP [10]. Thus high levels of a larger molecular weight form which persisted during Sandostatin therapy would presumably have little biological action.

This study suggests that VIPoma patients may expect many months of clinical remission during continuous Sandostatin treatment, even with disease progression that does not respond to conventional therapy. Sandostatin is well tolerated; patients readily accept the routine of multiple daily subcutaneous injections as a small price to pay for what is, initially at least, a spectacular symptomatic cure.

Glucagonoma and Gastrinoma

Details of these three patients are shown in Table 1. All had primary pancreatic tumors with multiple metastases. All had the characteristic migratory necrolytic rash of the glucagonoma syndrome [6, 9] and patient No. 5, with gastrin hypersecretion, also suffered recurrent peptic ulceration and diarrhea despite high-dose cimetidine (3–4 g/day). He had also previously undergone arterial embolization and streptozotocin treatment, which were unsuccessful.

After a single subcutaneous injection of Sandostatin (100 μg), elevated plasma levels of glucagon (and in case No. 5, of gastrin) fell substantially and remained below pre-injection levels for several hours. However, glucagon and gastrin levels were not normalized. During long-term therapy, this effect was less predictable, possibly owing to down-regulation of somatostatin receptors on the tumor or to tumor growth. Glucagon levels were not normalized and chronic Sandostatin administration had no apparent effect on immunoreactive plasma glucagon levels.

The clinical effects of Sandostatin were also hard to assess because of the well-described tendency of the glucagonoma rash to undergo spontaneous cycles of remission and relapse [6, 9]. Nevertheless, all three patients initially showed marked clearing of the rash after starting Sandostatin therapy. Further improvement was associated with increasing dosage, suggesting a true effect of Sandostatin. This is consistent with the observation that refractory glucagonoma rash can be cleared very rapidly after intravenous somatostatin infusion [8]. Other beneficial effects of Sandostatin included improvement of hypoproteinemia and nonspecific anemia (patient No. 6) and of glycemic control in the mildly diabetic patients (Nos. 5 and 6).

Patient 5 died, apparently of pulmonary embolism, a recognized complication of the glucagonoma syndrome [9]. The other two patients remained relatively well after 12–18 months of Sandostatin treatment. Tumor shrinkage during Sandostatin treatment was not documented in any patient.

In these patients, acute administration of Sandostatin suppressed pathologically elevated glucagon and gastrin levels, but with long-term therapy sustained suppression was less consistent. Sandostatin treatment appears to clear the glucagonoma rash; however, the natural variation in the severity and extent of the rash makes the present limited trials difficult to interpret.

Conclusions

The potent capacity of Sandostatin to suppress abnormal peptide hormone secretion from a variety of GEP tumors makes it a valuable new option in the treatment of these rare diseases, even when widespread metastatic disease is present and the patients are considered clinically to be 'end-stage' with respect to conventional treatment methods. Large-scale studies of longer duration will be essential to answer the important pathophysiological and clinical question of whether or not Sandostatin has any effect on tumor growth or, indeed, the ultimate prognosis of these syndromes.

Acknowledgements: We should like to thank the staff of the Francis Fraser Laboratories (in particular Mr. Jan Domin, Mr. Floyd Bailey and Miss Jenny Paterson) for performing many of the hormone assays, and Mrs. Jacqui Chatterton for her usual skill and efficiency in typing this manuscript.

References

1. Adrian T. E., Barnes A. J., Long R. J., O'Shaughnessy D. J., Brown M., Rivier J., Vale W., Blackburn A. M., Bloom S. R. (1981): The effect of somatostatin analogs on secretion of growth pancreatic and gastrointestinal hormones in man. J Clin Endocrinol Metab *53*:675–681
2. Allison D. J. (1978): Therapeutic embolization. Br J Hosp Med *20*:707–715
3. Bauer W., Briner U., Doepfner W., Haller R., Huguénin R., Marbach P., Petcher T. J., Pless J. (1982): A very potent and selective octapeptide analog of somatostatin with prolonged action. Life Sci *31*:1133–1140
4. Friesen S. R. (1982): Tumors of the endocrine pancreas. N Engl J Med *306*:580–590
5. Kraenzlin M. E., Ch'ng J. L. C., Wood S. M., Carr D. H., Bloom S. R. (1985): Long-term treatment of a VIPoma with somatostatin analogue resulting in remission of symptoms and possible shrinkage of metastases. Gastroenterology *88*:185–187
6. Mallinson C. N., Bloom S. R., Warin A. P., Salmon P. R., Cox B. (1974): A glucagonoma syndrome. Lancet *II*:1–5
7. Sabate M. I., Carlei F., Bloom S. R., Polak J. M. (1985): Endocrine tumours of the gut and pancreas. In: Polak J. M., Bloom S. R. (eds) Endocrine tumours. The pathology of regulatory peptide-producing tumours. Churchill-Livingstone, Edinburgh, pp 193–208
8. Sohier J., Jeanmougin M., Lombrail P., Passa P. (1980): Rapid improvement of skin lesions in glucagonomas with intravenous somatostatin infusions. Lancet *I*:40
9. Wood S. M., Polak J. M., Bloom S. R. (1983): The glucagonoma syndrome. In: Lefèbvre P. (ed) Handbook of experimental pharmacology IV. Springer, Berlin Heidelberg New York Tokyo
10. Wood S. M., Kraenzlin M. E., Adrian T. E., Bloom S. R. (1985): Treatment of patients with pancreatic endocrine tumours using a new long-acting somatostatin analogue: symptomatic and peptide responses. Gut *26*:438–444

11. Therapy of the Malignant Carcinoid Syndrome and Metastatic Islet Cell Carcinoma

L. K. Kvols

Division of Medical Oncology, Department of Oncology, Mayo Comprehensive Cancer Center, Mayo Clinic and Mayo Foundation, Rochester, Minnesota, USA

The variable symptom complexes associated with malignant carcinoid tumors and the peptide-producing metastatic islet cell carcinomas have posed therapeutic challenges to clinicians since they were first discussed in the medical literature more than three decades ago. These malignant diseases produce a constellation of clinical problems which create unique difficulties in management for the surgical and medical oncologist.

Surgical removal is frequently curative when the disease is detected at an early stage, and surgery may provide significant palliation for selected patients with metastatic disease. It is particularly important to consider early abdominal exploration in patients with symptoms of partial small bowel obstruction, since resection of the obstructing segment may give considerable relief. Metastatic disease often requires no treatment for months or even years in those patients whose disease is not seriously interfering with their lifestyle. Numerous therapeutic options are available for patients with troublesome or serious symptoms. They cover a therapeutic spectrum from simple oral medications to hepatic vascular occlusive procedures and aggressive cytotoxic chemotherapy regimens, alone or sequentially. Therefore the severity of the symptoms must be considered, as well as the effect of the disease on vital organ function, in order to select the most appropriate therapy.

The carcinoid syndrome is usually associated with carcinoid tumors of the small intestine which have metastasized to the liver. Less frequently, it is seen with primary tumors arising from other organs such as the lung, thymus, pancreas, stomach, or ovary. Episodic flushing and diarrhea are the most common initial symptoms.

Some patients may experience only flushing, whereas others may have only the diarrheal component of the syndrome. Occasionally, wheezing secondary to bronchospasm will be the presenting manifestation. The flushing symptoms run the gamut from an annoyance or embarrassment to complete incapacitation due to intense vasodilatation with associated pre-syncopal symptoms and troublesome palpitations. The flushing may be transient, lasting only seconds and confined to only the face and/or upper trunk, or it may persist for several minutes, or even up to an hour or more, and be more generalized. Flushing and diarrhea may occur spontaneously without a known precipitating factor, but patients will often relate the onset of these symptoms to ingestion of food or small amounts of alcohol. Because of the intensity of flushing after alcohol ingestion and the delay until this syndrome is clinically diagnosed, many individuals when first seen will relate that they have been avoiding all forms of alcohol for years. In some individuals, emotional factors such as feelings of anger or happiness will routinely cause flushing. While the diarrhea may be confined to the postprandial state, it may still manifest as a secretory diarrhea with its attendant dehydration and electrolyte aberrations, and it is often unresponsive to routine antidiarrhea medications. Patients often recognize their own threshold for exercise or the emotional factors which they must avoid to prevent the precipitation of incapacitating symptoms. In the later stages of the syndrome, signs and symptoms of congestive heart failure associated with right-sided valvular heart disease may dominate. Interestingly, when pulmonic stenosis is associated with tricuspid regurgitation and a coincident patent foramen ovale, the

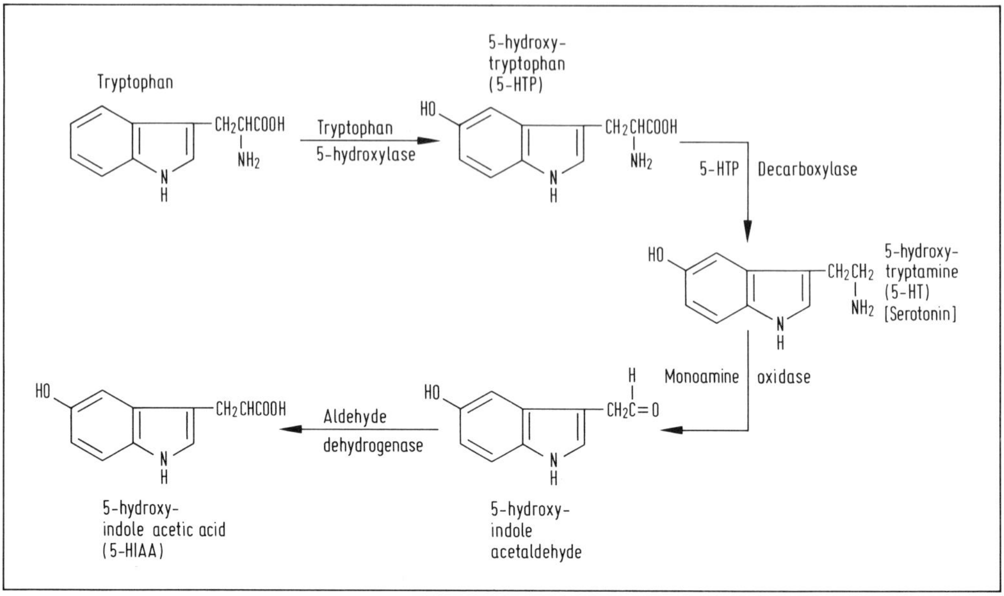

Fig. 1. Tryptophan metabolism

patient may develop arterial oxygen desaturation due to right-to-left shunt, and gradually the intense facial erythema may become dusky and cyanotic.

Although the precise pathophysiologic mechanisms of the syndrome have not been fully defined, increased serotonin production is almost always demonstrated and probably causes the diarrhea (Fig. 1). Increased urinary excretion of the serotonin metabolite, 5-hydroxyindoleacetic acid (5-HIAA), is clearly the most reliable and reproducible laboratory confirmation of the syndrome (Fig. 2). Occasionally the measurement of plasma levels of substance P and neurotensin will help in the diagnosis [12]. Histamines, substance P, and neurotensin may play a key role in the flushing of some patients, and recent studies with new pharmacologic assays are defining their importance [9, 56].

Tincture of opium, loperamide, or diphenoxylate often control mild diarrhea. While cyproheptadine at doses of 4 to 8 mg three times a day orally may control the diarrhea, it will rarely improve the flushing and will not decrease the levels of 5-HIAA, even though it has both anti-serotoninergic and anti-histaminic effects. Diarrhea in the carcinoid syndrome may sometimes be due to bile salt spillage and/or bacterial overgrowth, which require specific therapies. Mesenteric vascular ischemia due to the intense local fibrosis is commonly found upon exploratory laparotomy in patients with abdominal pain associated with the malignant carcinoid syndrome. Resection of these ischemic segments of intestine may be lifesaving and provide long-term palliation.

Numerous other treatment approaches have been tried to give symptomatic relief to these patients, including adrenergic antagonists, H-1 and H-2 histamine blockers, serotonin antagonists, bradykinin antagonists, and corticosteroids [45]. Some have been noted in anecdotal reports to be effective in occasional patients, but most produce distressing side effects and only infrequently and partially suppress the endocrine effects, without altering serotonin production. A first-generation specific 5-hydroxytryptamine M (neuronal) receptor antagonist was recently reported to improve diarrhea in three patients with carcinoid syndrome [1]. Further investigations of drugs in this class may be warranted.

The indolent and varied biologic behavior of carcinoid tumors, coupled with the limited efficacy of currently available anti-neoplastic drugs, demands careful selection of

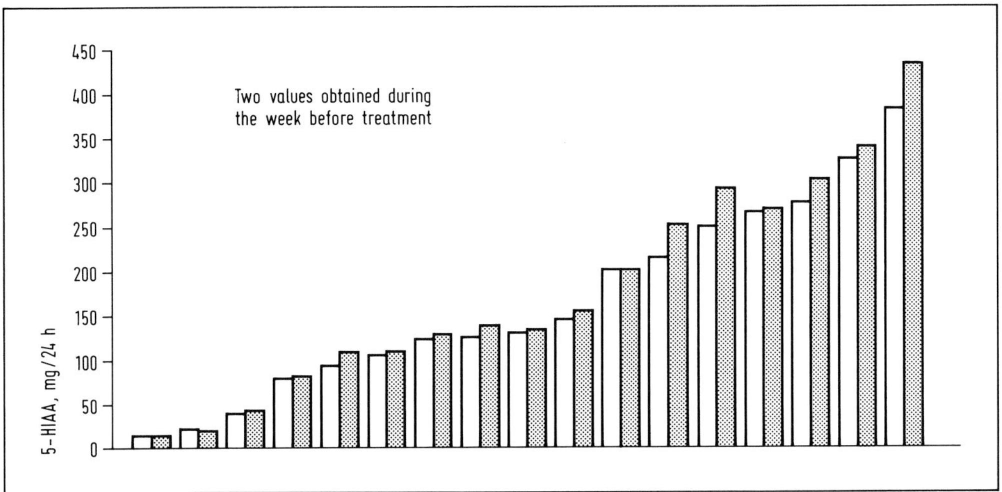

Fig. 2. Paired 24-h urinary 5-HIAA values collected within one week of each other in 17 patients receiving no intervening therapy

patients for chemotherapy trials. Aggressive treatment should not be used in patients in the early stages of their metastatic disease when they have no symptoms referable to their tumor or only minor symptoms associated with the syndrome. When, however, the symptoms interfere significantly with daily activities and do not respond to conventional pharmacologic agents, chemotherapy is indicated, as it is whenever a prognostic sign develops. Although the median survival time for patients with the malignant carcinoid syndrome is 38 months from the time of the first flush, this decreases to 14 months if the 5-HIAA is >150 mg/24 h and to only 11 months if carcinoid heart disease is evident [45].

Chemotherapy Trials in the Malignant Carcinoid Syndrome

The Mayo Clinic experience with single-drug trials is presented in Table 1 [45]. In 1975 Moertel first reported responses in six of nine carcinoid patients using the combination of 5-fluorouracil plus streptozotocin [44]. This combination was compared with cyclophosphamide plus streptozotocin in a randomized, multi-institutional trial performed by investigators in the Eastern Cooperative Oncology Group [47]. The objective response rates were 33% and 26% respectively (Table 2). More than 80 patients comprised the study population which yielded important and interesting data for analyses. While the response rate with the 5-fluorouracil and streptozotocin combination was somewhat better than with cyclophosphamide plus streptozotocin the difference was not statistically significant; neither were differences in duration of response, interval to progression, or survival. Response rates were more favorable in patients with a documented carcinoid syndrome and in those with a better performance status. With both regimens the response rate was significantly greater for small bowel carcinoids than for carcinoids of pulmonary or unknown origin.

On the basis of the results of this protocol, the Eastern Cooperative Oncology Group

Table 1. Single-agent chemotherapy – Mayo Clinic experience

Agent	Patients	Objective response	
		No.	Percentage
Doxorubicin	33	7	21
5-fluorouracil	19	5	26
DTIC	18	3	17
Dactinomycin	17	1	6
Cisplatin	15	1	7

DTIC = dimethyltriazenoimidazole carboximide

Table 2. Combination chemotherapy regimens for malignant carcinoid tumors

Regimen	Patients	Objective response	Author (ref.)
STZ* + 5-FU	42	14 (33%)	Moertel [47]
STZ + CTX	47	12 (26%)	Moertel [47]
STZ** + 5-FU	80	18 (23%)	Engstrom [11]

* Streptozotocin in five-day courses repeated every six weeks
** Streptozotocin in five-day courses repeated every 10 weeks

undertook a second protocol in which 5-fluorouracil and streptozotocin were again used, but the streptozotocin was given every 10 weeks rather than every 5 weeks as in the first protocol, in an attempt to decrease anorexia, nausea, and vomiting. The administration of 5-fluorouracil remained unchanged at every day for five days every five weeks. The comparative agent in this study was doxorubicin 60 mg/m^2 i.v. monthly, with heart disease as the only contraindication. Engstrom reported the results of this study for the Eastern Cooperative Oncology Group in 1984 [11]. Nausea and vomiting secondary to streptozotocin were not attenuated, and the response rate was lower, with only 18 of 80 (23%) fulfilling the criteria for response. The response rate for doxorubicin was 17 of 81 (23%). The median duration of response was 26 weeks for doxorubicin and 31 weeks for the combination. In contrast to the preceding study, the location of the primary tumor did not correlate with survival prognosis. Neither the amount of 5-HIAA in the urine at study entry nor the histologic classification of the tumor were prognostic for survival.

A weekly schedule of streptozotocin and doxorubicin has been reported to cause tumor regression in 4 of 10 carcinoid patients [20]. A phase II study of cisplatin therapy in patients with metastatic carcinoid tumor and the malignant carcinoid syndrome did not find it to be effective in the dose and schedule used [53]. A four-drug regimen of 5-fluorouracil, streptozotocin, doxorubicin, and cyclophosphamide does not appear to offer any clear-cut therapeutic advantage [7]. The phase II trial of single agent etoposide resulted in objective responses in only 2/17 patients with bronchial carcinoids [21].

Miscellaneous Treatment Approaches for the Carcinoid Syndrome

1. Parachlorophenylalanine

Parachlorophenylalanine has been shown to relieve diarrhea and to reduce urinary 5-hydroxyindoleacetic acid excretion, but rarely to control flushing. However, the hypersensitivity reactions and psychiatric disturbances associated with this agent preclude long-term clinical use [67].

2. Cyproheptadine

Cyproheptadine functions both as a histamine antagonist and as a serotonin antagonist. While it controls the diarrhea of the carcinoid syndrome, it rarely alters the flushing. Harris and Smith reported regression of a carcinoid tumor and a nonfunctioning apudoma in two of 12 patients treated with cyproheptadine [16]. They postulated that cyproheptadine might affect tumor growth by blocking the effects of amine hormones. A phase II study of this agent is currently under way at the Mayo Clinic to assess its anti-tumor effect in patients with measurable disease. In the first 16 patients treated no evidence of tumor mass shrinkage has been seen. Patients can usually tolerate oral doses of 8 mg three times a day without excessive sedation or dry mouth. Interestingly, many patients have gained weight on cyproheptadine, presumably because of its appetite-stimulating effect [46].

3. Tamoxifen

Investigators from Greece reported that the synthetic anti-estrogen, tamoxifen, caused symptomatic improvement in a patient with the carcinoid syndrome [69]. A second report on tamoxifen noted biochemical improvement (5-hydroxyindoleacetic acid decreased from 174 to 15 mg per 24 h), as well as objective tumor regression [55]. In a collaborative trial from the Mayo Clinic and the American Oncologic Hospital, 16 patients with metastatic carcinoid tumor were treated with tamoxifen (3 were known to be estrogen receptor-positive). None showed any evidence of objective improvement in malignant disease, as measured by reduced tumor size, or sustained reduction in levels of 5-hydroxyindoleacetic acid. All patients were treated for a minimum of eight weeks with divided daily doses of 20–40 mg. The median time to progression was 10 weeks, and the disease had progressed in all patients by 24 weeks [51].

4. *Interferon*

A report by Öberg and his associates has created interest in using interferon for the carcinoid syndrome [57]. Significant symptomatic improvement was noted in all 36 patients treated, and 5-hydroxyindoleacetic acid excretion was reduced in 15 (42%), but objective responses of tumor masses, based on the usual criteria, were seen in only 4 (11%). A study of higher dosages of interferon using recombinant DNA-produced alpha-interferon is now under way at the Mayo Clinic.

5. *Hepatic Arterial Devascularization*

Since 90% of the tumor cell's oxygenation is derived from the hepatic artery, whereas 50% of the oxygenation normal hepatocytes receive is from the portal system, the liver's unique dual blood supply has prompted investigators to take advantage of this therapeutically. Surgical ligation and percutaneous embolization have both been used successfully. Martin and his colleagues have reported on eight patients with the carcinoid syndrome who underwent hepatic artery ligation at the time of laparotomy [36]. The advantage of this surgical approach is that it permits the resection of the frequently obstructive ileal primary lesions or ischemic small intestine which was necessary in five of the six patients with small-bowel primaries in this group (Fig. 2). Facial flushing ceased in all patients and diarrhea was uniformly reduced by the time of hospital discharge. All patients became febrile and had striking increases in the SGOT values during the first postoperative week but recovered quickly thereafter. The duration of response ranged from three to ten months (median five months). Other investigators have confirmed that hepatic artery occlusion alone is effective in inducing tumor debulking in this disease [35, 43]. Because ligation-induced hepatic dysfunction is transient, ligation does not preclude future chemotherapy.

6. *Hepatic Artery Occlusion Followed by Combination Chemotherapy*

The early results of the Mayo Clinic trial of sequential hepatic artery occlusion and chemotherapy for metastatic carcinoid tumor have been reported previously [52]. Ten symptomatic patients with measurable hormonal and/or tumor parameters and proven hepatic dominant metastasis have been treated with hepatic artery occlusion by either surgical ligation or percutaneous embolization. Three weeks later, they were started on dimethyltriazenoimidazole carboximide (DTIC) 250 mg/m^2 × 5 days plus doxorubicin 60 mg/m^2 i.v., alternating every four weeks with 5-fluorouracil 400 mg/m^2 × 5 days plus streptozotocin 500 mg/m^2 × 5 days. Nine of the ten patients have had striking or complete relief of the carcinoid syndrome with urine 5-HIAA elevations reduced by 63 to 100%. The remaining patient had minor improvement for 12 months. Hepatic artery occlusion had side effects, as noted above in the earlier study. Chemotherapy produced its anticipated side effects, primarily vomiting and leukopenia. The early results with this program appear to show more frequent, more complete, and more lasting responses than in our prior experience with either hepatic artery occlusion or chemotherapy used alone.

7. *Somatostatin Analogue [Sandostatin® (Octreotide), SMS 201-995] Therapy*

Native somatostatin was reported to be effective in blocking the carcinoid flush induced by pentagastrin, in reducing circulat-

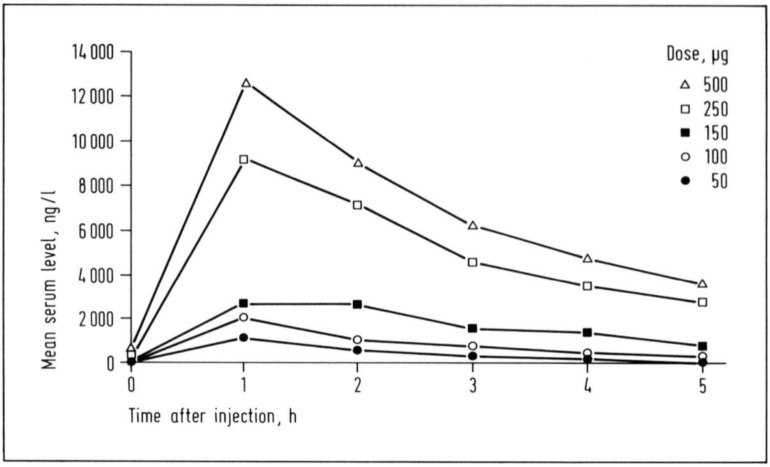

Fig. 3. Somatostatin analogue (SMS 201-995) in malignant carcinoid syndrome. Pharmacokinetics of the drug after variable doses. Mean values in nine patients

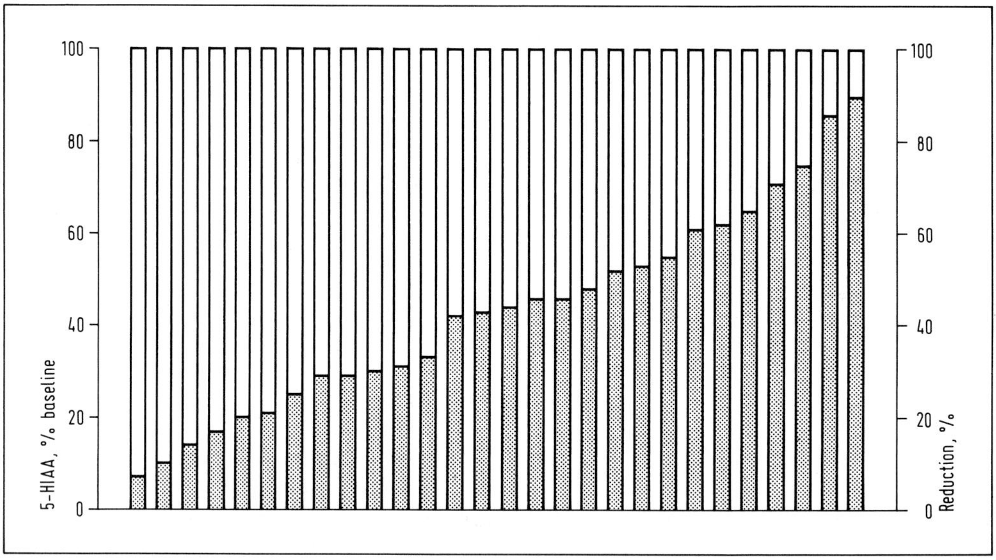

Fig. 4. Low-dose Sandostatin in malignant carcinoid syndrome

ing serotonin levels, and in controlling other symptoms associated with the carcinoid syndrome [15, 72]. The therapeutic usefulness of somatostatin was limited, since this agent had to be given by continuous intravenous infusion and had a half-life of less than two minutes. Sandostatin, a synthetic analogue of somatostatin, was found to be more specific and longer-acting in its inhibitory effects. This octapeptide retains in a conformationally stabilized form the pharmacophore presumed to be essential for the biological activity of this molecule. The presence of two D-amino acids which resist degradation by serum peptidases is in part responsible for the much longer half-life of this molecule after subcutaneous injection [3]. Dr Tom O'Dorisio, assisted by his staff at the Clinical Research Center at Ohio State University, and I have studied the serum levels of Sandostatin achieved after subcutaneous administration in nine patients with carcinoid or islet cell neoplasms and no prior exposure to the drug. The mean serum values in 9 patients treated with varying drug doses are depicted in Figure 3.

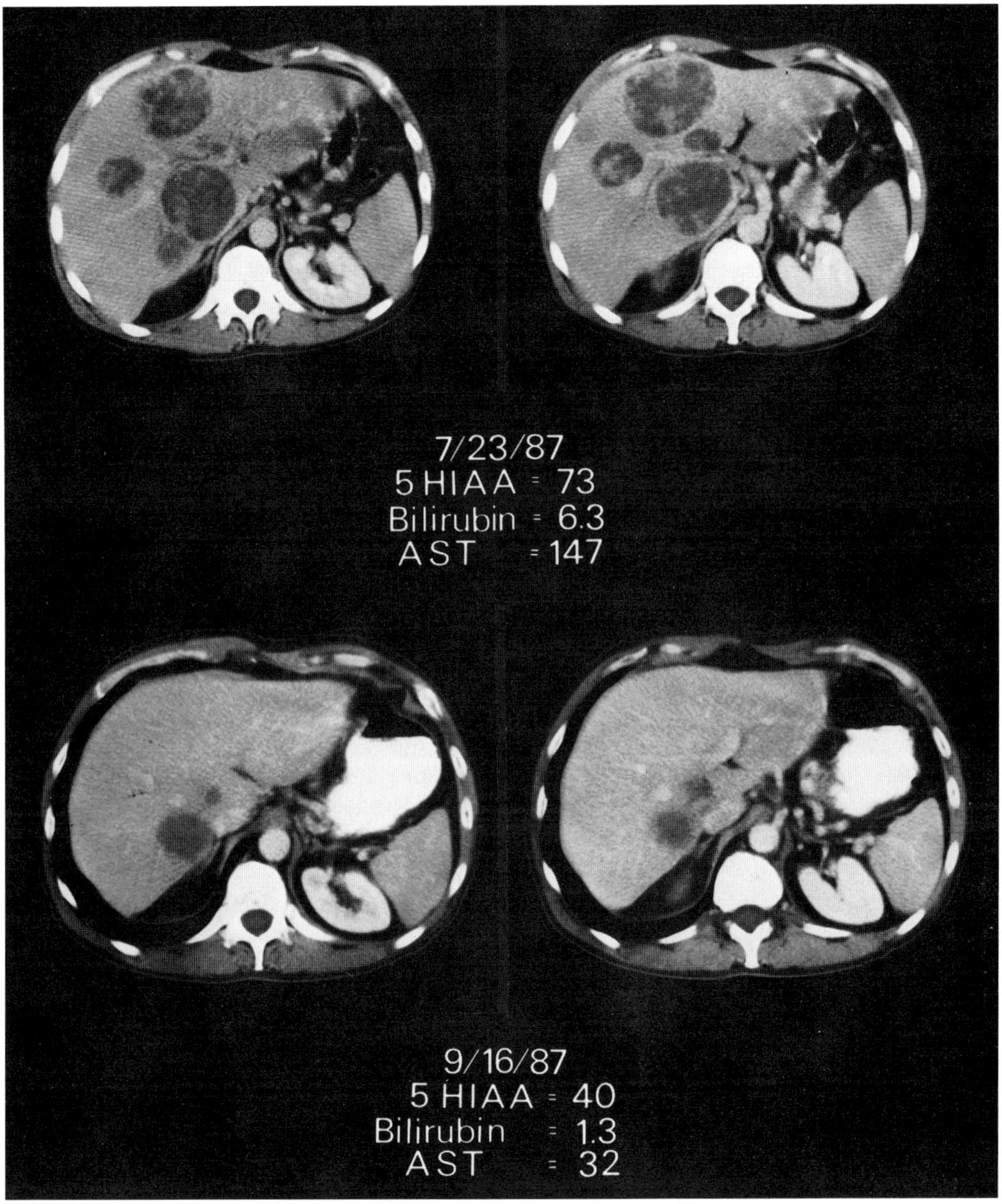

Fig. 5. Pre-treatment (top 2 panels) and post-treatment (bottom 2 panels) CT images of the liver in a patient treated with Sandostatin 500 µg t.i.d.

We have studied the chronic administration of Sandostatin in 53 patients with metastatic carcinoid tumor and the carcinoid syndrome using two separate protocols. The first 25 patients self-administered a dose of 150 µg three times daily by subcutaneous injection. Flushing and diarrhea associated with the syndrome were promptly relieved in 22 patients. Eighteen of the 25 patients (72%) had a 50% or greater decrease of their 5-HIAA level after therapy (Fig. 4). Resolution of hepatic pain, improvement in liver function tests and, in isolated instances, regression of measurable tumor masses raised the possibility of antineoplastic activity [29].

Since no clinically significant toxicity was seen, we elected to investigate the efficacy and toxicity of large doses. Twenty-eight patients with no prior exposure to somatostatin were prospectively entered in our next study and self-administered 500 µg three times daily by subcutaneous injection. Symptomatic improvement was once again achieved promptly in the majority of patients (flushing 24/25; diarrhea 20/24; wheezing 3/3). Symptoms commonly improved within the first few days of treatment. All 28 patients had a reduction in their 5-HIAA levels, and in 18/28 (64%) the reduction was greater than 50%. Twenty-three patients had tumor masses which could be assessed by bidimensional measurements and/or radiographic scanning. In this group 4/23 (17%) achieved objective partial regression i.e. >50% shrinkage of measurable tumor masses. Regression of tumor masses was seen as early as two months after starting treatment (Fig. 5). Treatment-induced steatorrhea was common at the 500 µg t.i.d. dosage (Fig. 6), and one patient developed gall bladder dilation, biliary sludge, and an asymptomatic gallstone. We have seen no evidence of hematologic, hepatic, neurologic or renal toxicity [33].

Sandostatin given by the methods we have employed is clearly effective in relieving symptoms in the majority of patients with the malignant carcinoid syndrome. The associated reduction in 5-HIAA excretion indicates that the clinical effectiveness of this agent is apparently not simply an end-organ effect but rather is related to inhibition of synthesis or release of serotonin and perhaps other biogenic amines and growth factors.

Interesting growth inhibition by Sandostatin has been demonstrated in two transplantable tumors. One is a rat chondrosarcoma which contains no somatostatin receptors, and the other is a hamster insulinoma which does contain the receptors [61]. Receptors for somatostatin have been identified in pituitary cells, brain synaptosome membranes, breast cancer, and pancreatic islet cells [41, 60, 62–64, 71, 73]. Whether the anti-neoplastic action of somatostatin is a direct effect, or an indirect effect through inhibiting growth hormone, insulin, or other tumor growth factor is unknown. Of note is that we have observed evidence of tumor regression in some of our patients. The optimal route, dose, and timing of Sandostatin necessary to cause tumor mass reduction in a higher percentage of patients certainly warrants further study.

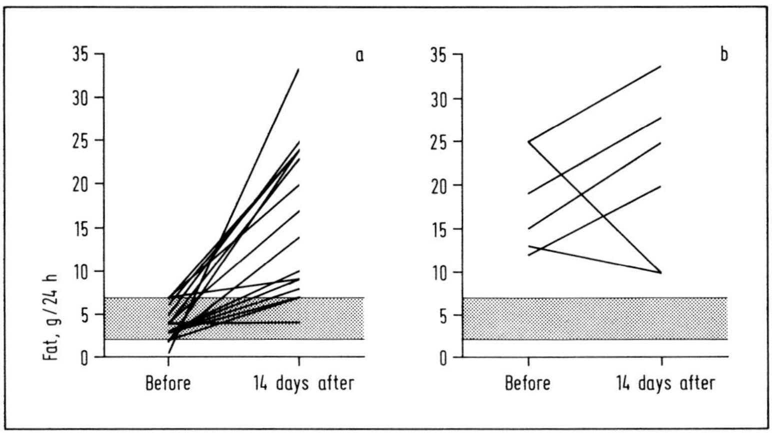

Fig. 6. High-dose somatostatin analogue (SMS 201-995) in malignant carcinoid syndrome. 72-h stool collection on a 100 g fat/day diet. Panel (a) is patients who had normal values before therapy and panel (b) is patients who had abnormal values before therapy. Normal range 2–7 g fat/24 h on a 100 g fat/day diet

Carcinoid Crisis

Carcinoid crisis is a serious, life-threatening complication of the carcinoid syndrome. Manifestations of the crisis may include hypotension or hypertension, prolonged cutaneous flushing, confusion, and, in its most severe form, coma. Carcinoid crisis has been reported to occur spontaneously, during diagnostic evaluation, and following initiation of chemotherapy [10, 27, 38]. Carcinoid crises may occur during induction of anesthesia or during the intra-operative period. Management of carcinoid crisis has been difficult because of the lack of response of the associated hemodynamic compromise to usual measures, including fluid and crystalloid replacement and vasopressors. Corticosteroids, aprotinin, ketanserin and tryptophan have been used, with questionable benefit [17, 42]. We have already reported the rapid reversal of life-threatening hypotension with Sandostatin during induction of anesthesia [34]. Subsequently, we observed three additional cases which emphasize the therapeutic usefulness of Sandostatin in the prevention and treatment of carcinoid crisis (Fig. 7) [32]. Our experience has been corroborated recently by other investigators [65]. The mechanism of action of somatostatin in this clinical situation is not completely defined. Somatostatin is known to alter calcium membrane permeability and to have an inhibitory effect on cAMP, resulting in lower intracellular calcium and cAMP levels [60]. Sandostatin has also been shown to prevent postprandial hypotension and, in some instances, orthostatic hypotension in patients with autonomic neuropathy [18, 19].

In patients with severe manifestations of the carcinoid syndrome, chemotherapy is initiated with substantially lower doses than normally used, because tumor lysis may cause sudden release of massive quantities of the vasoactive substances [47]. Carcinoid crises occurring with the administration of chemotherapy may be refractory to all standard treatment and result in death. Decreasing the initial dosage of chemotherapeutic agents by 50% for patients who demonstrate severe carcinoid syndrome or who have urinary 5-HIAA exceeding 150 mg/24 h is recommended, because patients are assumed to have an increased risk of chemotherapy-induced carcinoid crisis [4, 44]. Pretreating these patients with Sandostatin may allow full doses of cytotoxic drugs to be given.

We have used Sandostatin successfully to treat and prevent life-threatening carcinoid crisis. The drug should certainly be available

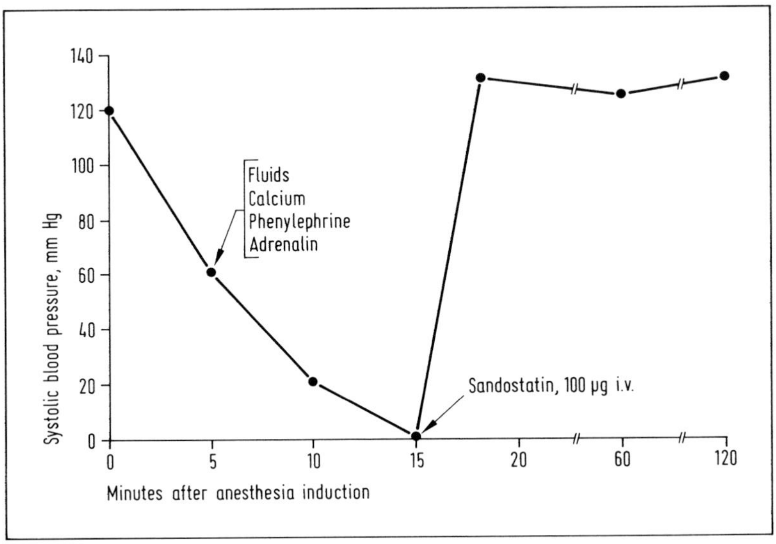

Fig. 7. Response of acute carcinoid crisis to intravenous Sandostatin

for emergency use in patients with malignant carcinoid syndrome who are undergoing surgery, commencing chemotherapy, and for treatment of spontaneously occurring carcinoid crisis. A dose of 250–500 μg administered subcutaneously *one to two hours* prior to induction of anesthesia should allow peak therapeutic serum levels to be achieved. In the acute situation we have safely administered intravenous doses of 100–500 μg intravenously. Our early clinical experience suggests that it may be prudent to begin therapy with Sandostatin using a dose of 150–250 μg subcutaneously every six to eight hours beginning 24–48 h prior to the induction of anesthesia or initiation of chemotherapy, in patients who have flagrant syndrome or who have previously had a hypotensive episode.

In summary, Sandostatin has proved to be a very useful addition to our therapeutic armamentarium for carcinoid patients. In the doses we used in our first study, it had only mild toxicity and, therefore, may be appropriate as early therapy in patients with symptomatic carcinoid syndromes but without an immediate threat from advancing tumor. Our studies have not attempted to establish the lowest dose level necessary to achieve symptomatic and biochemical control. Optimal therapy may require starting with low doses and increasing dose and/or frequency of administration until symptoms are controlled and maximum improvement of abnormal hormone levels without inducing clinically significant steatorrhea is observed. Patients in very poor clinical condition with dehydration, acidosis, or hypokalemia from a severe syndrome could be treated with Sandostatin initially to improve their status so that they could be safely treated with more aggressive approaches [26].

Islet Cell Cancer (ICC) of the Pancreas

Islet cell tumors of the pancreas may be nonfunctional, at least as defined and recognized by currently available assays, or they may produce a plethora of endocrine manifestations that can seriously disrupt the internal milieu. The course of these tumors may be very indolent; the cancer itself may produce minimal disability from the tumor burden per se, but patients may experience months or years of symptoms referable to the hypersecretion of hormones such as insulin, glucagon, vasoactive intestinal peptide, or gastrin. These tumors may cosecrete one or more of these hormones in non-physiologic quantities but the syndrome(s) resulting from the hypersecretion of one or more of the peptide hormones is often the component of the illness which most seriously interferes with the patient's life. The symptoms resulting from the hypersecretion of one or more peptides such as recurring hypoglycemia, painful rashes (Fig. 8), watery diarrhea, and refractory peptic ulceration may be disabling and difficult to control with currently available pharmacologic agents.

Because the rate of tumor growth is often slow, the standard approach to treating patients with metastatic islet cell carcinoma is to withhold any specific anti-tumor therapy until definite symptoms related to an enlarging tumor mass or serious symptoms related to hypersecretion of one or more of the various hormones associated with a recognized syndrome are seen. At that time chemotherapy with streptozotocin and 5-fluorouracil have been instituted. Although these drugs in combination have an expected response rate of up to 60%, often with a respectable duration of response (median 18 months), gastrointestinal and, occasionally, renal toxicity is often seen. Drugs which could control the problems of hormonal hypersecretion with less toxicity would be extremely beneficial since they may allow deferral of hepatic vascular occlusion or cytotoxic chemotherapy in selected patients.

Not until streptozotocin (STZ)-induced selective pancreatic beta-cell damage was observed was a chemotherapeutic agent identified which appeared to have specificity for metastatic ICC. The first report of clinical effectiveness of STZ in ICC was by Murray-Lyon and colleagues in 1968 [54]. Many anecdotal reports have since appeared suggesting the efficacy of STZ in this disease. Subsequently, a large series compiled by Broder and Carter from the National Cancer Institute confirmed the activity of STZ in ICC [5]. In this series, 37% of patients with measurable disease had an objective regres-

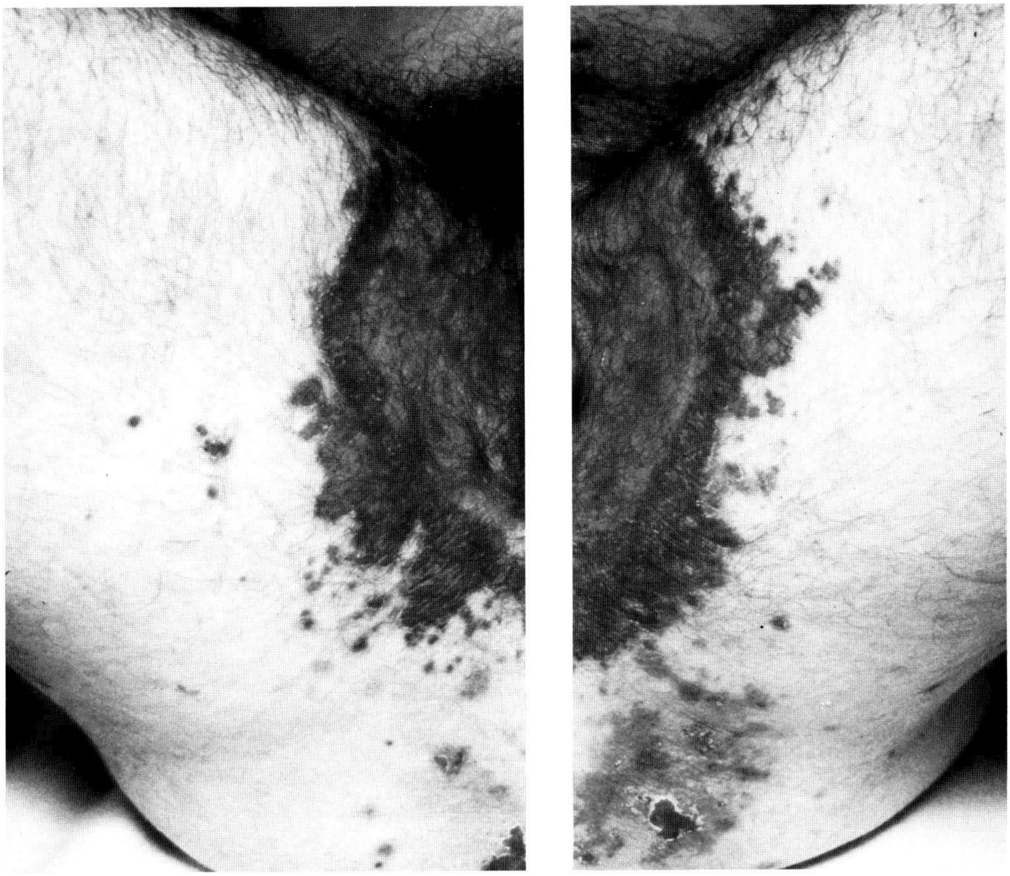

Fig. 8. Necrolytic migratory erythema in a patient with a glucagon-producing islet cell carcinoma

sion (greater than 50% reduction), and 54% of functional tumors had at least a 50% fall in biochemical parameters. At that time there was no consensus on the dosage or schedule of administration of STZ, and this series contained various methods of administration. In addition, the toxicity of STZ was often formidable, with frequent severe nausea and vomiting and less frequent nephrotoxicity and hepatotoxicity.

In 1971, the Mayo Clinic reported on the effectiveness of an intensive 5-day administration schedule of STZ, and this regimen was generally accepted as the standard mode of therapy [48].

Because of the lack of myelosuppression with STZ, combination with other drugs appeared feasible and early reports suggested an increased level of anti-tumor activity when combined with 5-FU [44]. A prospectively randomized study by the Eastern Cooperative Oncology Group published in 1980 compared STZ alone to the combination of STZ and 5-FU [49]. The combination had advantages over STZ alone in overall rates of response (63 versus 36%) and in the frequency of complete responses (37 versus 12%). The median duration of response was 17 months for all patients, and there was no apparent difference in the response of the various hormone-producing tumors. Although the difference was not statistically significant, those patients treated with the combination survived a median of 26 months compared with 16.5 months for the single drug.

Once again, toxicity was significant, with nausea and vomiting in over 80%, nephro-

Table 3. Chemotherapy experience with islet cell carcinoma

Regimen	Patients	Objective Response No.	Percentage	Author
Streptozotocin	17	7	41	Moertel
Adriamycin	20*	4	20	Moertel
Chlorozotocin	13†	7	53	Bukowski
STZ + 5-FU	29	19	66	Moertel
STZ + DOX	5	1	20	Kelsen

STZ = streptozotocin, DOX = doxorubicin, 5-FU = 5-fluorouracil
* Previously treated patients
† No prior chemotherapy patients

Table 4. Eastern Cooperative Oncology Group randomized trial in islet cell carcinoma

Treatment arm	Regimen
Group A	5-FU 400 mg/m^2 days 1–5, q 6 weeks STZ 500 mg/m^2 days 1–5, q 6 weeks
Group B	DOX 50 mg/m^2 day 1, q 3 weeks STZ 500 mg/m^2 days 1–5, q 6 weeks
Group C	CZT 150 mg/m2 day 1, q 7 weeks*

5-FU = 5-fluorouracil, STZ = streptozotocin, DOX = doxorubicin, CZT = chlorozotocin
* On progression, CZT patients are randomized to receive treatment with either arm A or arm B

toxicity developing in 30%, and a single case of fatal hepatotoxicity. The drug combination was associated with more leukopenia (73 versus 5%), and one treatment-related death was due to sepsis. This study confirmed the effectiveness of STZ and 5-FU combinations but also indicated a need for ongoing studies to identify less toxic, equally active programs.

Other combinations with STZ have been used, and Kelsen et al. have reported a program of weekly STZ and DOX where 1 of 5 ICC patients had an objective remission [20]. Since this treatment was associated with only minor myelosuppression, the dosage of adriamycin was to be escalated in future patients to try to improve the response rate. Single-agent adriamycin has also been reported to have definite activity with 4 responses in 20 previously treated patients [50]. Table 3 summarizes the above-mentioned chemotherapy experience with ICC.

A current Eastern Cooperative Oncology Group study (Table 4) is comparing STZ + 5-FU with STZ + DOX and with the new nitrosourea, chlorozotocin (CZT). CZT is a drug structurally similar to STZ but with considerably less gastrointestinal toxicity and increased myelosuppression. CZT can be given at full doses on a single day every 6–7 weeks, whereas STZ needs to be given over 5 days; also, CZT appears to be less nephrotoxic. This drug has been evaluated in a phase II trial by the Southwest Oncology Group.

Among 17 patients with ICC receiving either 200 mg/m^2 or 100 mg/m^2 every 6 weeks, there were 2 complete and 5 partial responses [6]. No responses were seen among the 4 previously treated patients, suggesting a similar mechanism of action and cross resistance to STZ. If the anti-tumor activity of CZT is proved to be equal to that of STZ, the improved tolerance of CZT may make it the preferred nitrosourea in metastatic ICC.

Kessinger and colleagues identified DTIC as an effective drug in the treatment of malignant glucagonoma resistant to STZ in 1979 [22]. This report was followed by several isolated reports confirming activity of DTIC in untreated and a few previously treated patients with metastatic malignant glucagonoma [2, 25, 37, 59, 70]. In 1983 Kessinger et al. expanded their experience to include 5 additional ICC patients among a series of APUD (amine precursor uptake and decarboxylation) tumors treated with DTIC [23]. In this group one complete tumor regression, and one complete and two partial biochemical remissions were noted. Almost all reported responding cases of ICC treated with DTIC are malignant glucagonomas [28]. This high level of response possibly represents some reporting bias. Nevertheless, this activity has prompted some authors to recommend DTIC as the drug of choice for malignant glucagonoma [2, 23, 25, 59]. A prospective trial of this agent in ICC is being done by the Eastern Cooperative Oncology Group at this time.

Anecdotal reports of other chemotherapeutic agents used in ICC have been less encouraging. A single response to actinomycin D and steroids has been reported; while etoposide (VP 16) has been found to be ineffective in a report on 2 patients [13, 14]. The combination of DOX and cisplatin used in patients with APUD tumor resulted in two minor responses in patients with ICC lasting 52 and 23 weeks [68]. Experience with cisplatin alone is limited, and further studies are needed to identify its level of anti-tumor activity.

Experience with hepatic artery occlusion (HAO) in ICC is much less than with carcinoid but has shown early promise. Moertel and colleagues have treated three functioning ICC patients with HAO followed by chemotherapy. All have had dramatic hormonal response and two have had striking tumor regressions; a further two with nonfunctional tumors have had only minor improvements [52].

Somatostatin analogues have been shown to have some very exciting applications in the treatment of the plethora of endocrine manifestations of ICC which affect the function of the gastrointestinal tract [30]. This therapy was not associated with any side effects and appeared ideally suited for the long-term control of symptoms. We expanded our initial series and in 1987 reported our experience treating 22 ICC patients, many of whose tumors were producing multiple hormones. Figures 9–11 display the relative frequency with which we saw major reductions in excessive hormone production [31]. Interestingly, examples of a disparity in hormonal responsiveness within an individual patient have been noted. One such patient presented with Verner-Morrison syndrome due to overproduction of vasoactive intestinal peptide (VIP). His serum VIP was 420 pg/ml (normal <75 pg/ml). He also had a high glucagon level and severe dermatitis characteristic of necrolytic migratory erythema (Fig. 8). With Sandostatin treatment, the VIP level decreased to 42 pg/ml and persisted in this range for one year, with excellent symptomatic control of diarrhea (Fig. 12). The necrolytic dermatitis partially resolved and became less painful for two months, coincident with a fall in circulating glucagon. However, after initially falling to 25% of baseline, the glucagon rose steadily, the necrolytic migratory erythema again became severe, and after 270 days of treatment, progressive malignant hepatomegaly developed. Maton and his co-investigators also found this hormonal therapy effective in controlling the symptoms of a patient with pancreatic cholera [40]. Kraenzlin has described a case of malignant VIPoma which had excellent symptomatic control and an accompanying fall in VIP levels associated with regression of hepatic metastases after 14 months of treatment [24]. Similarly, Clements has described a case of metastatic VIPoma which regressed after 9 months of treatment with Sandostatin [8]. Santangello reported a case with excellent symptomatic control without tumor regression for 9 months [66].

Insulinomas, like VIPomas, may be one of the islet cell carcinomas that are more sensitive to the action of somatostatin analogue. Three of four cases in whom insulin was the sole or dominant hormone being produced have shown remarkable improvement in symptoms that parallels the normalization of serum insulin, but as yet have not shown tumor regression. Osei and O'Dorisio have also reported a case of malignant insulinoma stable for 20 weeks on Sandostatin, with similar impressive reductions in circulating insulin levels [58]. Sandostatin may be effective when conventional agents such as diazoxide and thiazide diuretics have failed.

After one month of Sandostatin treatment, six of the nine patients with an active Zollinger-Ellison syndrome had symptomatic improvement and a fall in serum

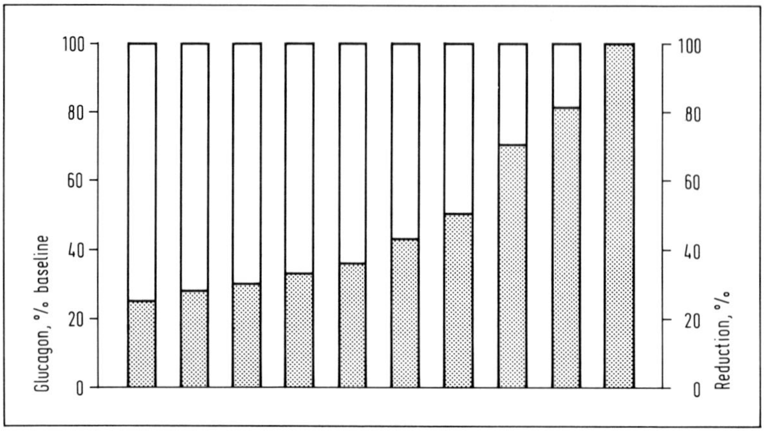

Fig. 9. Effect of Sandostatin on glucagonomas. Lowest post-treatment value in 10 patients

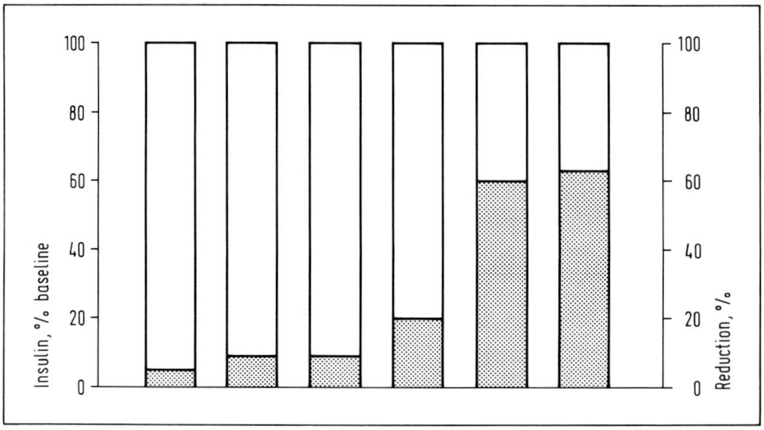

Fig. 10. Effect of Sandostatin on insulinomas. Lowest post-treatment value in 6 patients

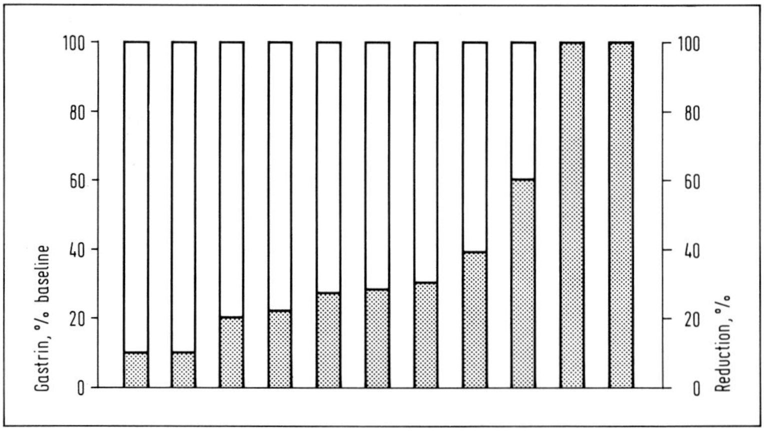

Fig. 11. Effect of Sandostatin on gastrinomas. Lowest post-treatment value in 11 patients

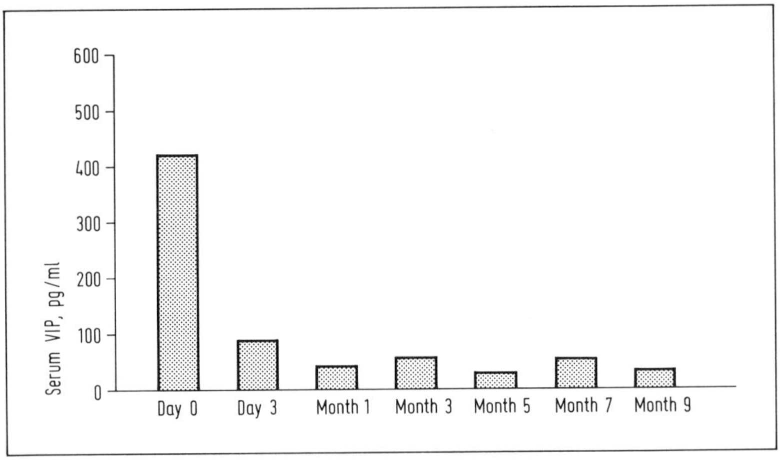

Fig. 12. Serum VIP levels in a patient on Sandostatin 150 μg t.i.d.

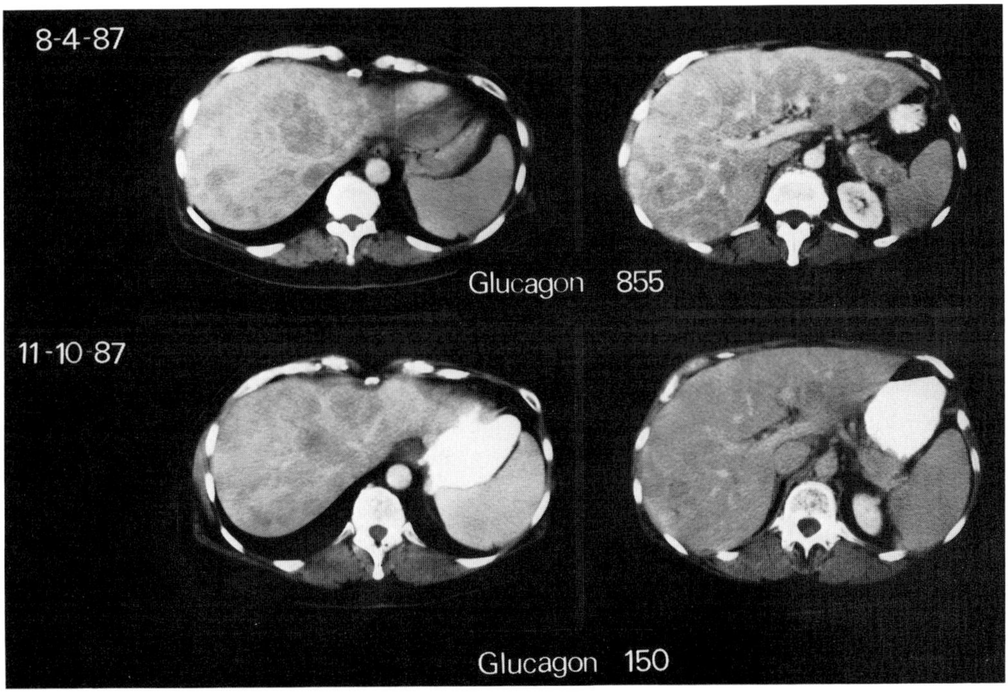

Fig. 13. Pre-treatment (top 2 panels) and post-treatment (bottom 2 panels) CT images of the liver in a patient with a glucagonoma treated with Sandostatin 500 μg t.i.d.

gastrin. In three of the responding patients, major (25–50%) reductions in their daily dosages of H-2 blockers were possible. Four of the six responding patients were later found to have worsening malignant hepatomegaly, despite decreases in serum gastrin levels. This emphasizes the need for serial assessment of the tumor mass with ultrasound or CT scans.

Two of our three patients with predominantly malignant glucagonoma had rapid progression of disease and died within 2 months of starting Sandostatin therapy. The other patient, who had lost 15 kg during the six months prior to starting Sandostatin therapy, experienced rapid resolution of his anorexia and gained 5 kg after one month of therapy. After 5 months his glucagon levels had fallen to less than 30% of baseline but hepatic metastases had progressed. The response to Sandostatin therapy of a patient with a glucagon-producing islet cell carcinoma is depicted in Figure 13. She also had striking reversal of the anorexia which so frequently accompanies this syndrome, and gained weight.

Sandostatin has given the medical oncologists, gastroenterologists, and endocrinologists a major and often stunningly effective new way to treat these very difficult and challenging cases. Unfortunately, we have observed only two cases of objective regressions with Sandostatin therapy in more than 30 patients with metastatic islet cell cancer. Experience to date would therefore suggest that Sandostatin would not be the treatment of choice in the patient who is ill predominantly from the tumor mass per se. On the other hand, if the major clinical problem is due to hypersecretion of one of the myriad of peptides which these malignant cells may produce, and the tumor is not exhibiting an aggressive growth pattern, a therapeutic trial of Sandostatin may effectively control the hormonal-mediated syndromes. The exact role of somatostatin analogues in the overall management of patients with functioning islet cell tumors remains to be determined, but symptomatic control can be remarkable.

Considerable progress in the treatment of ICC has been made, and multicenter cooperative studies have played a major role in the identification of new, effective and less toxic drug combinations. Further work is still needed to determine what role agents such as Sandostatin will play as possible adjunctive therapy in the overall management of this disease.

References

1. Anderson JV, Coupe MO, Morris JA, Hodgson HJF, Bloom SR: Remission of symptoms in carcinoid syndrome with a new 5-hydroxytryptamine M receptor antagonist. Br Med J *294*:1129, 1987
2. Awrich AE, Peetz M, Fletcher WS: Dimethyltriazenoimidazole carboximide therapy of islet cell carcinoma of the pancreas. J Surg Oncol *17* (4):321–326, 1981
3. Bauer W, Briner U, Doepfner W, et al.: SMS 201-995. A very potent and selective octapeptide analogue of somatostatin with prolonged action. Life Sci *31*:1133–1140, 1982
4. Bonomi P, Hovey C, Dainauskas JR, Slayton R, Wolter J: Management of carcinoid syndrome. Med Pediatr Oncol *6*:77–83, 1979
5. Broder LE, Carter SK: Pancreatic islet cell carcinoma. II. Results of therapy with streptozotocin in 52 patients. Ann Intern Med *79*:108–118, 1973
6. Bukowski RM, McCracken JD, Balcerzak SP, Fabian CJ: Phase II study of chlorozotocin in islet cell carcinoma. A Southwest Oncology Group Study. Cancer Chemother Pharmacol *11* (1):48–50, 1983
7. Bukowski RM, Johnson KG, Peterson RF, Stephens RL, Rivkin SE, Neilan B, Costanzi JH: A phase II trial of combination chemotherapy in patients with metastatic carcinoid tumors. A Southwest Oncology Group Study. Cancer *60* (12):2891–2895, 1987
8. Clements D, Elias E: Regression of metastatic VIPoma with somatostatin analogue SMS 201-995. Lancet April: 874–875, 1985
9. Conlon JM, Deacon CF, Richter G, Stockmann F, Creutzfeldt W: Circulating tachykinins (Substance P, neurokinin A, neuropeptide K) and the carcinoid flush. Scand J Gastroenterol *22* (1):97–105, 1987
10. Dery R: Theoretical and clinical consideration in anaesthesia for secreting carcinoid tumors. Can Anaesth Soc J *18* (3):245–263, 1971
11. Engstrom PF, Lavin PT, Folsch E, Moertel CG, Folsch E, Douglas HO: Streptozotocin plus fluorouracil versus doxorubicin therapy for metastatic carcinoid tumors. J Clin Oncol *2*:1255–1259, 1984
12. Feldman JM, O'Dorisio TM: Role of neuropeptides and serotonin in the diagnosis of carcinoid tumors. Am J Med *81*:41–48, 1986
13. Fennelly JJ, Cantwell B, Fielding JF, Fitzgerald O, Collins PG, Buchanan KD: Metastatic pancreatic vipoma: a case report of clinical response following treatment with corticosteroids and actinomycin D. Clin Oncol *8* (2):167–170, 1982
14. Fiore JJ, Kelsen DP, Cheng E, Dukeman M: Phase II trial of VP-16 in apudomas. Proc Am Assoc Cancer Res *15*:174, 1984
15. Frolich JC, Bloomgarden ZT, Oates JA, et al.: The carcinoid flush: provocation by pentagastrin and inhibition by somatostatin. N Engl J Med *299*:1055–1057, 1978
16. Harris AL, Smith IE: Regression of carcinoid tumor with cyproheptadine. Br Med J *285* (5340):475, 1982
17. Harris AL, Smith IE: Tryptophan in the treatment of carcinoid crisis. Chemother

Pharmacol *10*:137–139, 1983

18. Hoeldtke RD: Treatment of postprandial hypotension with a somatostatin analogue SMS 201-995. Am J Med *81* (6 B):83–87, 1986
19. Hoeldtke RD, O'Dorisio TM, Boden G: Prevention of postprandial hypotension with somatostatin. Ann Intern Med *103*:889–890, 1985
20. Kelsen DP, Cheng E, Kemeny N, Magill GB, Yagoda A: Streptozotocin and adriamycin in the treatment of apud tumors (carcinoid, islet cell, and medullary carcinomas of the thyroid). Proc Am Assoc Cancer Res *23*:433, 1982
21. Kelsen D, Fiore J, Heelan R, Cheng E, Magill G: Phase II trial of etoposide in apud tumors. Cancer Treat Rep *71* (3):305–307, 1987
22. Kessinger A, Lemon HM, Foley JF: The glucagonoma syndrome and its management. J Surg Oncol *9*:419–424, 1977
23. Kessinger A, Lemon HM, Foley JF: Therapy of malignant apud cell tumors: Effectiveness of DTIC. Cancer *51*:790–794, 1983
24. Kraenzlin ME, Ch'ng JC, Wood SM, Carr DH, Bloom SR: Long term treatment of a vipoma with somatostatin analogue resulting in remission of symptoms and possible shrinkage of metastases. Gastroenterology *88*:185–187, 1985
25. Kurose T, Seino Y, Ishida H, Fujita J, et al.: Successful treatment of metastatic glucagonoma with dacarbazine. Lancet *1* (8377): 621–622, 1984
26. Kvols LK: Metastatic carcinoid tumors and the carcinoid syndrome: A selective review of chemotherapy and hormonal therapy. Am J Med *81*:49–55, 1986
27. Kvols LK, Buck M: Chemotherapy of metastatic carcinoid and islet cell tumors. A review. Am J Med *82* (5 B):77–83, 1987
28. Kvols LK, Buck M: Chemotherapy of endocrine malignancies: A review. Semin Oncol *14* (3):343–353, 1987
29. Kvols LK, Moertel CG, O'Connell MJ, Schutt AJ, Rubin J, Hahn RG: Treatment of the malignant carcinoid syndrome: evaluation of a long acting somatostatin analogue. N Engl J Med *315*:663–666, 1986
30. Kvols LK, Schutt AJ, Buck M, Rubin J, Moertel CG: Treatment of metastatic islet cell carcinomas with a long acting somatostatin analogue (SMS 201-995). Proc Am Soc Clin Oncol *5*:85, 1986
31. Kvols LK, Buck M, Moertel CG, Schutt AJ, Rubin J, O'Connell MJ, Hahn RG: Treatment of metastatic islet cell carcinoma with a somatostatin analogue (SMS 201-995). Ann Intern Med *107*:162–168, 1987
32. Kvols LK, Maples WJ, O'Connell MJ: Carcinoid crisis: Successful treatment and prevention with somatostatin analogue (SMS 201-995). Proc Am Soc Clin Oncol *6*:96, 1987
33. Kvols LK, Moertel CG, Schutt AJ, Rubin J: Treatment of the malignant carcinoid syndrome with a long acting somatostatin analogue (SMS 201-995): Preliminary evidence that more is not better. Proc Am Soc Clin Oncol *6*:95, 1987
34. Marsh HM, Martin JK Jr, Kvols LK, Gracey DR, Warner MA, Warner ME, Moertel CG: Carcinoid crisis during anesthesia: Successful treatment with a somatostatin analogue. Anesthesiology *66* (1):89–91, 1987
35. Martensson H, Nobin A, Bengmark S, Lunderquist A, Owman T, Sanden A: Embolization of the liver in the management of metastatic carcinoid tumors. J Surg Oncol *27*:152–158, 1984
36. Martin JK, Moertel CG, Adson MA, Schutt AJ: Surgical treatment of functioning metastatic carcinoid tumors. Arch Surg *118*:537–542, 1983
37. Marynick SP, Fagadau WR, Duncan LA: Malignant glucagonoma syndrome: response to chemotherapy. Ann Intern Med *93*:453–454, 1980
38. Mason RA, Steane PA: Carcinoid syndrome: its relevance to the anaesthetist. Anaesthesia *31*:228–242, 1976
39. Maton PN, Camilleri M, Griffin G, Hodgson H, Allison DJ, Chadwick VS: The role of hepatic arterial embolization in the carcinoid syndrome. Br Med J *287*:932–935, 1983
40. Maton PN, O'Dorisio TM, Howe BA, McArthur KE, Howard JM, Cherner JA, Malakey TB, Collen MJ, Gardner JD, Jensen RT: Effect of a long-acting somatostatin analogue (SMS 201-995) in a patient with pancreatic cholera. N Engl J Med *312* (1):17–21, 1985
41. Mauer R, Reubi JC: Somatostatin receptors. JAMA *253*:2741, 1985
42. Miller R, Patel AU, Warner RRP, Parns IH: Anaesthesia for the carcinoid syndrome: A report of nine cases. Can Anaesth Soc J *25* (3):240–244, 1978
43. Mitty HA, Warner RRP, Newman LH, Train JS, Parnes IH: Control of carcinoid syndrome with hepatic artery embolization. Radiology *155*:623–626, 1985
44. Moertel CG: Clinical management of advanced gastrointestinal cancer. Cancer *36*: 675–682, 1975
45. Moertel CG: Treatment of the carcinoid tumor and the malignant carcinoid syndrome. J Clin Oncol *1*:727, 1983
46. Moertel CG: An odyssey in the land of small tumors. J Clin Oncol *5*:1503–1522, 1987

47. Moertel CG, Hanley JA: Combination chemotherapy trials in metastatic carcinoid tumor and the malignant carcinoid syndrome. Cancer Clin Trials *2*:327–334, 1979
48. Moertel CG, Reitemeier RJ, Schutt AJ, Hahn RG: Phase II study of streptozotocin (NSC-85998) in the treatment of advanced gastrointestinal cancer. Cancer Chemother Rep *55*:303–307, 1971
49. Moertel CG, Hanley JA, Johnson LA: Streptozotocin alone compared with streptozotocin plus fluoruracil in the treatment of advanced islet-cell carcinoma. N Engl J Med *303*:1189–1194, 1980
50. Moertel CG, Lavin PT, Hahn RG: Phase II trial of doxorubicin therapy for advanced islet cell carcinoma. Cancer Treat Rep *66* (7):1567–1569, 1982
51. Moertel CG, Engstrom PF, Schutt AJ: Tamoxifen therapy for metastatic carcinoid tumor: A negative study. Ann Intern Med *100*:531–532, 1984
52. Moertel CG, May GR, Martin JK, Rubin J, Schutt AJ: Sequential hepatic artery occlusion (HAO) and chemotherapy for metastatic carcinoid tumor and islet cell carcinoma (ICC). Proc Am Soc Clin Oncol *4*:80, 1985
53. Moertel CG, Rubin J, O'Connell MJ: Phase II study of cisplatin therapy in patients with metastatic carcinoid tumor and the malignant carcinoid syndrome. Cancer Treat Rep *70* (12):1459–1460, 1986
54. Murray-Lyon IM, Eddelston ALWF, Williams R, et al.: Treatment of multiple hormone producing malignant islet cell tumour with streptozotocin. Lancet *2*:895–898, 1968
55. Myers CF, Ershler WB, Tannenbaum MA, et al.: Tamoxifen and carcinoid tumor. Ann Intern Med *96*:383, 1982
56. Norheim I, Theodorsson-Norheim E, Öberg K: Tachykinins are a new family of peptides important for the diagnosis and treatment of carcinoids. Lakartidningen *84* (9):63–632, 1987
57. Öberg K, Norheim I, Lind E, Alm G, Lundqvist G, Wide L, Jonsdottir B, Magnusson A, Wilander E: Treatment of malignant carcinoid tumors with human leukocyte interferon: Long-term results. Cancer Treat Rep *70* (11):1297–1304, 1986
58. Osei K, O'Dorisio TM: Malignant insulinoma: effects of a somatostatin analog (201-995) on serum glucose, growth and gastroentero-pancreatic hormones. Ann Intern Med *103*:223–225, 1985
59. Prinz RA, Badrinath K, Banerji M, Sparagana M, Dorsh TR, Lawrence AM: Operative and chemotherapeutic management of malignant glucagon producing tumors. Surgery *90* (4):713–719, 1981
60. Reichlin S: Somatostatin. N Engl J Med *309*:2741, 1985
61. Reubi JC: A somatostatin analogue inhibits chondrosarcoma and insulinoma tumour growth. Acta Endocrinol *109*:108–114, 1985
62. Reubi JC, Häcki WH, Lamberts SW: Hormone-producing gastrointestinal tumors contain a high density of somatostatin receptors. J Clin Endocrinol Metab *65* (6):1127–1134, 1987
63. Reubi JC, Heitz PU, Gyr K: Vasoactive intestinal peptide producing tumour contains high density of somatostatin receptors. Lancet *1* (8535):741–742, 1987
64. Reubi JC, Maurer R, von Werder K, Torhorst J, Klijn JG, Lamberts SW: Somatostatin receptors in human endocrine tumors. Cancer Res *47*:551–558, 1987
65. Roy RC, Carter RF, Wright PD: Somatostatin, anaesthesia, and the carcinoid syndrome. Peri-operative administration of a somatostatin analogue to suppress carcinoid tumour activity. Anaesthesia *42* (6): 627–632, 1987
66. Santangello WC, O'Dorisio TM, Kim JG, Severino G, Krejs GJ: Pancreatic cholera syndrome: effect of a synthetic somatostatin analog on intestinal water and ion transport. Ann Intern Med *103*:363–367, 1985
67. Sjoerdsma A, Lovenberg W, Engelman K, et al.: Serotonin now; clinical implications of inhibiting its synthesis with parachlorophenylalanine. Ann Intern Med *73*:607–629, 1970
68. Sridhar KS, Holland JF, Brown JC, Cohen JM, Ohnuma T: Doxorubicin plus cisplatin in the treatment of apudomas. Cancer *55*:2634–2637, 1985
69. Stathopoulous GP, Karvountzis GG, Yiotis J: Tamoxifen in carcinoid syndrome. N Engl J Med *305*:52, 1981
70. Strauss GM, Weitzman SA, Aoki TT: Dimethyltriazenoimidazole carboximide therapy of malignant glucagonoma. Ann Intern Med *90*:57–58, 1979
71. Sullivan SJ, Schonbrunn A: Characterization of somatostatin receptors which mediate inhibition of insulin secretion in RinM5F insulinoma cells. Endocrinology *121* (2):544–552, 1987
72. Thulin L, Samnegard H, Tyden G, Long D, Efendic S: Efficacy of somatostatin in a patient with carcinoid syndrome. Lancet *2*:43, 1978
73. Wilson DM, Hoffman AR: Reduction of pituitary size by the somatostatin analogue SMS 201-996 in a patient with an islet cell tumour secreting growth hormone releasing factor. Acta Endocrinol *113* (1):23–28, 1986

12. Sandostatin® in the Treatment of Advanced Malignancies

U. Sagman, S. Fine

Ontario Cancer Institute, The Princess Margaret Hospital, Toronto, Ontario, Canada

The efficacy of Sandostatin® (octreotide) was evaluated in a group of patients with treatment-resistant aggressive malignancies manifested by rapidly enlarging metastases and associated endocrine syndromes. The malignancies included carcinoid and pancreatic endocrine tumors of the gastroenteropancreatic (GEP) system, as well as hormone-sensitive tumors (breast cancer) and neuroendocrine tumors of non-GEP origin (medullary carcinoma of thyroid and small cell lung cancer). The latter group was specifically included to permit evaluation of the effects of Sandostatin on both gastrointestinal and endocrine physiology.

Patients and Treatment

Sandostatin was administered subcutaneously to 12 patients with advanced metastatic malignancies: medullary thyroid carcinoma (2 patients); small cell lung cancer (1); VIPoma (1); metastatic apudoma (1); breast cancer (1) and primary carcinoid tumors of bowel (4), ovary (1), and lung (1).

Diagnosis was confirmed by histopathology: selected specimens underwent immunohistochemical staining and tumor deposits were monitored with radiology scans, including CT scans. The presence of tumor-elaborated peptides was also monitored.

Sandostatin treatment was initiated at a dose of 150 µg every 12 h and rapidly titrated to a dose that provided symptomatic control (achieved within days). This resulted in an average maintenance daily dose of 1 mg, (500 µg 12-hourly), with a range of 300 µg to 3 mg. Patient characteristics, maintenance dose and weeks of therapy are given in Table 1.

The efficacy of Sandostatin therapy was assessed on the basis of the patients' symptomatic responses i.e., control of symptoms and a measurable change in tumor deposits. The objective measurements were based on the following definitions: regression (RG) was defined as a 50% or greater reduction in measurable tumor deposits, no change (NC) as a less than 50% reduction with no evidence of new deposits, or progression (PG) as a 25% or greater increase in tumor dimension or the appearance of new lesions.

Results

The symptomatic and objective responses to Sandostatin therapy are outlined in Table 1. Several facets of Sandostatin therapy are illustrated in the patient with a life-threatening metastatic VIPoma, previously resistant to other therapy, who has been maintained for more than 108 weeks on Sandostatin. All functional manifestations of the syndrome rapidly disappeared and the unremitting voluminous diarrhea, severe acidemia and hypokalemia were controlled dramatically with Sandostatin therapy (Fig. 1). Within 4 weeks of the initiation of therapy a reduction in the plasma concentration of tumor-associated peptides, including VIP, was evident, along with tumor regression which has been sustained for two years. Of particular note, is the observation that temporary withdrawal of Sandostatin after 18 months of therapy resulted in rapid re-appearance of all presenting symptoms of the pancreatic cholera syndrome.

Response in the patients with the carcinoid syndrome was variable, though flushing and diarrhea were readily controlled initially in all patients. Four of the patients

Table 1. Efficacy of somatostatin analogue Sandostatin® (SMS) in advanced malignancies

Sex	Age	Disease [1]	Weeks on SMS [2]	Maintenance dose (q 12 h)	Symptoms controlled [3]	Measurable tumor [4]
F	60	MTC	10+	500 μg	D	PG
M	48	MTC	6	500 μg	D	NE
M	51	SCLC	4	500 μg	NONE	PG
F	60	VPM	108+	150 μg	WHDA, W	RG
F	32	MAP	2	500 μg	NONE	PG
F	39	BST	11	500 μg	W	PG
M	60	CTB	12	1500 μg	F, D	PG
F	73	CTB	20	250 μg	F, D, W	PG
M	60	CTB	30+	500 μg	F, D, W	NC
M	58	CTB	42+	500 μg	F, D, W	NC
F	52	CTO	33+	750 μg	F, D, W	NC
F	73	CTL	5+	500 μg	F, D, W	PG

[1] MTC = medullary thyroid carcinoma
SCLC = small cell lung cancer
VPM = VIPoma
MAP = metastatic apudoma
BST = breast cancer
CTB = carcinoid tumor of the bowel
CTO = carcinoid tumor of the ovary
CTL = carcinoid tumor of the lung

[2] + = ongoing treatment

[3] WDHA = watery diarrhea, hypokalemia and achlorhydria syndrome
F = flushing
D = diarrhea
W = weight loss

[4] RG = regression
NC = no change
PG = progression
NE = not evaluable

(two with a carcinoid of the bowel, one with a lung carcinoid and one with an ovarian carcinoid) have had a sustained response to treatment and are currently maintained on a self-administered regimen. One patient with a carcinoid of the bowel improved with a gradual increase in doses over 12 weeks, but at a total daily dose of 3 mg he became refractory to treatment. Measurable tumor size was relatively refractory to Sandostatin, but in three patients further tumor growth appeared to be arrested. One of these patients had manifested relentless tumor progression prior to Sandostatin administration, in spite of aggressive management with multiple surgical interventions, extensive chemotherapy and dose-limiting radiotherapy. We have not witnessed any significant correlation between hormone or amine output and clinical response or tumor growth.

In two patients with medullary carcinoma of the thyroid associated with severe diarrhea, symptoms were controlled dramatically with Sandostatin. Symptoms improved in one of these patients despite tumor progression. Elevated plasma levels of calcitonin and carcinoembryonic antigen were not changed with therapy, nor were the urinary levels of 5-HIAA.

Sandostatin was not effective in the patient with a rapidly progressive, metastatic apudoma occupying the entire abdominal cavity with multiple metastatic sites. Likewise, a 4 weeks' course of Sandostatin therapy in a patient with small cell lung cancer did not halt the progression of the tumor.

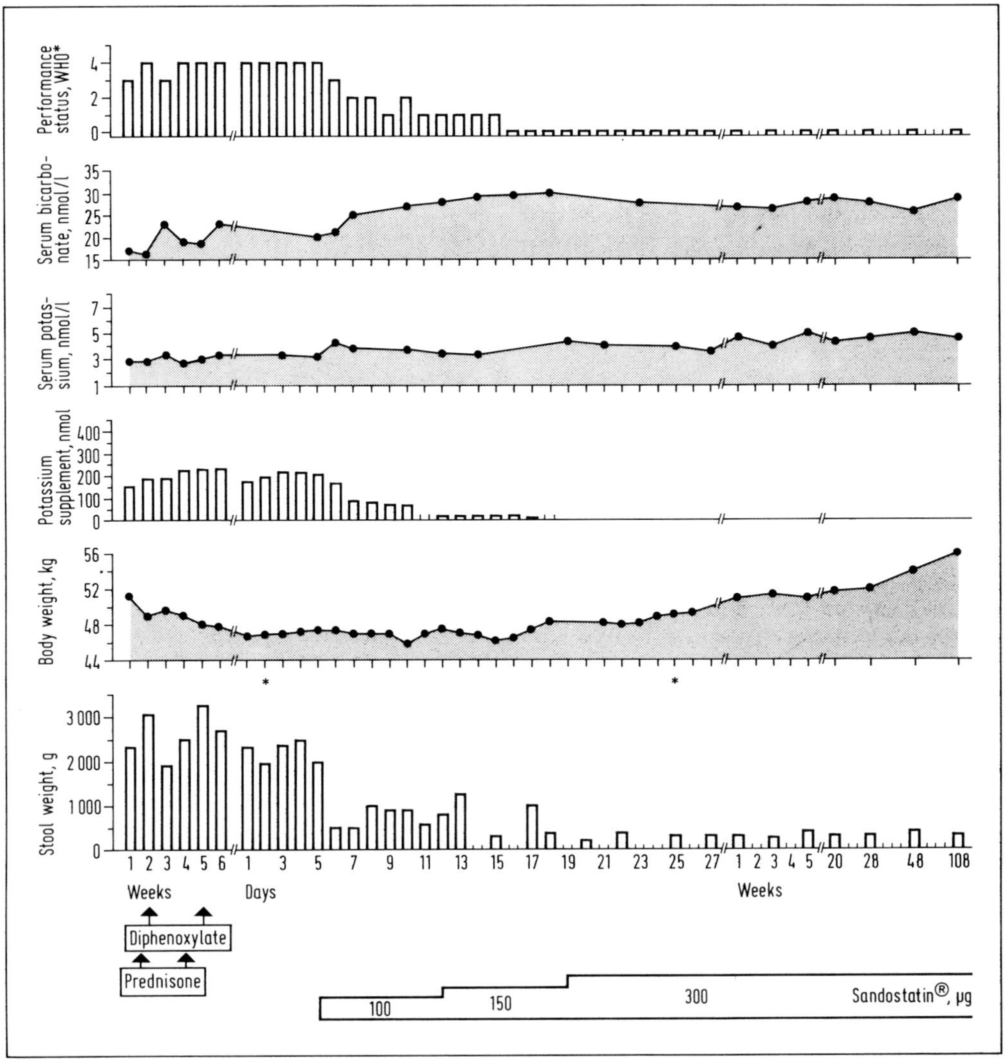

Fig. 1. Effect of Sandostatin on the course of a patient with VIPoma and the pancreatic cholera syndrome. Drug was administered as follows: 50 µg b.i.d. days 1–7, 50 µg t.i.d. days 8–14, 150 µg b.i.d. day 15 and thereafter. (* WHO, World Health Organization Criteria [6])

One patient with breast cancer, unresponsive to previous therapy, experienced weight gain and an improved sense of well-being, but no objective tumor response was apparent.

Overall, the patients tolerated Sandostatin therapy well. Four patients experienced discomfort at the injection site during the initial days of therapy. Mild hyperglycemia was noted in two patients, but glucose intolerance was not seen in any. No thyroid function abnormalities developed. Long-term monitoring to evaluate alterations in gastrointestinal physiology have revealed no evidence of malabsorption or steatorrhea. To date, none of the patients has required pancreatic enzyme replacement.

Discussion and Conclusions

Sandostatin has proved to be a major therapeutic advance in the treatment of patients with neuroendocrine tumors. In some patients in whom conventional treatment modalities failed survival has been directly related to Sandostatin therapy. Our experience demonstrates that this new agent is not only efficacious in the symptomatic control of life-threatening complications (some advanced neuroendocrine and hormone-sensitive tumors) but has also been associated with tumor regression in a few cases. In addition, the acute and long-term safety of Sandostatin indicates its important position in the therapeutic armamentarium for neuroendocrine neoplasms.

As part of our ongoing studies with Sandostatin, we are addressing several issues pertaining to its clinical applications. First, we are attempting to define the spectrum of malignancies which will respond to Sandostatin therapy. It is increasingly apparent that Sandostatin exhibits broad inhibitory functions. As such, the factors governing the clinical spectrum from symptomatic control to potential tumor regression need to be clarified. Already established as an anti-secretory agent in select endocrine malignancies [7], Sandostatin has an anti-growth potential that has been exemplified in vivo [3] and in vitro [4], in both human and animal systems. The range of targets for these demonstrable antiproliferative effects includes pancreatic malignancies of exocrine source [4], human endocrine malignancies of pancreatic and possible pituitary origin [2], a human breast-cancer cell line [5] and a tumor model exhibiting receptors to somatostatin (insulinoma), and one without such receptors (chondrosarcoma) [3]. Furthermore, the illustration [1] that somatostatin inhibits the binding of the oncogene-encoded epidermal growth factor (EGF) to its receptor may therefore focus its spectrum to that of an anti-oncogene. That phorbol esters (tumor promoting agents) inhibit the receptor binding of somatostatin [8] further corroborates a role for somatostatin and its analogue(s) in the modulation of carcinogenesis.

The empirical approach to Sandostatin administration in this study has been satisfactory, though optimal dose and scheduling of drug administration have not been fully evaluated. In our experience, gradual dose titration resulted in progressive amelioration of symptoms in responding patients. This may attest to a direct dose-response relationship. As with the introduction of any new agent initial management attempted to optimize a therapeutic index so that the patient would benefit from treatment and yet not encounter unacceptable toxicity. While the doses used did produce a good symptomatic response and perhaps favorably affected the tumor burden, higher doses might have produced greater benefits without adverse effects.

In agreement with other reports, the adverse effects of Sandostatin were infrequent and predominantly transient. Having established the excellent acute tolerability of Sandostatin, we are continuing to assess the long-term effects of Sandostatin therapy.

Since the natural history of endocrine tumors and their respective clinical features are highly variable, caution must be exercised when interpreting response to treatment. Conventional definitions of tumor response may not be applicable in this setting. Hence both objective and subjective responses to treatment must be documented and correlated with biological parameters.

Finally, we believe that further studies must be made to clarify the basic mechanism of action of Somatostatin, to identify markers of potential response to treatment, and to merge insights from basic biology with clinical experience.

References

1. Ghirlanda G, Uccioli L, Perri F, Altomonte L, Bertoli A, Manna R, Fruti L, Greco AV: Epidermal growth factor, somatostatin, and psoriasis. Lancet 1983: *1*; 65
2. Lamberts SWJ, Uitterlinden P, Verschoor L, Krijin J, Dungen V, Del Pozo: E: Long-term treatment of acromegaly with the somatostatin analogue SMS 201-995. N Engl J Med 1985: *313*; 1576–1580
3. Reubi JC: A somatostatin analogue inhibits chondrosarcoma and insulinoma tumor growth. Acta Endocrinol 1985: *109*; 108–114
4. Schally AV, Comaru-Schally AM, Redding TW: Antitumor effects of analogs of hypothalamic hormones in endocrine-dependent cancers. Proc Soc Exp Biol Med 1984: *1975*; 259–281
5. Setyone-Han B, Henkelman MS, Foekens JA, Klign JGM: Direct inhibitory effects of

somatostatin (analogues) on the growth of human breast cancer cells. Cancer Res 1987: *47*; 1556–1570

6. WHO handbook for reporting results of cancer treatment. Publication No. 48. World Health Organization, Geneva, Switzerland, 1979
7. Wood SM, Kraenzlin ME, Adrian TE, Bloom SR: Treatments of patients with pancreatic endocrine tumors using a new long-acting somatostatin analogue; symptomatic and peptide responses. Gut 1985: *26*; 438–444
8. Zeggori M, Susini C, Viguerie W, Esteve JP, Vaysse W, Ribet A: Tumor promoter inhibition of cellular binding of somatostatin. BBRC 1985: *128*; 850–857

13. Treatment of Malignant Neuroendocrine Gut and Pancreatic Tumors with Sandostatin®

K. Öberg [1], B. Eriksson [1], I. Norheim [2]

[1] Ludwig Institute for Cancer Research and [2] Department of Internal Medicine, University Hospital, Uppsala, Sweden

Malignant neuroendocrine gut and pancreatic tumors present as specific clinical syndromes. Although these neoplasms advance slowly, the associated excess hormone production can result in severe symptoms. Clinical syndromes such as Zollinger-Ellison's, Verner-Morrison's, and carcinoid syndromes are related to the peptide secretions of these tumors. Most patients who present with clinical symptoms have metastases at the time of diagnosis. The ultimate treatment for malignant neuroendocrine gut and pancreatic tumors has still to be elucidated. Surgery has always been considered the primary treatment modality for these tumors [11], but when metastases have appeared, cure cannot be achieved. Resections of primary tumors and liver metastases, and other debulking procedures may lead to short remissions.

Chemotherapy results in symptomatic response in about 60% of patients with malignant endocrine pancreatic tumors [3, 7], but in only about 10 to 30% of patients with carcinoid tumors [5, 6].

Streptozocin alone, or in combination with 5-FU or adriamycin, is the only agent with proven effect in neuroendocrine gut and pancreatic tumors. Human leucocyte interferon has been shown by objective response to be effective in about 77% of patients with malignant endocrine pancreatic tumors [1], and in about 50% of patients with malignant carcinoid tumors [8]. Most patients treated with both chemotherapy and interferons achieve significant reductions in tumor-secreted peptides; in a few, the size of the tumor is reduced. Complete remissions are rare.

The naturally occurring peptide, somatostatin, exerts both endocrine and paracrine control on different cell systems. Known as the 'great inhibitor' of various peptide hormones, somatostatin notably inhibits hormone synthesis and release and also blocks hormonal effects at the end organs [10]. The new analogue of somatostatin, Sandostatin® (octreotide), also known as SMS 201-995, has a prolonged plasma half-life which enhances its use clinically. Sandostatin has been reported to have up to a 70% objective response rate in patients with neuroendocrine gut and pancreatic tumors [4, 12]. Tumor size has been reduced in only a few patients. The mechanisms by which Sandostatin could be inhibiting tumor cell growth have to be investigated.

We report here our experience with both short- and long-term Sandostatin treatment in a substantial number of patients with neuroendocrine gut and pancreatic tumors.

Patients

Thirty-seven patients who had either carcinoid tumors with liver metastases (n = 28), or pancreatic (n = 9) tumors were given Sandostatin therapy. Twenty of the 28 carcinoid patients had a mid-gut tumor, and were included in the acute study of flush provocation, comparing placebo and a single 5 μg s.c. dose of Sandostatin. These patients were then entered in the long-term study of efficacy and safety, in which they received 50 μg Sandostatin s.c. twice a day for three months.

The nine patients with malignant, endocrine, pancreatic tumors were started on 50 μg Sandostatin twice daily; in three, the dose was increased during the first two months. Seven of these patients had undergone surgery to remove the tumors. Liver metastases were present in eight of these patients.

Evaluation of Tumor Response

An *objective response* was defined as a 50% or greater reduction in tumor markers and/or tumor size. *Stable disease* was defined as a less than 50% reduction in tumor markers and/or tumor mass and no new metastases. *Progressive disease* was defined as a 25% increase in tumor markers and/or tumor mass or the appearance of new metastases.

Results

Acute Study: Mid-Gut Carcinoid Patients

In this double-blind, single-dose, crossover study the effects of a 50 μg s.c. Sandostatin dose and placebo were compared in 20 carcinoid patients in whom a cutaneous flush was stimulated by an intravenous injection of pentagastrin 0.6 μg/kg. Each patient received the placebo and Sandostatin on separate days, 45 min prior to the pentagastrin challenge. Blood samples were drawn for analyses of tachykinins 0, 1.5, 3, 5, 15 and 45 min post-challenge. The patient graded the intensity of his or her flush on a scale from 0 to 10. With placebo, the median degree of flush was 8.5 interquartile range (IQR 4–10) as compared to 2 (IQR 0–4) with Sandostatin. The median increase in tachykinins with placebo was 140.5%, with a maximum at 3 min ($p < 0.001$). In contrast with Sandostatin there was a significant ($p < 0.01$) decline in tachykinins compared with the basal level prior to the Sandostatin dose [9].

Long-Term Sandostatin Treatment in Carcinoid Patients

The same carcinoid patients were entered in the open, long-term study of Sandostatin 50 μg twice daily for three months. Nineteen of the 20 patients could be evaluated: 5 (26%) had an objective response, 13 (73%) had stable disease, and only one showed progressive disease. In six of these patients, following the initial three months of therapy, the dose of Sandostatin was increased to 100 μg three times daily, and treatment was continued for another three months. At the end of the second three months of Sandostatin therapy, two additional patients showed an objective response bringing the total with an objective response to 7 of 19 (37%). The objective response in all patients was a decrease in tumor markers, but one patient also showed a significant reduction of tumor size. A subjective response of less diarrhea and/or cutaneous flushing was noted in 13 patients (73%).

An additional 8 patients with malignant carcinoid tumors were treated with Sandostatin for up to 2½ years. The objective response rate within this group was equal to that obtained in the other carcinoid patients. Two case histories from this group provide excellent experience of the therapeutic benefits of Sandostatin.

Case History I

Patient I had a bronchial carcinoid with liver metastases, and severe flushing attacks. In concert with several infectious episodes, she developed a severe carcinoid crisis, and Sandostatin therapy was initiated in September 1984. After an initial, hepatic artery infusion with Sandostatin 50 μg/h for 4 h, the crisis resolved. She was then maintained on 100 to 200 μg Sandostatin t.i.d. During Sandostatin maintenance therapy, she again experienced carcinoid crisis which responded to either intra-arterial or intravenous infusions of Sandostatin 50 μg/h for from 4 to 8 h. She could then be maintained on Sandostatin 200 μg three times a day. She has been maintained on this dose for 2½ years, during which time the liver metastases have not increased in size.

Case History II

Patient II is a 68-year-old woman with a mid-gut carcinoid tumor, who developed right heart failure associated with the carcinoid syndrome. Her heart and lung functions were severely impaired, and she underwent surgery to replace the right heart valves. Post-operatively, she developed severe bronchoconstriction necessitating maintenance on a respirator for 14 days. Treatment with Sandostatin 50 μg t.i.d. was started, and 24 h later she was able to breathe on her own. After two weeks in the hospital, she was discharged on Sandostatin 100 μg b.i.d. Throughout one year on this Sandostatin regimen, her clinical condition has been good.

Long-Term Treatment with Sandostatin in Patients with Malignant Endocrine Pancreatic Tumors

Four of the nine (44.4%) patients with malignant endocrine pancreatic tumors, showed an objective response to 50 μg Sandostatin b.i.d. The mean duration of response was 10 months (range 5–16 months). The four patients, one with the Zollinger-Ellison syndrome and 3 with the Verner-Morrison syndrome, showed a reduction of tumor markers by more than 50%. Although no patient had a significant reduction of tumor mass, tumor mass did not increase during the observation time (mean 6 months) in any patient. Two of the nine patients had stable disease for a mean of 5 months; the remaining 3 patients had progressive disease [2].

In one patient with a malignant insulinoma, blood glucose levels fell dramatically after the first day of Sandostatin therapy in the hospital, and alternate-day treatment had to be initiated. One patient with endogenous somatostatin production showed complete resistance to Sandostatin therapy; even at an intravenous dose of 2400 μg/day clinical symptoms did not respond. The symptoms of the 9 patients improved in 6 (66%).

Adverse Effects

The side effects of Sandostatin treatment were remarkably few. Abdominal discomfort and borborygmia were reported by half the patients. Patients with malignant carcinoid tumors showed increased diarrhea when Sandostatin therapy was started, but this responded to the addition of pancreatic enzymes in most patients. A slight increase in fasting blood glucose levels was found in 4 of the 9 patients with endocrine pancreatic tumors. One patient with an insulin-treated diabetes mellitus required a higher insulin dose. Pain at the site of injection was a complaint in patients receiving higher doses.

Discussion

The new somatostatin analogue Sandostatin has demonstrated beneficial effects in the management of malignant neuroendocrine tumors [4, 12]. In our study, clinical symptoms improved in more than half our patients. However, we were not able to demonstrate as high an objective tumor response as in other studies, possibly because we used lower doses, or our patient population was different, or our patients had more advanced disease.

We did observe that higher doses were required over time to control peptide levels, and some patients seemed to develop tachyphylaxis, which may be due to down-regulation of somatostatin receptors. We also observed that symptomatic improvement persisted despite increasing peptide levels, and that it occurred without an accompanying decrease in tumor markers. This discrepancy between objective and symptomatic responses may be a reflection of the stronger and longer-lasting effect of Sandostatin on the peripheral target organs.

The two case histories described dramatically the benefits of Sandostatin treatment of patients with malignant neuroendocrine tumors. Both would have died without Sandostatin therapy.

Conclusion

We conclude that Sandostatin is an excellent drug for the acute treatment of severe symptoms due to excessive secretion of humoral agents from neuroendocrine gut and pancreatic tumors. The drug is also an important adjunct to other treatments in the long-term management of neuroendocrine tumors. With recent advances in therapeutic modalities, including embolization, interferon and Sandostatin therapy, the survival of patients with neuroendocrine gut and pancreatic tumors has been extended. At present a permanent cure cannot be achieved in most patients, necessitating alternating between different treatment modalities.

References

1. Eriksson B, Öberg K, Alm G, Lundqvist G, Magnusson A, Wide L, Wilander E: Treatment of malignant endocrine pancreatic tumors with human leukocyte interferon. Lancet 1986; *ii*:1307–1309
2. Eriksson B, Öberg K, Andersson T, Lundqvist G, Wide L, Wilander E: Treatment of malignant endocrine pancreatic tumors with a new somatostatin analogue, SMS 201-995. Scand J Gastroenterol 1988; *23*: 508–512
3. Johansson H, Boström H, Öberg K: Treatment of malignant endocrine pancreatic tumors. Results from an Uppsala material. Ups J Med Sci 1984; [Suppl] *39*:179–189
4. Kvols LK, Moertel CG, O'Connell MJ, Schutt AJ, Rubin J, Hahn RG: Treatment of the malignant carcinoid syndrome; evaluation of a long-acting somatostatin analogue. N Engl J Med 1986; *315*, 11:663–666
5. Legha SW, Valdiveso M, Nelson RS, Benjamin RS, Bodey GP: Chemotherapy for metastatic carcinoid tumors. Experiences with 32 patients and a review of the literature. Cancer Treat Rep 1977; *61*:1699–1703
6. Moertel CG, Hanley JA: Combination chemotherapy trials in metastatic carcinoid tumor and the malignant carcinoid syndrome. Cancer Clin Trials 1979; *2*:327
7. Moertel CG, Hanley JA, Johnson LA: Streptozocin alone compared with streptozocin plus fluorouracil in the treatment of advanced islet cell carcinoma. N Engl J Med 1980; *303*:1189
8. Öberg K, Norheim I, Lind E, Jonsdottir B, Magnusson A, Lundqvist G, Wide L, Alm G: Treatment of malignant carcinoid tumors with human leukocyte interferon. Long-term results. Cancer Treat Rep 1986; *70*:1297–1304
9. Öberg K, Norheim I, Theodersson E, Ahlmann H, Lundqvist G, Wide L: The effects of octreotide on basal and stimulated hormone levels in patients with carcinoid syndrome. J Clin Endocrinol Metab (in press)
10. Reichlin S: Somatostatin. N Engl J Med 1983; *309*:1495–1501, 1556–1563
11. Welbourn RB: Apudomas of the gut. Am J Surg 1977; *133*:13–22
12. Wood SM, Kraenzlin ME, Adrian TE, Bloom SR: Treatment of patients with pancreatic endocrine tumors using a new long-acting somatostatin analogue; symptomatic and peptide responses. Gut 1985; *26*:438–444

14. Sandostatin® and Gastroenteropancreatic Endocrine Tumors – Therapeutic Characteristics

M. J. Dunne [1], R. Elton [2], T. Fletcher [3], P. Hofker [2], J. Shui [2]

[1] AIDS Unit, Department of Health, London, UK, [2] Sandoz Pharmaceuticals Corporation, East Hanover, New Jersey, USA, and [3] Clinical Research Unit London (CRUL), Sandoz House, Feltham, UK

Introduction

Somatostatin

Although its existence had been suggested by earlier work, somatostatin was conclusively identified by Guillemin and associates in 1972 during a search for growth hormone-releasing factors in hypothalamic extracts [6]. Growth hormone release-inhibitory activity was found to be due to a cyclic peptide named somatostatin or somatotropin release inhibitory factor (SRIF). Somatostatin was detected soon afterwards in the D-cells of the pancreatic islets [20] and in the D-cells of the stomach and small intestine.

Somatostatin-related peptides constitute a family that includes the originally identified peptide (somatostatin 14), an extended peptide (somatostatin 28) and larger prohormone forms. It has an extensive distribution throughout the body, including the brain and central nervous system, the peripheral nervous system, the gastrointestinal tract and various exocrine and endocrine glands [26].

Human pharmacological effects of somatostatin are diverse and include: inhibition of growth hormone (GH) and thyroid-stimulating hormone (TSH) release from the anterior pituitary gland; inhibition of insulin and glucagon release from the pancreas; and inhibition of release of a variety of peptides from the gastrointestinal tract, e.g. vasoactive intestinal peptide (VIP), gastrin, etc.

Potential therapeutic application of somatostatin is limited by its short plasma half-life of about 3 min, which necessitates administration by constant infusion.

Sandostatin (SMS 201-995, octreotide) is a synthetic cyclic octapeptide analogue of somatostatin with the following amino acid sequence [25]:

(D)Phe – Cys – Phe – (D)Trp – Lys – Thr – Cys – Thr – ol

In contrast to somatostatin, Sandostatin has an extended plasma half-life of approximately 1–2 h after subcutaneous and intravenous administration and a considerably prolonged duration of action.

In studies in healthy volunteers, Sandostatin has been shown to be a powerful inhibitor of stimulated release of GH, TSH, insulin, glucagon, gastrin and other gastrointestinal peptides [19, 33], with seemingly greater relative potency as an inhibitor of GH secretion.

Because somatostatin has been reported to have beneficial clinical effects in patients with a variety of gastroenteropancreatic (GEP) endocrine tumors [31], the therapeutic characteristics of Sandostatin treatment in patients with GEP tumors have been evaluated, and are the subject of this review.

Materials and Methods

Study Design

GEP endocrine tumors associated with characteristic syndromes are extremely rare and are estimated to occur with an approximate incidence of 1–2 per million, in Western societies. This, together with the clinical heterogeneity of the different tumor sub-categories, would make prospective controlled clinical trials in each type impossible or extremely prolonged, with the exception perhaps of carcinoid tumors in the largest referral centers. The information presented here is therefore based largely on uncontrolled assessments of safety and efficacy of Sandostatin in the management of patients with GEP endocrine tumors, treated on a compassionate need or named-patient basis in several centers. The one exception to this is the Mayo Clinic Center which treated 26 of the 85 patients with carcinoid tumors presented here, following a standard treatment protocol. The individual results from this center are presented elsewhere in this publication (see Kvols L, chapter 11), but, for the purposes of this survey, have been incorporated, in part, into the general body of data presented here.

Patient Inclusion Criteria

Patients with an identified primary GEP tumor or metastatic lesion and associated clinical syndrome were included. The classification was based on the predominant peptide secreted, although multiple peptide secretion is frequently a characteristic of such tumors. The tumor was identified at operation, biochemically and/or radiologically. Patients enrolled in the United States met the criteria for compassionate need, i.e. they had a requirement for therapy that could not be met by existing medical or surgical modalities and they had been exposed to other therapeutic options (which included surgical intervention, hepatic artery embolization, cytotoxic chemotherapy, or medical symptomatic treatment) prior to exposure to Sandostatin. The majority of patients enrolled outside the United States also fulfilled these criteria.

Data Recording and Analysis

Standard general case-report forms, appropriate for the various tumor sub-categories, were provided for recording background information, diagnosis, symptoms and clinical features, physical examinations, co-existent diseases, prior treatments and concomitant medications, routine laboratory tests of safety, efficacy parameters and the occurrence of adverse events. Evaluations were required prior to commencement of therapy, after three to seven days of treatment, and monthly thereafter. If therapy was discontinued, a final evaluation, which included laboratory safety tests, was to be completed.

Because of considerable heterogeneity in recording of data, particularly clinical efficacy (for example, diarrhea was variably reported volumetrically as litres per day or gravimetrically, descriptively as mild, moderate or severe or by appearance and frequency), a case-report form for internal use was established, on which the severity of the presenting clinical and biochemical features was converted to standard nomenclature. Further evaluations of clinical and biochemical responses to treatment were similarly converted and standard ratings established versus baseline and versus previous evaluations. The scale used to quantify the change was:

1 = symptom resolution or normalization of marker,
2 = symptom improvement or reduction of marker of 10% or greater,
3 = no change,
4 = symptom worse or increase in marker of 10% or greater,
5 = new symptom.

A mean rating between 1.5 and 2.4 was classified overall as 'improved', between 2.5 and 3.4 as 'no change'. Mean ratings above and below these ranges were considered as worse or resolved respectively. This evaluation of change facilitated assessments of efficacy in comparison with the baseline pretreatment condition and also assessments of continuing efficacy by means of current rating versus previous. In evaluating the 'overall condition' response (defined as a composite of changes in the predominant symptoms, biochemical responses and other information provided by the treating physician), a 2 (improved) was the best possible rating in view of the continuing presence of the tumor.

To ensure consistency of the internal ratings, sessions were held in which all assessors reviewed the same cases and finally, an outside consultant (Dr. Thomas M. O'Dorisio) independently reviewed the patient records, rated them and compared the ratings with those obtained internally.

Sandostatin Administration

Sandostatin was provided in ampules containing 50, 100 or 500 μg/ml. Recommendations for drug administration were on the basis of dose titration for individual patients, with a starting dose of 50 μg twice daily and escalation of the dosage and frequency of administration (depending on tolerability), until the required therapeutic effect was achieved. One research group (the Mayo Clinic) chose a fixed dosage escalation to a standard maintenance dose of 150 μg t.i.d. from day 7 of therapy.

Evaluation Parameters

The main parameter of evaluation of efficacy was the clinical effect of Sandostatin on symptoms (diarrhea, flushing, rash, abdominal pain, neuroglycopenia, etc.), rated against status at baseline and at previous evaluation as outlined above. Biochemical evidence of efficacy was determined by changes in circulating levels or urinary excretion of relevant tumor markers (VIP, gastrin, glucagon, insulin, PP, urinary 5-HIAA excretion, etc.), also rated as outlined above. Reports of any effect of treatment on tumor mass or metastatic disease assessed radiologically were also noted.

Safety was assessed by periodic determination of clinical chemistry and hematology parameters and by standard recording of adverse reactions. Since such laboratory tests were sometimes abnormal in association with the underlying clinical syndrome (for example, hypokalemia as a result of chronic secretory diarrhea associated with VIPoma), an improvement in status or a return to normal was an integral factor in assessing overall efficacy. Changes in laboratory values related to metastatic disease (for example, abnormal liver function tests), to the malignant state (for example, anemia), or to prior therapy (particularly cytotoxic chemotherapy) made some interpretations difficult.

Adverse reactions were recorded with reference to their nature, severity, relationship to medication, date of onset, duration, course, whether treatment of the event was required and response to such treatment.

Results

Quality of Data

Because of the diverse origins of the data (from 40 investigators in the United States and from 38 investigators in 12 countries outside the United States), inherent inconsistencies in the data were related mainly to availability, methodology and standardization of the analysis of tumor markers, peptides and other laboratory tests, and to clinical heterogeneity and patient diversity with respect to symptoms, severity of disease, previous therapies, etc., even within tumor subgroups. Nevertheless, a total of 173 patients have been evaluated for efficacy, with a distribution between subgroups as outlined in Table 1.

Efficacy

Because response to Sandostatin varied with category of tumor, each of the seven subgroups is considered separately.

Carcinoid Tumors

A total of 85 patients (47 US of which 26 were treated at the Mayo Clinic, 38 non-US) were evaluated for efficacy. A summary of the combined US/non-US efficacy results is given in Figures 1 and 2.

Table 1. Sandostatin in gastroenteropancreatic endocrine tumors, combined efficacy data

Tumor type	US	Non-US	Total
Carcinoid	47	38	85
VIPoma	12	13	25
Glucagonoma	9	7	16
Gastrinoma	14	12	26
Insulinoma	3	12	15
GRFoma	4	–	4
PPoma	2	–	2
Overall total			173

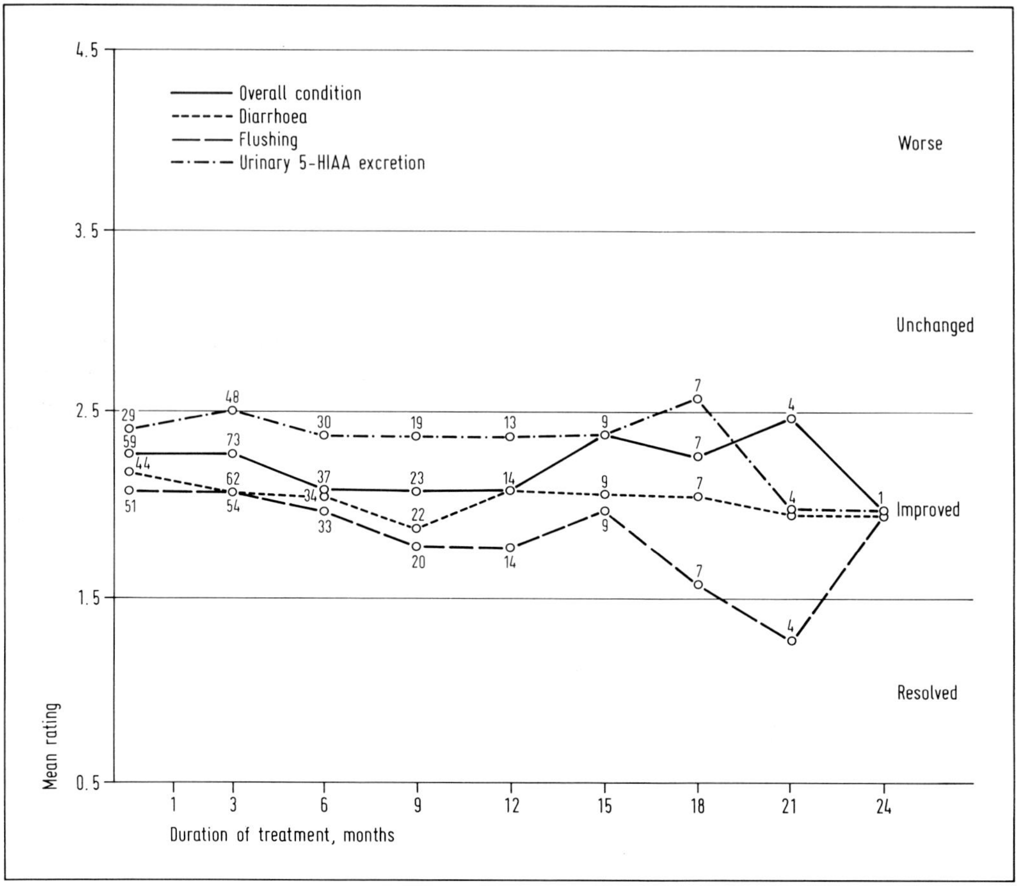

Fig. 1. Sandostatin® in carcinoid tumors: combined efficacy data; mean rating vs baseline. (Patient numbers indicated at each evaluation point)

Dosage: A dichotomy existed between the doses of Sandostatin administered at the Mayo Clinic (mean daily dose 479 µg after one month) and elsewhere (mean 283 µg). The Mayo Clinic apart, doses ranged between 100 and 1500 µg per day.

Duration of treatment: At the time of evaluation, duration ranged from less than two weeks (mostly in patients in whom therapy had been discontinued owing to lack of efficacy) to twenty-four months of therapy. A total of 27 patients were treated for six months or longer and 12 patients for twelve months or longer.

Discontinuation of therapy: A total of 28 patients (16%) had their therapy discontinued, 21 for lack of efficacy. In 3 patients, therapy was stopped owing to progression of malignancy. These patients subsequently died. Three patients died owing to extensive malignancy whilst on treatment and one patient failed to comply with therapy.

Symptom response:

● Diarrhea

A total of 74 patients had diarrhea at the onset of therapy. Symptom response, as measured by the mean rating of the symptom, was achieved within the first two weeks of therapy. Of the evaluable patients seen at this time, the mean response was 2.1 calculated from 20 US patients and 2.4 calculated from 21 non-US patients. The mean rating was unchanged up to one year or longer in the US patients; in the non-US patients it reached the US mean of 2.1 within a similar time frame.

Comparison of the visit-to-visit ratings suggests that the majority of patients maintained their response or achieved further improvements with time.

Inspection of individual responses during the first two weeks revealed that 29 of 44 (66%) patients either improved or had resolution (5 of 44, 11%) of their diarrhea. At six months' therapy, 25 of 34 (74%) had improvement or resolution, and at twelve months', the corresponding figures were 12 of 14 (86%). Over the evaluation period, 7 (9%) patients experienced worsening of diarrhea, reflecting the advanced stage and progression of their malignant disease.

● Flushing

A total of 73 patients experienced flushing as part of their syndrome prior to starting Sandostatin therapy. The mean response rating in the first two weeks of therapy compared with pretreatment values was 2.0 calculated from 23 evaluable US patients and 2.3 calculated from 28 non-US patients.

In the US patients, the response was basically unchanged over twenty-four months of treatment; in the non-US patients, the mean response rating reached 2.0 at month 3, though at later time points, visit-to-visit comparisons were variable, suggesting the possibility of symptomatic breakthrough in some patients.

Examination of the individual responses during the first two weeks revealed that flushing improved in 40 of 51 (78%) patients, and resolved in 5 of 51 (10%). At six months' therapy, 28 of 33 (85%) had improvement or resolution and at twelve months', the corresponding figures were 13 of 14 (93%).

Over the entire evaluation period, 5 patients experienced worsening of their flushing episodes.

Biochemical marker response – urinary 5-HIAA excretion: A total of 60 patients had elevated urinary 5-HIAA excretion levels prior to starting treatment. The mean response rating in the first two weeks of therapy was 2.4 calculated from 21 evaluable US patients and 2.5 calculated from 8 non-US patients, indicating a marginal improvement or no change overall. Similar ratings were made at later times.

Comparison of the visit-to-visit data suggests that the responses remained stable.

Examination of the individual responses over the treatment time showed a reduction in urinary 5-HIAA excretion levels in 35 of 60 (58%) but only 3 patients showed levels in the normal range. In 14 patients (23%) levels were unchanged and in 15 (22%) they were increased above pretreatment values.

Tumor size response: In the majority of cases where documentation had been presented, no predictable anti-tumor action or effect on tumor size, growth or progression of metastases was shown. Tumor shrinkage was reported in 2 patients (one US, one non-US) only.

Overall condition response: By combining the responses identified above as an overall condition response, a mean rating (using the end-point assessment) of 2.4 for the US series and 2.3 for the non-US series was obtained. An examination of the overall response by category from the pooled data indicated that Sandostatin treatment was associated with improvement within the first two weeks in 41 of 59 carcinoid patients (69%). At later assessments, similar responses were observed, and over the entire study period, 60 of 84 patients (71%) had improved, 17 of 84 (20%) were unchanged and 7 of 84 (8%) had deteriorated.

VIPoma

A total of 25 patients (12 US, 13 non-US) were evaluated for efficacy. A summary of the combined US, non-US data is given in Figures 3 and 4.

Dosage: The mean dosage used to treat these patients was 250 μg after one month but, as in the carcinoids, considerable variability was seen, dosage ranging between 50 μg administered on alternate days to more than 1000 μg daily.

Duration of treatment: At the time of evaluation this ranged from less than one month to more than twenty-four months of therapy. A total of 13 patients were treated for six

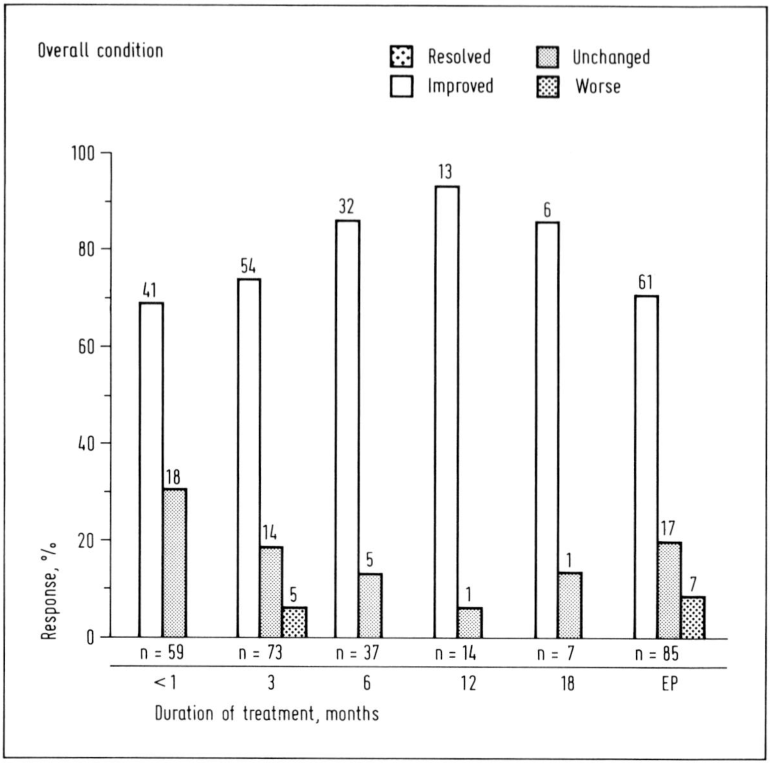

Overall condition
Resolved
Improved
Unchanged
Worse
100
80
60
40
20
0
Response, %
41
18
54
14
5
32
5
13
1
6
1
61
17
7
n = 59
n = 73
n = 37
n = 14
n = 7
n = 85
<1
3
6
12
18
EP
Duration of treatment, months

a

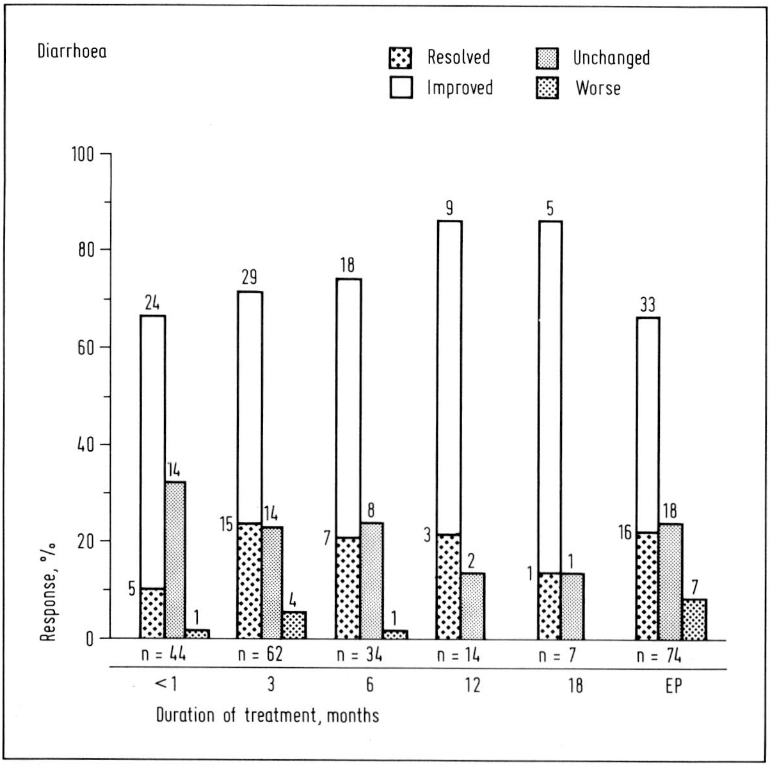

Diarrhoea
Resolved
Improved
Unchanged
Worse
100
80
60
40
20
0
Response, %
24
5
14
1
29
15
14
4
18
7
8
1
9
3
2
5
1
1
33
16
18
7
n = 44
n = 62
n = 34
n = 14
n = 7
n = 74
<1
3
6
12
18
EP
Duration of treatment, months

b

c

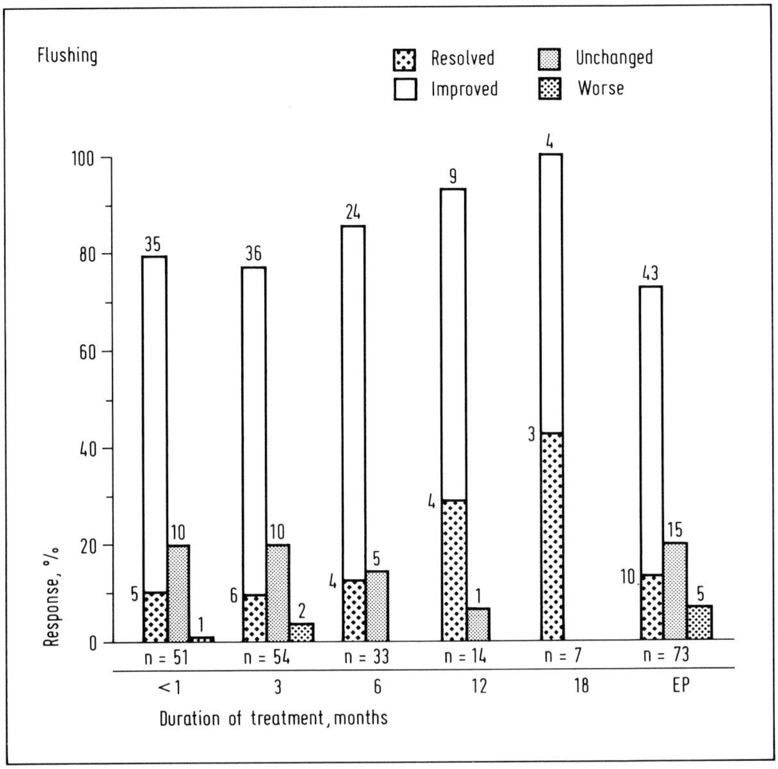

d

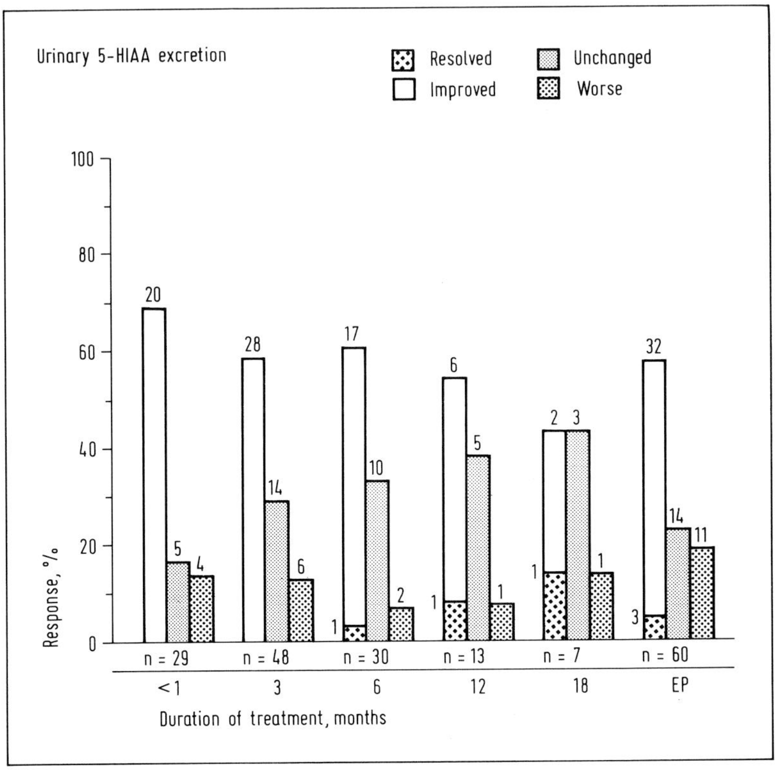

Fig. 2a–d. Sandostatin® in carcinoid tumors: combined efficacy data; categorical rating vs baseline (EP = endpoint evaluation)

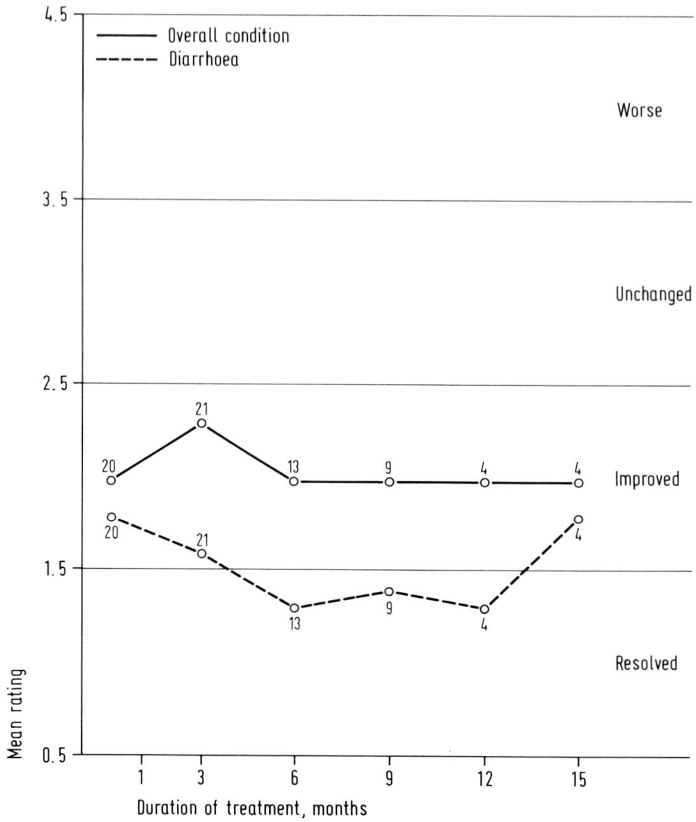

Fig. 3. Sandostatin® in VIPoma: combined efficacy data; mean rating vs baseline. (Patient numbers indicated at each evaluation point)

months or longer and 4 patients for twelve months or longer.

Discontinuation of therapy: Therapy was discontinued in 4 patients only, in 2 of them because of return of symptoms which were not suppressible by increasing doses of Sandostatin. Four patients died owing to progression of extensive malignancy.

Symptom response:

● Diarrhea

A total of 25 patients had diarrhea at the onset of therapy; 19 of 20 evaluable patients showed an improvement of this symptom within one month, the mean rating being 1.8 calculated from the pooled data. Over the first twelve-month period, the mean rating was unchanged and comparison of the visit-to-visit ratings suggested that, in the majority of patients, the response was maintained.

Inspection of the individual responses during the first three months revealed that a total of 18 of 21 (86%) improved or had resolution (12 of 21, 57%) of their diarrhea. In the majority this was evident within the first three days of treatment. At six months, 13 of 13 had improvement or resolution and at twelve months, the corresponding figures were 4 of 4 patients.

Over the evaluation period, 2 (8%) patients experienced worsening of their diarrhea, which manifested itself as a sudden return of severe symptoms after a period of initial control which was not responsive to increasing doses of the drug. In one case, the phenomenon occurred in the presence of disease progression in a patient with extensive malignancy.

a

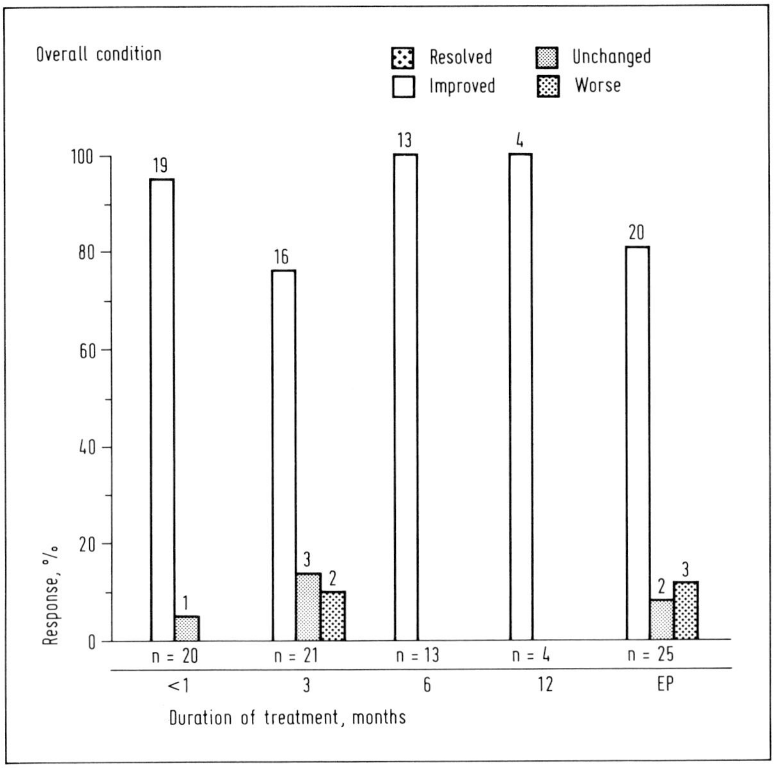

b

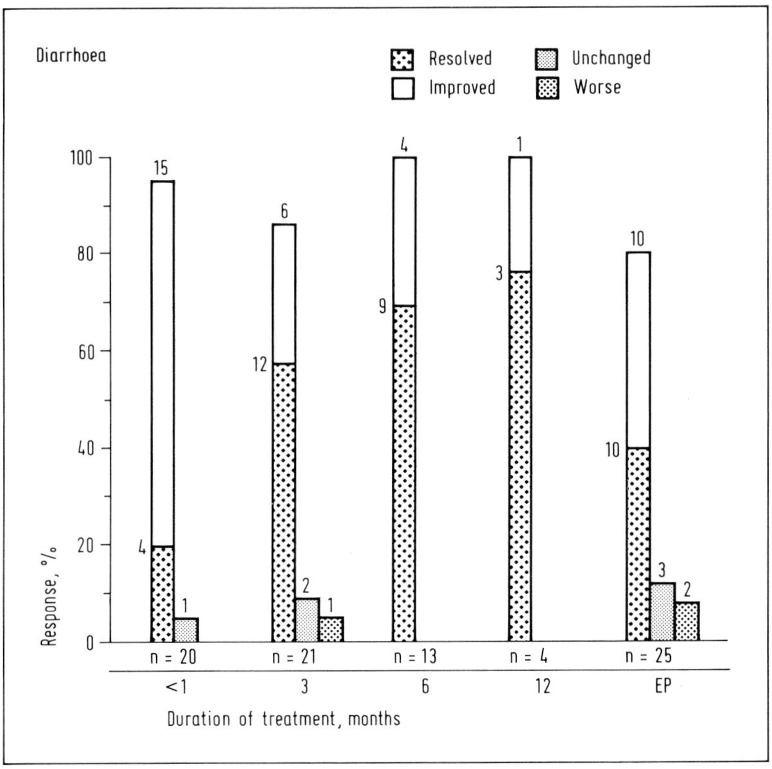

Fig. 4a–c. Sandostatin® in VIPoma: combined efficacy data; categorical rating vs baseline (EP = end-point evaluation)

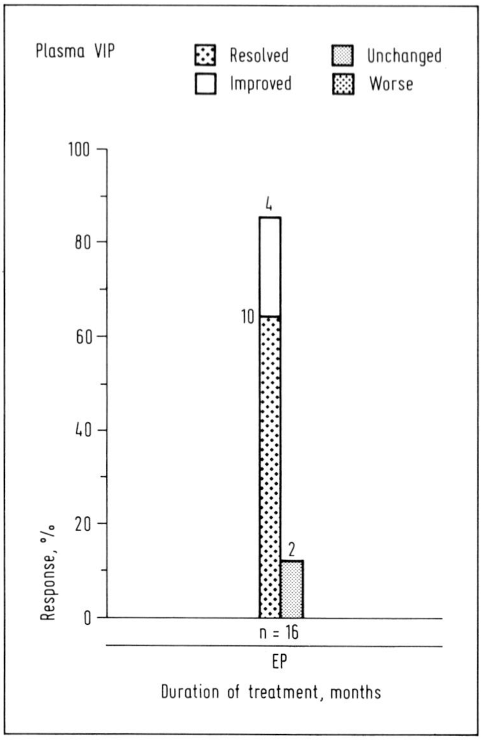

Fig. 4c

Biochemical response:

● Electrolyte supplementation/hypokalemia

A total of 15 patients required electrolyte supplementation prior to starting Sandostatin. Further evidence for efficacy in this indication arises from the observation that serum or plasma potassium levels and other electrolyte abnormalities were restored to normal or maintained within the normal reference range on withdrawal of parenteral supplements in 13 patients.

● Tumor marker – plasma VIP levels

A total of 20 patients had elevated circulating levels of VIP recorded prior to treatment. Examination of the individual responses over the treatment period showed a reduction in VIP levels in 14 of 16 (88%) evaluable patients, levels within the normal reference range being achieved in 10 of 16 (63%). In 2 patients (12%) levels were unchanged or showed considerable fluctuation; both were poorly responsive to Sandostatin overall.

Tumor size response: As in the case of the carcinoid tumors, no predictable anti-tumor action or effect on tumor size, growth or progression of metastases was evident. Apparent shrinkage of metastases evaluated by various radiological methods was reported in 4 non-US patients at some point during treatment.

Overall condition response: By combining the responses as a general overall response and using the end-point assessment, a mean rating of 2.4 for the US patients and 2.2 for the non-US patients was obtained. An examination of the overall response by category at one or more intervals suggested that 20 of 25 (80%) patients improved, 2 of 25 (8%) were unchanged and 3 (12%) had deteriorated. The overall responses seemed to improve after four months, probably reflecting the fact that only responsive patients remained on therapy.

Glucagonomas

A total of 16 patients (nine US, seven non-US) were evaluated for efficacy and a summary of the combined data is given in Figures 5 and 6.

Dosage: The mean dosage employed to treat these patients over the treatment period was between 200 and 300 µg daily but again, individual variability was considerable.

Duration of treatment: At the time of evaluation, this ranged up to twenty-one months of therapy.

A total of 5 patients were treated for six months or longer and a total of 4 for twelve months or longer.

Discontinuation of therapy: A total of 5 patients had their therapy discontinued, in 3 cases owing to lack of efficacy. In one patient, treatment was stopped because of the occurrence of adverse effects and one patient had therapy discontinued in favor of elective surgery to resect the tumor. This patient had not been operated on previously because of extensive rash, which resolved on Sandostatin.

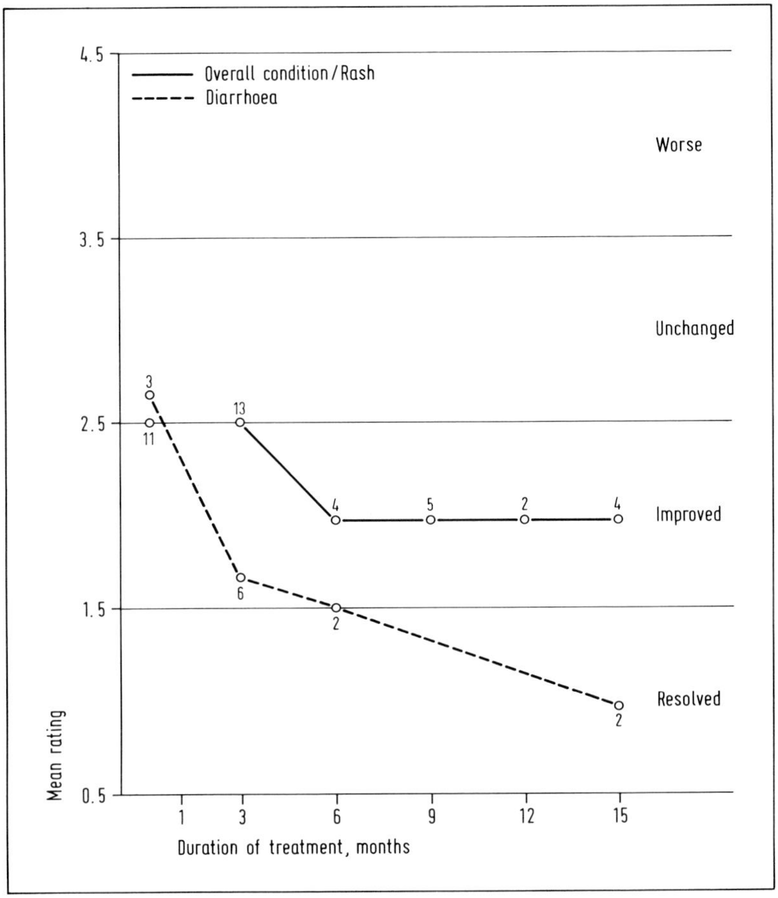

Fig. 5. Sandostatin® in glucagonoma: combined efficacy data; mean rating vs baseline. (Patient numbers indicated at each evaluation point)

Symptom response:

● Necrolytic migratory erythema

A total of 16 patients had the characteristic glucagonoma rash as a feature of their disease. Six of 11 evaluable patients showed an initial improvement in this symptom, 5 were unchanged, the mean rating in the first two weeks of therapy being 2.2 calculated from 5 US patients and 2.7 calculated from 6 non-US patients. Over a 6-month period, the rating reflected that responsive patients only remained on therapy.

Individual responses in the first two weeks of treatment revealed that a total of 6 of 11 (55%) patients improved or had a resolution of their rash. At six months 4 of 4 had improvement or resolution and at twelve months' treatment, the corresponding figures were 3 of 3 patients. Over the total evaluation period 3 (19%) of patients exhibited a return or worsening of their rash.

● Diarrhea

A total of 6 patients had diarrhea as part of their syndrome. The mean rating of this symptom over the first three months of therapy was 1.7; the categorical response (endpoint evaluation) showed that, in 2 of 6 patients, diarrhea improved and in the 4 remaining patients it resolved.

Biochemical response:

● Diabetes mellitus

A total of 4 non-US patients had mild diabetes mellitus as part of their syndrome. Little effect of treatment on this feature was observed at least as evidenced by improved glucose control or reduced insulin requirements.

● Tumor marker – plasma glucagon levels

Prior to starting Sandostatin, 6 non-US patients had elevated circulating levels of

a

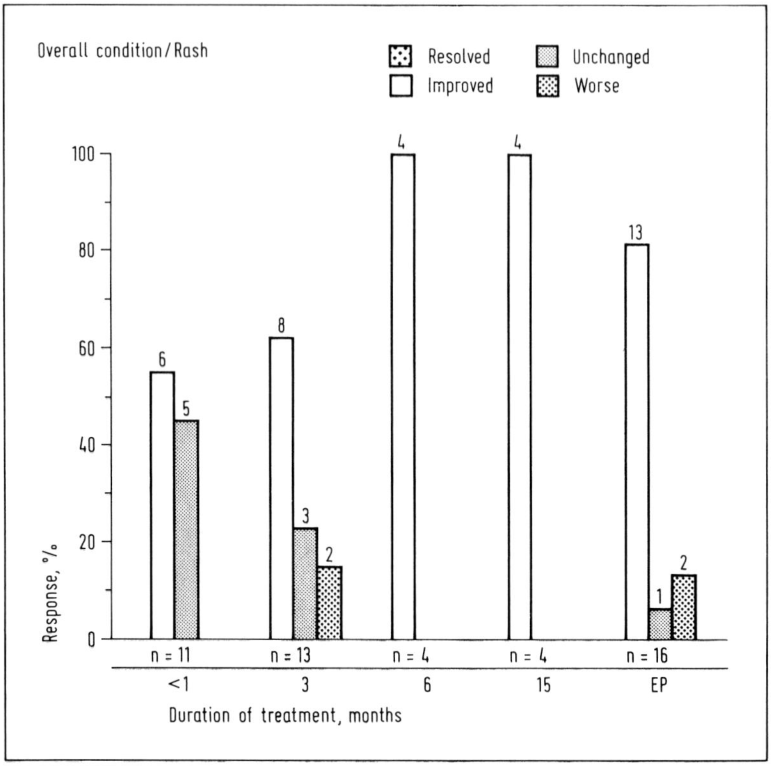

b

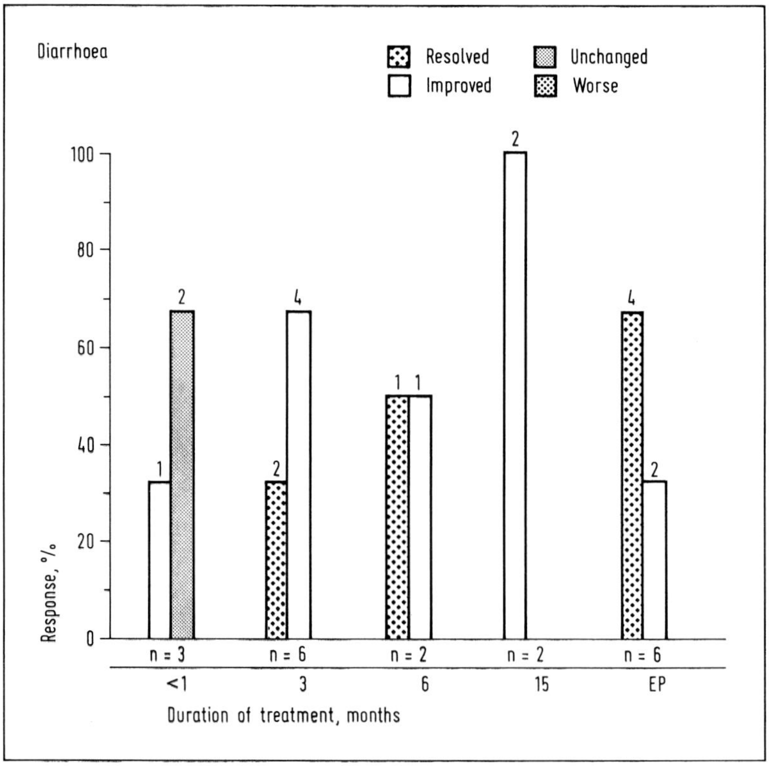

Fig. 6a and b. Sandostatin® in glucagonoma: combined efficacy data; categorical ratings vs baseline (EP = end-point evaluation)

glucagon which were not reduced with treatment. However, the rash often improved without a reduction in circulating glucagon levels.

Overall condition response: Of the 16 patients included, 11 were evaluable over the first three months of therapy. The mean rating of 2.5 at the end of month 3 indicated borderline benefit of therapy. Thereafter, with considerably reduced patient numbers, the mean rating improved, indicating the withdrawal of non-responsive patients. Inspection of patients according to response indicated that 50% (approximately) improved in the early part of the treatment period, when patient numbers were greatest.

Gastrinomas
Efficacy and safety of Sandostatin were evaluated by periodic assessment of 26 patients (14 US, 12 non-US) with gastrinomas. A summary of the combined data is given in Figures 7 and 8. This was a somewhat heterogeneous group of patients, in that symptomatology was highly variable and included abdominal pain or discomfort, diarrhea, weight loss, flushing, fatigue and lethargy. These patients were probably atypical in that the majority remained symptomatic despite treatment with other agents.

Dosage: In this category, the mean dosages were lower than in others and ranged from 170 μg (up to one month) to 250 μg/day at six months; the lack of response seen in some patients may therefore reflect inadequate dosing.

Duration of treatment: This ranged from less than one month to nine months of therapy. At the time of evaluation, a total of 6 patients had been treated for six months or longer and 3 patients for nine months.

Discontinuation of therapy: A total of 16 patients had their therapy discontinued in the majority owing to ineffectiveness, and 2 patients died from their malignancy.

Symptom response:
● Diarrhea
For this symptom, the mean rating calculated from 7 evaluable patients in the first three months of treatment was 1.8, and 2.2 for 10 patients at the end-point evaluation. The categorical responses showed that, within the first three months, diarrhea resolved in 3 patients, improved in 2 and was unchanged in 2.

● Abdominal pain
A total of 12 patients had abdominal pain as part of their gastrinoma syndrome. Inspection of the individual responses indicated that 6 of 12 (50%) patients had improvement or resolution of their pain or discomfort over the treatment period.

Biochemical response:
● Plasma gastrin
A total of 26 patients had elevated plasma gastrin levels prior to Sandostatin therapy.

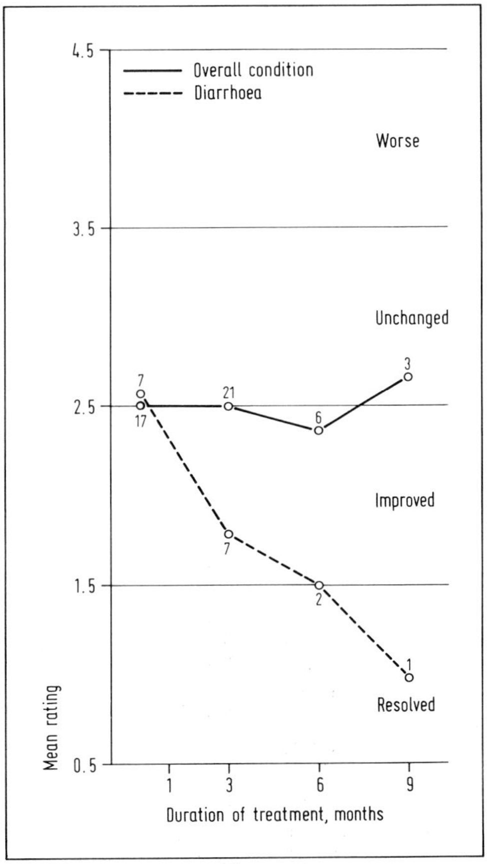

Fig. 7. Sandostatin® in gastrinoma: combined efficacy data; mean rating vs baseline. (Patient numbers indicated at each evaluation point)

a

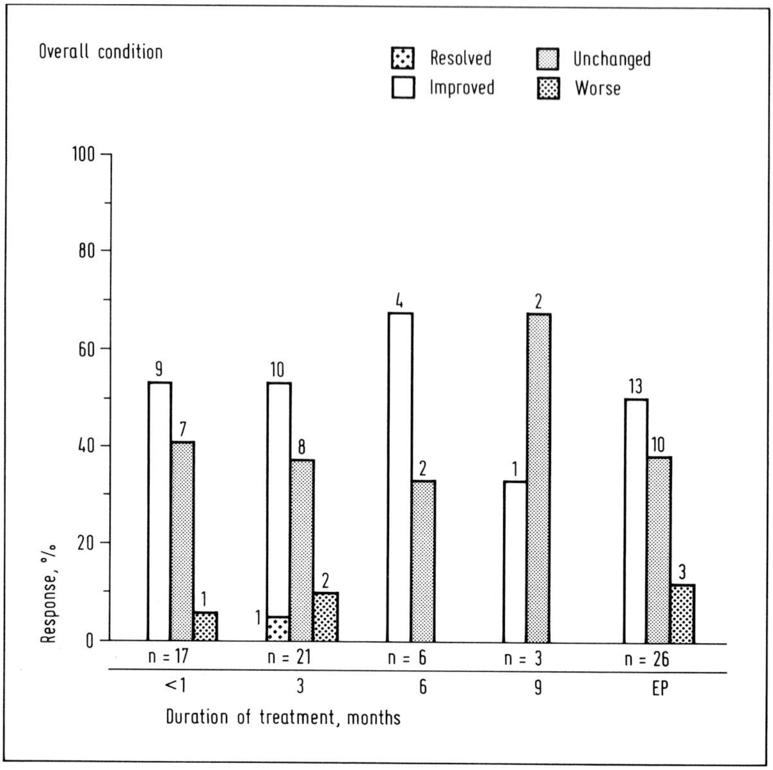

b

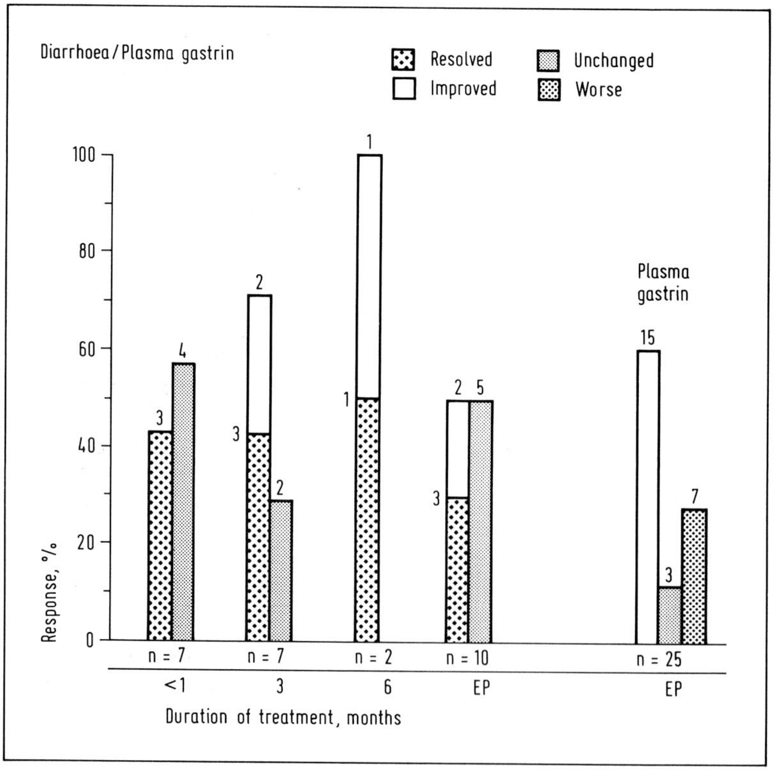

Fig. 8 a and b. Sandostatin® in gastrinoma: combined efficacy data; categorical ratings vs baseline (EP = end-point evaluation)

Levels were suppressed in 15, unchanged or variable in 3 and elevated above baseline in 7 patients. There was no consistent relationship between clinical response to Sandostatin and pretreatment circulating gastrin levels though the data would suggest that the patients who responded best were generally those who showed a marked suppression of plasma gastrin levels.

● Overall condition response
The mean rating of the overall response during the first two weeks of Sandostatin therapy was 2.5 for the 17 patients assessed. This was a marginal response which was essentially unchanged at later time periods. Examination of the categorical responses revealed that approximately 50% of the collective were rated as improved at each evaluation interval.

Insulinomas
Data from 15 patients (3 US, 12 non-US) were available for evaluation of efficacy (Figures 9 and 10). Of the collective, 7 patients were considered to have a single and benign tumor and 8 patients to have malignant and metastatic tumor.

Dosage: In US-treated patients, this ranged from 220 µg daily average at two weeks up to 675 µg after ten months. One patient treated for twenty-two months received 900 µg daily. Non-US patients received mean daily doses of 200 µg.

Duration of treatment/discontinuation of therapy: Treatment extended to twenty-four months. Ten patients were treated for less than three months; in 3 of these who had benign disease treatment had been administered in the pre-operative period to stabilize the patients in preparation for surgery. In 7 patients, therapy was discontinued owing to lack of efficacy within this period, and in 2 additional patients, at later time intervals; in 3 of these patients only, treatment continued beyond four months.

Symptom response:
● Hypoglycemia/overall condition
Hypoglycemia was the cardinal feature in all patients; the overall condition response closely reflected the hypoglycemia response. The mean rating of 2.1 within the first month includes the 3 patients with benign disease who responded pre-operatively; the mean rating of 2.6 at three months reflects their withdrawal. The improvement in mean ratings at later intervals is due to the discontinuation of therapy for non-responders.

Inspection of the categorical responses indicated an improvement in symptoms or glycemic control in approximately 50% within the first three months of therapy. At the end-point evaluation, 3 patients were rated as unchanged but 4 patients were rated as worse (see Discussion and Conclusions).

Biochemical response:
● Plasma insulin levels
Availability of evaluable data was limited and indicated that a sustained suppression

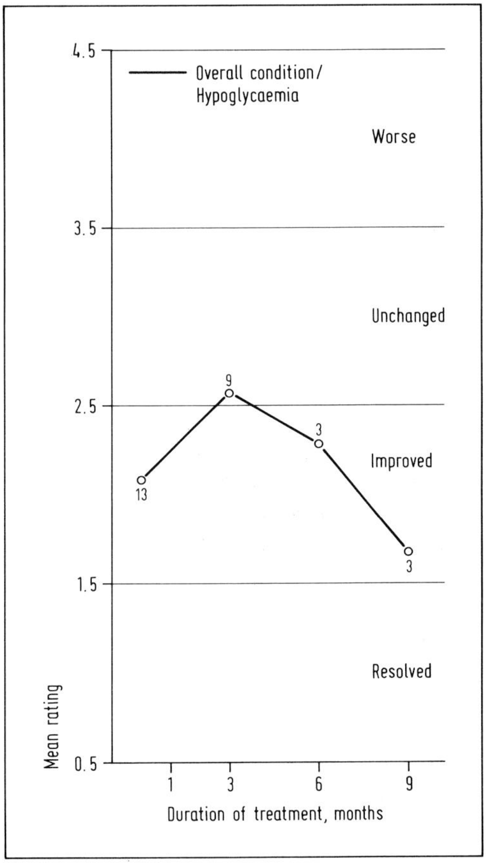

Fig. 9. Sandostatin® in insulinoma: combined efficacy data; mean rating vs baseline. (Patient numbers indicated at each evaluation point)

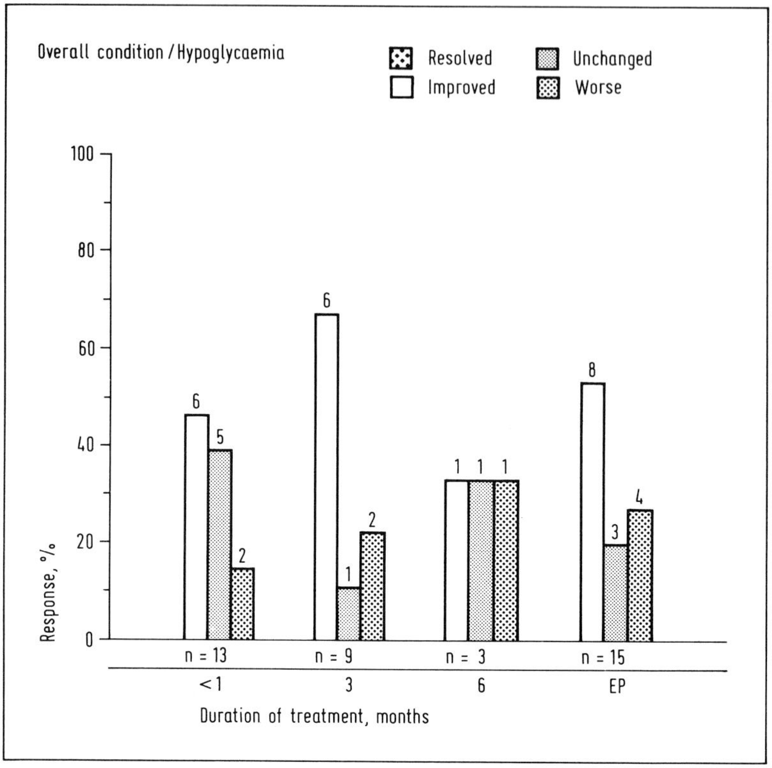

Fig. 10. Sandostatin in insulinoma: combined efficacy data; categorical rating vs baseline (EP = endpoint evaluation)

of circulating insulin levels was an inconsistent and unpredictable characteristic of treatment which did not correlate with a clinical response.

GRFomas

Four patients with clinical symptoms associated with excessive growth hormone secretion secondary to GRF-secreting tumors of the pancreas were evaluated over periods of up to eighteen months. Mean daily dosage over time was 350 µg, ranging from 200 to 600 µg. There was a tendency to escalate the dosage to the higher end of the range after one year of treatment.

Symptomatic improvement was achieved in 3 of the 4 patients and was associated with decrease in growth hormone and/or somatomedin-C. The one patient who failed to respond did not have changes in growth hormone levels.

PPomas

Only 2 patients with pure pancreatic polypeptide-secreting tumors have been identified in this series. These patients were treated for periods up to five weeks, when data collection was discontinued. The daily dosage ranged from 250–320 µg.

Although the physiological action of pancreatic polypeptide remains to be elucidated, both of these patients experienced diarrhea. Therapy with Sandostatin resulted in a diminution of diarrhea in both and was associated with decreases in serum levels of the peptide to within the normal range.

Safety and Adverse Reactions

Since the majority of patients reported herein had metastatic disease and were severely ill prior to starting Sandostatin therapy, uniform and rigorous collection of safety data was often not feasible and was influenced by the medical needs of the patients. Laboratory parameters were difficult to assess, owing to the co-existence of malignancy, e.g. biochemical measurements of hepatic dysfunction may reflect the presence of

Table 2. Adverse reactions in GEP tumor patients and healthy volunteers

Adverse reaction	GEP tumors n = 196*	Volunteers n = 264	Total n = 460
Abdominal discomfort	8	62	70
Nausea	17	51	68
Diarrhea	12	47	59
Injection-site pain	16	25	41
Loose stools	6	31	37
Fatty stools	7	19	26
Headache	3	22	25
Dizziness	3	21	24
Flushing	1	21	22
Vomiting	5	1	6
Flatulence	1	5	6
Other	31	43	74
Total adverse reactions	110	348	458
Number of patients/volunteers with adverse reactions	66/196 (34%)	131/264 (50%)	197/460 (43%)

* Includes 23 patients not evaluated for efficacy

metastases, concomitant or previous therapies (hepatic artery ligation, cytostatic agents, hyper-alimentation) or intercurrent medical conditions. Renal function may be affected by hydration status, particularly in patients with secretory diarrhea, by treatment with nephrotoxic drugs and by concomitant diseases, e.g. diabetes mellitus.

The data collected and evaluated support the basic safety of the drug with chronic administration at doses up to 1500 µg daily. Although there were isolated reports of hepatic and renal dysfunctions and of hematological abnormalities associated with Sandostatin treatment, these events were unpredictable and treatment-limiting organ toxicity was not reported. The anticipated changes associated with the pharmacological actions of the drug, i.e. postprandial hyperglycemia or impairment of glucose tolerance (due to suppression of pancreatic insulin release) and fat malabsorption (the pathogenesis of which is probably complex and related to inhibition of exocrine pancreatic function, gall bladder paresis and endocrine factors) [18], were documented but did not limit the use of the drug in this group of patients.

Adverse reactions to acute and chronic Sandostatin administration have been assessed in a total of 196 patients (110 US, 86 non-US) and in a total of 264 normal volunteers; the most frequently reported effects are shown in Table 2. Pain at the site of injection and effects relating to the gastrointestinal tract (nausea, abdominal discomfort, flatulence, fatty stools, diarrhea) dominated. Of the patients with GEP endocrine tumors, 66 (34%) reported a total of 110 reactions. In contrast, 131 of 264 (50%) volunteers reported a total of 348 reactions, reflecting perhaps the pharmacological potency of Sandostatin in a young healthy population not experiencing a therapeutic effect. Reactions were graded mild in 53 (48%), moderate in 42 (38%), severe in 15 (14%); where stated, relationship to Sandostatin was considered probable or certain in 55 (58%), uncertain in 32 (33%) and negative in 9 (9%). The course of the reactions ranged from spontaneous disappearance to persistent but tolerated, e.g. injection site pain, fatty stools in some patients. The occurrence of stools resembling steatorrhea had been noted in a number of volunteer studies; this effect of treatment was confirmed in the patients, 25 (13%) reporting the occurrence of diarrhea, loose stools or fatty stools, elevated faecal fat levels being demonstrated in 9 non-US patients.

Discussion and Conclusions

Rationale

Natural somatostatin inhibits the release of a variety of gastrointestinal regulatory peptides [2–4, 15, 28]. Its therapeutic potential has been extensively investigated with variable results, in a number of GEP tumors [31]. Whatever its potential, long-term management of these tumors with natural somatostatin is impractical because of the compound's very short plasma half-life, which necessitates continuous parenteral administration.

Although surgery, hepatic artery embolization, chemotherapy and medical symptomatic therapy are of undoubted value in the management of such patients in terms of palliation and, sometimes, cure, the natural progression of the disease process frequently leads to severe, and often uncontrollable, symptoms due to peptide secretion by the tumor. A requirement for alternative or supplementary therapy has been defined: "There is therefore a definite place for antisecretory therapy, to be used either to suppress peptide-related metabolic abnormalities while curative treatment is attempted, or in the long-term, when that fails" [34].

Sandostatin fulfils such requirements in many respects.

Efficacy

Using the methods of evaluation of uncontrolled data derived from diverse sources, it is evident that in this group of patients (the majority of whom had malignant tumors, remained severely and distressingly symptomatic despite previous therapies including surgery, chemotherapy, medical symptomatic treatment, and had few or no remaining therapeutic options), Sandostatin therapy was associated with symptomatic benefit and an improved quality of life. There was a sustained profound improvement in diarrhea in most patients with VIPoma and the carcinoid syndrome and a less rapid and less marked improvement in the necrolytic migratory rash of the glucagonoma syndrome and an improvement in other features of the carcinoid syndrome in most patients.

The therapeutic benefit in patients with gastrinoma and insulinoma was less obvious and may reflect heterogeneity in the patient population, intrinsic non-responsiveness, and inadequate or inappropriate dosing. However, responsive patients within these categories also showed a sustained improvement. From very small numbers of patients, a therapeutic benefit of Sandostatin is also indicated in patients with tumors secreting GRF or PP.

The responses to Sandostatin treatment outlined here are similar to those reported in the literature [1, 5, 7, 8, 13, 16, 17, 22–24, 32, 34, 35]; the homogeneous results in 25 patients with the carcinoid syndrome reported by Kvols et al. [16], showing a symptomatic response in 22 and a significant reduction in urinary 5-HIAA excretion levels in 18, may reflect careful patient selection, and a more defined management protocol. (This series is elaborated upon elsewhere in this volume.) Once established, it would seem that the clinical response is maintained over long periods although sudden escape associated with return of symptoms has been described [14].

The variability in response seen in some tumor subgroups may be related to degree and extent of malignant disease, varying doses of Sandostatin, or inadequate tumor responsiveness to Sandostatin due possibly to non-expression of somatostatin receptors, and to patients' compliance and tolerability.

It is interesting that, VIPomas and possibly gastrinomas excepted, there was little correlation between levels of tumor marker and symptomatic response to Sandostatin. In many tumors, the pathogenic relationship of the marker to the typical clinical features is unclear. However, in some responsive patients with insulinoma, the improvement in glycemic control in the absence of detectable suppression of circulating immunoreactive insulin levels remains to be explained. It is tempting to speculate that Sandostatin may act not only to inhibit release of the bioactive tumor product (recognized or not), but also to alter the circulating molecular form (for example, to a larger, less bioactive variety); to inhibit the action of the bioactive product at the end organ, or even to act directly on the end organ to produce a pharmacological effect contrary to that of the tumor product (for example, by affecting fluid and electrolyte transport in the jejunum or inhibiting acid secretion in the stomach). The identification of the presence of somatostatin receptors in high density on a gastrinoma [27], however, would suggest that the prime site of action is the tumor itself.

Although tumor stasis or even shrinkage on Sandostatin treatment has been reported in the literature [7, 8, 16, 29, 30, 34], results from this collective would indicate that these are inconsistent and unpredictable phenomena. The nature of such findings has been debated and from anecdotal data it has been suggested that Sandostatin treatment may result in tumor infarction through an effect on tumor blood supply [30].

Safety

From a consideration of the somatostatinoma syndrome [3] and the pharmacological effects of infused somatostatin, certain adverse effects of Sandostatin administration might be anticipated. For some patients, subcutaneous injection poses a problem (injection-site pain is presumably related to the injected volume and acidity of the solution). Although steatorrhea has been reported in some patients, to date no deleterious consequences have been ascribed to this with chronic Sandostatin treatment. Administration of pancreatic enzymes may help alleviate this phenomenon [30].

Other gastrointestinal side effects and impairment of glucose tolerance may be reduced by avoiding food around the time of drug administration, i.e. by injecting between meals.

In patients with insulinoma who are poorly responsive to Sandostatin, administration of drug may exacerbate the hypoglycemia, owing to suppression of release of counterregulatory hormones, particularly glucagon. Prior to starting chronic therapy, therefore, each patient should be exposed to escalating test doses of Sandostatin under close clinical supervision, in order to establish the response pattern. This is usually manifest within 72 h.

The possibility of endogenous anti-Sandostatin antibody formation has been investigated. Results of assays performed in 20 patients treated for at least six months showed a borderline positive result in one patient only (T. O'Dorisio, personal communication). Another study in 7 patients treated for nine to twenty-six months failed to detect antibodies [11].

From a consideration of the clinical features of the somatostatinoma syndrome, the occurrence of gallstones in patients treated chronically with Sandostatin might be anticipated. Although not described in this collective, such an association has been made in a patient with a thyrotropin-secreting pituitary adenoma [9]; increasing experience with long-term treatment and use of high doses of Sandostatin should clarify the incidence of this feature. Significant suppression of thyroid function with chronic treatment has not been described.

Dosage

Dosage ranged from 50 μg/day to 1500 μg/day in those patients continuing on therapy. This variation may reflect severity of symptoms, desired symptomatic control, degree and extent of malignancy, tumor sensitivity and tolerability. In some patients there was a tendency for dosage to increase with time, as symptoms recurred and malignancy progressed.

Future Perspectives

Gastroenteropancreatic endocrine tumors are rare, but are of particular interest because of the association of characteristic symptoms with bioactive peptide over-production. Somatostatin inhibits release of peptides of the gastroenteropancreatic endocrine system. Sandostatin, with a similar spectrum of pharmacological activity but with the advantage of longer duration of effect, is a rational and effective adjunct to the therapeutic options available to patients with these tumors.

It is possible, however, that the application of Sandostatin tumor therapy may extend beyond the endocrine neoplasms considered to date.

The development and progression of certain tumors in animals may be dependent on the endocrine milieu. Malignant rat chondrosarcomas, for example, seem to require GH, GH-related growth factors (e.g. somatomedins), insulin and glucocorticoids [21].

Administration of somatostatin analogues to rats has been associated with reduced progression of Swarm sarcoma, an effect also seen with Sandostatin in rats with chondrosarcoma. Such anti-tumor effects may be mediated by inhibition of GH, somatomedins and insulin release. Gastrointestinal peptides may also have a tropic effect on bowel cancers. If so, there may be a rationale for the use of somatostatin analogues which are potent inhibitors of the release of such peptides. It has also been postulated that somatostatin analogues might be useful in treating oncogene-induced tumors, perhaps by reversing the stimulatory effect of epidermal growth factor (EGF), a peptide with potent mitogenic activity [10]. Such effects have yet to be described in man.

To date, use of Sandostatin has been limited mainly to the treatment of end-stage patients as 'anti-secretory' therapy, in an effort to control their distressing symptoms. The application of Sandostatin in the preoperative preparation of patients scheduled for curative or palliative surgery or for chemotherapy and the combination of Sandostatin with other therapies (endocrine, antineoplastic and medical symptomatic) remain to be investigated. In particular, the combination of potent somatostatin analogues with analogues of LHRH in the treatment of pancreatic carcinoma, a tumor which may, in part, be sex-hormone dependent, has been proposed [12].

Already, Sandostatin has an established role in the management of symptomatic patients with GEP endocrine tumors; its final optimal therapeutic profile in these and other conditions remains to be defined.

References

1. Altimari A. F., Bhoopalam N., O'Dorisio T., Lange C. L., Sandberg L., Prinz R. A.: Use of somatostatin analogue (SMS 201-995) in the glucagonoma syndrome. Surgery 1986; *100*:989–996
2. Bloom S. R., Mortimer C. H., Thorner M. O., Hall R., Gomez-Pan A., Roy V. M., Russell A. C. G., Coy D. H., Kastin A. J., Schally A. V.: Inhibition of gastrin and gastric acid secretion by growth hormone release inhibiting hormone. Lancet 1974; *II*:1106–1109
3. Bloom S. R., Polak J. M.: Glucagonomas, VIPomas and somatostatinomas. Clin Endocrinol Metab 1980; *9*:285–297
4. Boden G., Sivitz M. C., Owen O. E.: Somatostatin suppresses secretin and pancreatic exocrine secretion. Science 1975; *190*:163–165
5. Bonfils S., Ruszniewski P., Costil V., Lancournet H., Vatier J., Rene E., Mignon M.: Prolonged treatment of Zollinger-Ellison syndrome by long-acting somatostatin. Lancet 1986; *1*:554–555
6. Brazeau P., Vale W., Burgus R., Ling N., Butcher M., Rivier J., Guillemin R.: Hypothalamic polypeptide that inhibits the secretion of immunoreactive pituitary growth hormone. Science 1973; *179*:77–79
7. Ch'ng J. L. C., Anderson J. V., Williams S. J., Carr D. H., Bloom S. R.: Remission of symptoms during long-term treatment of metastatic pancreatic endocrine tumors with long-acting somatostatin analogue. B Med J 1986; *292*:981–982
8. Clements D., Elias E.: Regression of metastatic VIPoma with somatostatin analogue SMS 201-995. Lancet 1985; *1*:874–875
9. Comi R. J., Gesundheit N., Murray L., Gorden P., Weintraub B. D.: Response of thyrotropin-secreting pituitary adenomas to a long-acting somatostatin analogue. N Engl J Med 1987; *317*:12–17
10. Defeudis F. V., Moreau J.-P.: Studies on somatostatin analogues might lead to new therapies for certain types of cancer. Trends Pharmacol Sci 1986; *7*:384–386
11. Fuessl H. S., Domin J., Anderson J. V., Bloom S. R.: Chronic administration of the somatostatin analogue SMS 201-995 does not lead to endogenous antibody formation. Aliment Pharmacol Ther 1987; *1*:45–50
12. Gonzalez-Barcena D., Rangel-Garcia N. E., Perez-Sanchez P. L., Gutierrez-Damperio C., Garcia-Carrasco F., Comaru-Schally A. M., Schally A. V.: Response to D-Trp-6-LH-RH in advanced adenocarcinoma of the pancreas. Lancet 1986; *2*:154
13. Juby L. D., Burke D. A., Axon A. T. R.: Somatostatin analogue SMS 201-995 long-term therapy for VIPoma. Postgrad Med J 1987; *63*:287–289
14. Koelz A., Kraenzlin M., Gyr K., Meier V., Bloom S. R., Heitz P., Stalder H.: Escape of the response to a long-acting somatostatin analogue (SMS 201-995) in patients with VIPoma. Gastroenterology 1987; *92*:527–531

15. Koerker D. J., Ruch W., Chideckel E.: Somatostatin: Hypothalamic inhibitor of the endocrine pancreas. Science 1974; *184*:484
16. Kvols L. K., Moertel C. G., O'Connell M. J., Schutt A. J., Rubin J., Halin R. G.: Treatment of the malignant carcinoid syndrome. Evaluation of a long-acting somatostatin analogue. N Engl J Med 1986; *315*:663–666
17. Kvols L. K., Buck M., Moertel C. G., Schutt A. J., Rubin J., O'Connell M. J., Hahn R. G.: Treatment of metastatic islet cell carcinoma with a somatostatin analogue (SMS 201-995). Ann Intern Med 1987; *107*:162–168
18. Lembke B., Creutzfeldt W., Schleser S., Ebert R., Shaw C., Koop I.: Effect of the somatostatin analogue Sandostatin (SMS 201-995) on gastrointestinal, pancreatic and biliary function and hormone release in normal man. Digestion 1987; *36*:103–124
19. Lightman S. L., Fox P., Dunne M. J.: The effect of SMS 201-995, a long-acting somatostatin analogue on anterior pituitary function in healthy male volunteers. In: Bloom S. R., Greenwood C. (eds) Proceedings of somatostatin 85. Scand J Gastroenterol 1986; *21* [Suppl 119]:84–95
20. Luft R., Efendic S., Hokfelt T., Johansson O., Arimura A.: Immunohistochemical evidence for the localization of somatostatin-like immunoreactivity in a cell population of the pancreatic islets. Med Biol 1974; *52*:428–430
21. McCumbee W. D., McCarty K. S. Jr, Lebowitz H. E.: Hormone responsiveness of a transplantable rat chondrosarcoma. II. Evidence for in vivo hormone dependence. Endocrinology 1980; *106*:1930–1940
22. Marsh H. M., Martin J. K., Kvols L. K., Gracey D. R., Warner M. A., Warner M. E., Moertel C. G.: Carcinoid crisis during anaesthesia: Successful treatment with a somatostatin analogue. Anaesthesiology 1987; *66*:89–91
23. Maton P. N., O'Dorisio T. M., Brent A., Howe B. S., McArthur E., Howard J. M., Cherner J. A., Malarkey T. B., Collen M. J., Gardner J. D., Jensen R. T.: Effect of a long-acting somatostatin analogue (SMS 201-995) in a patient with pancreatic cholera. N Engl J Med 1985; *312*:17–21
24. Osei K., O'Dorisio T. M.: Malignant insulinoma: Effects of a somatostatin analogue (compound 201-995) on serum glucose, growth and gastroenteropancreatic hormones. Ann Intern Med 1985; *103*:223–225
25. Pless J., Bauer W., Briner U., Doepfner W., Marbach P., Maurer R., Petcher T. J., Reubi J. C., Vonderscher J.: Chemistry and pharmacology of SMS 201-995, a long-acting octapeptide analogue of somatostatin. In: Bloom S. R., Greenwood C. (eds) Proceedings of somatostatin 85. Scand J Gastroenterol 1986; *21* [Suppl 119]:54–64
26. Reichlin S.: Somatostatin. N Engl J Med 1983; *309*:1459–1501 and 1556–1563
27. Reubi J. C.: Somatostatin receptors as markers for endocrine tumors. JAMA 1987; *257*:3277
28. Schlegel W., Raptis S., Harvery R. F., Oliver J. M., Pfeiffer E. F.: Inhibition of cholecystokinin-pancreozymin release by somatostatin. Lancet 1977; *ii*:166–167
29. Shepherd J. J., Senator G. B.: Regression of liver metastases in a patient with gastrin-secreting tumor treated with SMS 201-995. Lancet 1986; *ii*:574
30. Vinik A. I., Tsai S. T., Moattari A. R., Cheung P., Eckhauser F. E., Cho K.: Somatostatin analogue (SMS 201-995) in the management of gastroenteropancreatic tumors and diarrhea syndromes. Am J Med 1986; *81* [Suppl 6B]:23–40
31. Weil C.: Gastroenteropancreatic endocrine tumors. Klin Wochenschr 1985; *63*:433–459
32. Von Werder K., Losa M., Muller O. A., Schweiberer L., Fahlbusch R., Del Pozo E.: Treatment of metastasising GRF-producing tumor with a long-acting somatostatin analogue. Lancet 1984; *11*:282–283
33. Williams G., Fuessl H., Kraenzlin M., Bloom S. R.: Postprandial effects of SMS 201-995 on gut hormones and glucose tolerance. In: Bloom S. R., Greenwood C. (eds) Proceedings of somatostatin 85. Scand J Gastroenterol 1986; *21* [Suppl 119]:73–83
34. Wood S. M., Kraenzlin M. E., Adrian T. E., Bloom S. R.: Treatment of patients with pancreatic endocrine tumors using a new long-acting somatostatin analogue: Symptomatic and peptide responses. Gut 1985; *26*:438–444
35. Wormann B., Kutz K., Ottenjann R.: Treatment of relapsing bleeding peptic ulcers with the somatostatin analogue SMS 201-995 in a patient with Zollinger-Ellison syndrome. Hepatogastroenterology 1985; *32*:152–153

15. Consensus

T. M. O'Dorisio

The Ohio State University, College of Medicine, Columbus, Ohio, USA

First and most important in the evaluation of any treatment modality is the assessment of its efficacy, defined as therapeutic success. During the final consensus round table discussion, the therapeutic success with Sandostatin® that had been described during the meeting by all participants was reviewed in respect to several important questions regarding Sandostatin administration, efficacy and safety. During this discussion, five key consensus statements were formulated which are presented here along with a review of the data comprising the basis upon which the consensus was reached.

1. Sandostatin as symptomatic therapy improves the patient's quality of life

It was concluded that Sandostatin is a unique peptidomimetic agent which often dramatically ameliorates the debilitating symptoms of patients suffering from clinically expressed endocrine tumors of the GEP system. Specifically, the symptoms of secretory diarrhea and flushing associated with carcinoid syndrome and VIPoma/watery diarrhea syndrome were reported to be abolished or significantly improved (reduced by more than 50%) by Drs Dunne, Elton and colleagues. In addition Dr Kvols noted that 17% of his patients with malignant carcinoid tumors achieved objective tumor regression (defined as 50% shrinkage of measurable tumor mass). In the context of his review, Dr Kvols reported his own findings demonstrating that carcinoid crisis, often associated with induction of anesthesia and manifesting as profound hypotension, is readily reversible with intravenous Sandostatin therapy. Dr Kvols also reported that Sandostatin is effective in stabilizing a debilitated patient with carcinoid syndrome who may need surgical or chemotherapeutic intervention.

While VIPoma is rarer than the other GEP endocrine tumors (discussed below), its clinical manifestation, watery diarrhea, is often fulminant and life-threatening. Dr Williams and his colleagues noted that their studies suggested that "VIPoma hypoglycemia and insulinoma studied and evaluated thus far responded to Sandostatin". However, there have been fewer dramatic responses of malignant insulinoma patients, as noted by Dr O'Dorisio. Dr Lamberts suggested that the number of somatostatin binding sites on an insulinoma tumor may determine, in part, its responsiveness to Sandostatin therapy. He went on to propose that the type of somatostatin binding site (somatostatin-28 vs somatostatin-14) may predict tumor response.

Although the number of somatostatin-treated patients with glucagonoma syndromes (manifesting with severe migratory necrolytic rash) has, to date, been small, a response rate of over 50% has been observed. As Dr Williams noted in his discussion, although glucagon levels fall substantially (albeit not to within normal limits) with a single injection of Sandostatin, nevertheless, "all tumor patients initially showed marked clearing of their rash after starting Sandostatin therapy. Further, improvement was associated with increasing the dosage, a true effect of Sandostatin on the rash of glucagonoma. This is consistent with the observations that refractory glucagonoma rash can be cleared very rapidly after intravenous somatostatin (native) infusion".

Finally, the consensus committee examined the treatment of the newest member of the GEP endocrine tumor family, GRFoma. Of the four evaluable patients with clinical symptoms of excess growth hormone secretion (most often in the form of acromegaly) 75% evinced a diminution in the concentrations of growth hormone and/or somatomedin-C.

Following a thorough review of all the data presented on the various clinically expressed GEP tumors and their response to Sandostatin, the group agreed that a physician can indeed determine the success and failure of Sandostatin therapy in terms of its impact on the patient's quality of life, defined by his or her ability to conduct and maintain normal daily activities.

2. Sandostatin is a very safe agent with no clear contraindications

Sandostatin has been used safely in patients of all ages, including neonates and octogenarians. The consensus group agreed that, to date, no restrictions on the use of Sandostatin in any age group have been indicated. The second point of agreement regarding the safety of Sandostatin relates to the absence of contraindications (the exceptions being the rare hypersensitivity to Sandostatin or a patient with *severe* hepatic or renal failure). In addition, the potential for drug-drug interaction appears to be quite small. However, the consensus group did suggest the following general precautionary measures:

● *Diabetes mellitus.* As noted by Dr Dunne, "caution should be observed when using Sandostatin in insulin-dependent diabetes patients because the drug will reduce insulin requirements [by inhibiting counter-regulatory hormones preferentially] ... There is [therefore] a real danger of precipitating hypoglycemia attacks in these patients". Dr Lamberts also suggested that "if you are treating an insulinoma [patient], it is wise to give the first [few] doses [of Sandostatin] in a hospital setting with an indwelling infusion of glucose because some patients might have a paradoxic reaction to Sandostatin [again, by preferential inhibition of the counter-regulatory hormones]".

● *VIPoma/watery diarrhea syndrome and potassium supplementation.* Dr Lamberts cautioned that "since all VIPoma patients are on potassium supplements, they too should be given Sandostatin [initially] in a hospital setting so that potassium supplementation could be quickly stopped, avoiding hyperkalemia [secondary to Sandostatin's inhibition of aldosterone secretion]".

● *Carcinoid syndrome and intestinal obstruction.* There was agreement that carcinoid syndrome patients presenting with acute abdominal pain may be at increased risk of intestinal obstruction when Sandostatin therapy is initiated. Dr Kvols noted a "malignant carcinoid patient who developed a paralytic ileus after receiving 100 μg of Sandostatin." Dr Williams reinforced Dr Kvols' comment by noting that "motility stasis [induced by Sandostatin] could lead to paralytic pseudo-hernia".

● *Drug-drug interaction.* The consensus group noted that Sandostatin is remarkably free of drug-drug interactions, with the following few exceptions. Dr Gyr advises "caution when using Sandostatin with other antimotility drugs. Patients may expect many months of clinical remission during continuous Sandostatin treatment even with disease progression that does not respond to conventional therapy". The consensus group concluded that, outside the carcinoid syndrome group, VIPoma/watery diarrhea syndrome patients display the most dramatic response to Sandostatin therapy even after all other treatment modalities, including extensive surgery and chemotherapy, have failed.

While the goal of the committee was better delineation of the role of Sandostatin in the management of patients with symptomatic carcinoid syndrome and VIPoma/watery diarrhea syndrome, the therapeutic use of Sandostatin in other symptomatic GEP endocrine tumors was also addressed. The committee agreed that conventional H_2 blockade therapy for gastric acid hypersecretion is often more than adequate in patients with symptomatic gastrinomas. However, Sandostatin has been shown to be quite effective in some patients refractory to maximum doses of the H_2 blockers. As reported by Dr J. A. Chayvialle, "Sandostatin dramatically improved the control of acid hypersecretion in two patients with high residual basal rates while on large doses of ranitidine". He further noted that "Sandostatin normalized plasma gastrin concentration in 4 of 9 patients". In this regard, the consensus group addressed the potential benefit of lowering gastrin levels in gastrinoma patients whose symptoms have been effectively controlled by conventional therapy. As Chayvialle concluded, "Sandostatin may be especially valuable in those responsive (malignant) gastrinoma patients, since chronic potent inhibition of gastrin release might prevent or delay fundic EC cell hyperplasia".

The committee concurred with the combined European/USA data on insulinoma compiled by Drs Dunne, Elton and colleagues; specifically, slightly under 50% of the insulinoma patients with symptomatic hypoglycemia will respond to Sandostatin. In this regard, the committee noted that because of the effect of Sandostatin on the GI tract (generalized hypomotility), the absorption and kinetics of concurrently administered oral medicines may be altered (slower absorption and delayed peak absorption may be observed). Dr O'Dorisio pointed out that "in the case of oral cyclosporin A therapy, absorption may be abnormal because of the exocrine insufficiency associated with higher doses of Sandostatin thereby affecting the fat soluble absorption of cyclosporin A". In the instance of chemotherapy, Dr Dunne pointed out that "to date, there has been no data to enable us to say that administration of Sandostatin in conjunction with cytotoxic agents is safe".

3. Sandostatin is remarkably free of side effects

Although the combined experience in Europe and the USA (as shown by Dunne, Elton and colleagues) suggested a high proportion (43%) of side effects for both patients and volunteers using Sandostatin, none of the side effects was considered severe enough to justify discontinuation.

4. Sandostatin can be easily administered over a large dosage range

It was felt by the group that the initial dose of Sandostatin should be about 50 μg/injection and that to begin with at least two injections should be given daily. Sandostatin can be given as frequently as every 3 h if symptoms are shown to abate with the lower dose but 'breakthrough' has been noted. If higher doses are used (100–300 μg/injection), it would probably not be necessary to give more than two injections daily, since the higher doses would ensure a higher trough level prior to the next injection. It was also noted that Sandostatin is a very stable agent which remains biologically active at room temperature for many weeks. The group agreed that as multidose vials become more readily available, patients can use them at room temperature as needed (eg for travel), but that the vials should be refrigerated when the patients are at home.

Regarding the injection site, Dr Kvols' unpublished work suggests that "the difference in peak [Sandostatin] levels after injection into the abdomen versus the arm was not significant". Dr Williams concurred and further pointed out "whichever injection site was less painful or more convenient, that is the site to be recommended". Dr O'Dorisio noted that "burning at the site of injection with Sandostatin could often be alleviated by bringing Sandostatin in the syringe to room temperature prior to injection".

5. Sandostatin does not appear to be immunogenic

Although the issue of antibody formation during chronic Sandostatin therapy could not be fully discussed, the experience from both Europe and the USA suggests that Sandostatin is not immunogenic and that antibody formation does not appear to be a problem. However, the issue of tachyphylaxis (or down-regulation or 'tolerance') in response to long-term Sandostatin was raised. It was felt that because of the structure of Sandostatin, long-term use could indeed be associated with a 'tolerance' effect and that dose escalation, or even withdrawal and support for a time before re-institution at lower doses, may be necessary and beneficial.

16. Future Directions

T. M. O'Dorisio

The Ohio State University, College of Medicine, Columbus, Ohio, USA

The rapidly accruing literature on Sandostatin indicates that it may be effective outside its current area of application, the treatment of symptomatic endocrine tumors of the GEP system. The following brief remarks and suggested future directions for Sandostatin represent ideas and comments from clinical research protocols and from reports on special applications presented in either abstract or publication form.

Future directions of Sandostatin in both the clinical and basic research arenas may include careful investigation of the reported observations that Sandostatin lowers the peptide levels of many neuroendocrine tumors by as much as 100% (more often between 40% and 60%). The information garnered from several published studies demonstrating the lowering of high circulating tumor peptide levels suggests that Sandostatin affects tumor peptide release and/or synthesis. A further implication is that Sandostatin may inhibit tumor growth by reducing the blood flow to the tumor, or perhaps more directly by binding to the tumor tissue. Future studies should address these potentially important actions of Sandostatin.

The use of Sandostatin in combination with known chemotherapeutic agents or, particularly, agents known to be biologic response modifiers (eg interferon, tumor necrosis factor and interleukin-2) needs to be further developed and tested in well-controlled clinical studies.

Observations of an analgesic effect, particularly in the headache of acromegaly, imply an action of Sandostatin independent of its effect on tumor growth hormone release, since the headache is reduced very rapidly. This analgesic effect of Sandostatin may be useful in combating the pain of certain arthritic states, migraine headache and, perhaps, even the painful neuropathy associated with such disease states as diabetes mellitus. Clinical trials directed not only at the secretory diarrhea associated with neuroendocrine tumors, but also in states such as acquired immune deficiency syndrome and graft-versus-host disease of bone marrow transplant, and, perhaps, even the serious secretory diarrhea associated with vibrio cholera, are also recommended. Although one mechanism of native somatostatin (the action on the inhibitory subunit of adenylate cyclase) has been confirmed with in vitro studies, complete studies regarding other mechanisms of Sandostatin have yielded no clear results to date. Ultimately, all secretory diarrhea states mediated by the cAMP system may well be found to respond to Sandostatin therapy. Studies of the effect of Sandostatin in the potentially important indications of psoriasis, orthostatic hypotension and postprandial hypotension, particularly in diabetic hypotension, are being conducted. Studies addressing the effects of Sandostatin on portal hypotension, gastritis and esophageal variceal bleeding are currently under way in both Europe and the USA.

Another area of study relates to the use of Sandostatin alone or with known chemotherapeutic agents for the treatment of nonendocrine cancers. The potential effect of Sandostatin in combination with such agents or with biologic response modifiers needs to be determined. Only in the most carefully designed and controlled clinical research settings will we be able to establish Sandostatin clearly as an effective anti-tumor agent. Because of the very high native somatostatin concentrations in the CNS and the large number of somatostatin receptors in CNS tissue, the potentially important therapeutic role of Sandostatin in CNS tumors and in central and peripheral neurologic disease states needs to be examined carefully.

Finally, the role of Sandostatin in blunting angiogenesis in proliferative retinopathy needs to be carefully explored and its potential usefulness in preventing or delaying *early retinopathy* in insulin-dependent diabetic patients determined.

Bibliography

I. VIPoma

Achord, J. L.: Secretin, Cholecystokinin, and Vasoactive Intestinal Polypeptide in Pancreatic Cholera. Ann Intern Med 105 (4):632–633, 1986

Anderson, J. V., Bloom, S. R.: Long-Term Therapy with a Somatostatin Analogue (SMS 201-995) in a Series of Patients with Vasoactive Intestinal Peptide Secreting Pancreatic Tumours. Can J Physiol Pharmacol 64 [Suppl]: 9 (Abstr. No. 119), 1986

Benson, G. D., et al: Control of Watery Diarrhoea Syndrome in a Patient with a Vasoactive Intestinal Peptide-Secreting Tumour, Using SMS 201-995 and Dexamethasone. Scand J Gastroenterol 21 [Suppl 119]:170–176, 1986

Bloom, S. R., et al: Effect of Chronic Administration of a Long-Acting Somatostatin Analogue on Glucose Homeostasis. Diabetologia 27:258 (Abstr. No. 47), 1984

Clements, D., Elias, E.: Regression of Metastatic Vipoma with Somatostatin Analogue SMS 201-995. Lancet 1 (8433):874–875, 1985

Jensen, R. T.: Somatostatin. Biomed Pharmacother 39:399, 1985

Juby, L. D., et al: Somatostatin Analogue SMS 201-995 Long Term Therapy for Vipoma. Postgrad Med 63:287–289, 1987

Koberstein, B., et al: [Hypokalemia and Intestinal Pseudoobstruction Surgically Confirmed VIPoma[sic] Indicating Somatostatin Therapy.] Med Klin 83 (7):251–256, 1988

Koelz, A., et al: Escape of the Response to a Long-Acting Somatostatin Analogue (SMS 201-995) in Patients with VIPoma. Gastroenterology 92:527–531, 1987

Kraenzlin, M. E., et al: Can Inhibition of Hormone Secretion be Associated with Endocrine Tumour Shrinkage? Lancet 2:1501, 1983

Kraenzlin, M. E., et al: Remision of Symptoms and Shrinkage of Metastasis with Long Term Treatment with Somatostatin Analogue. Gut 25 (5):A 576 (Abstr. No. F 92), 1984

Kraenzlin, M. E., et al: Long-Term Treatment of a VIPoma with Somatostatin Analogue Resulting in Remission of Symptoms and Possible Shrinkage of Metastases. Gastroenterology 88 (1):185–187, 1985

Krejs, G. J.: VIPoma Syndrome. Am J Med 82 [Suppl 5 b]:37–48, 1987

Maton, P. N., et al: Effect of a Long-Acting Somatostatin Analogue (SMS 201-995) in a Patient with Pancreatic Cholera. N Engl J Med 312 (1):17–21, 1985

Maton, P. N., et al: Successful Therapy of Pancreatic Cholera with the Long-Acting Somatostatin Analogue SMS 201-995. Relation Between Plasma Concentrations of Drug and Clinical and Biochemical Responses. Scand J Gastroenterol 21 [Supp 119]:181–186, 1986

Öberg, K., et al: WDHA Syndrome Caused by a Ganglioneuroblastoma Producing Vasoactive Intestinal Polypeptide and Neuropeptide Y. Treatment with SMS 201-995, a Somatostatin Analogue. Scand J Gastroenterol 21 [Suppl 119]:228–229, 1986

Reubi, J. C., et al: Vasoactive Intestinal Peptide Producing Tumour Contains High Density of Somatostatin Receptors. Lancet 1:741–742, 1987

Rood, R. P., et al: Pancreatic Cholera Syndrome Due to a Vasoactive Intestinal Polypeptide-Producing Tumor: Further Insights Into the Pathophysiology. Gastroenterology 94:813–818, 1988

Sagman, U., Fine, S.: Demonstration of Tumor Regression with Somatostatin Analogue (SMS 201-995) in a Patient with Pancreatic Cholera. Can J Physiol Pharmacol [Suppl]:66 (Abstr. No. 244), 1986

Santangelo, W. C.: Effect of a Somatostatin Analogue on Intestinal Water and ION Transport in Pancreatic Cholera Syndrome. Gastroenterology 88 (5):1570, 1985

Santangelo, W. C., et al: Pancreatic Cholera Syndrome: Effect of a Synthetic Somatostatin Analog on Intestinal Water and ION Transport. Ann Intern Med 103 (3):363–367, 1985

Santangelo, W. C., et al: VIPoma Syndrome: Effect of a Somatostatin Analogue on Intestinal Water and ION Transport. Regul Pept [Suppl 3]:S 53, 1985

Santangelo, W. C., et al: Long-Term Treatment of a Child with Pancreatic Cholera Syndrome with Somatostatin Analog (SMS 201-995). Can J Physiol Pharmacol [Suppl]:66–67 (Abstr. No. 245), 1986

Santangelo, W. C., et al: VIPoma Syndrome: Effect of a Synthetic Somatostatin Analogue. Scand J Gastroenterol 21 [Suppl 119]:187–190, 1986

Smith, S. S., et al: Watery Diarrhea, Hypokalemia, Achlorhydria Syndrome in An Infant: Effect of the Long-Acting Somatostatin Analogue SMS 201-995 on the Disease and Linear Growth. J Pediatr Gastroenterol Nutr 6:710–716, 1987

II. Carcinoid Tumors

Ahlman, H., et al: Use of a Somatostatin Analogue in Association with Surgery and Hepatic Arterial Embolisation in the Treatment of the Carcinoid Syndrome. Br J Cancer 56 (6):840–842, 1987

Anderson, J. V., et al: Remission of Symptoms in Carcinoid Syndrome With a New 5-Hydroxytryptamine M Receptor Antagonist. Br Med J 294 (6580):1129, 1987

Brabant, G., et al: Treatment of Carcinoid Syndrome and VIPoma with a Long-Acting Somatostatin Analogue (SMS 201-995). Scand J Gastroenterol 21 [Suppl 119]:177–180, 1986

Clements, D., et al: SMS 201-995 and Endocrine Tumours. Scand J Gastroenterol 21 [Suppl 119]:251–255, 1986

Conlon, J. M., et al: Circulating Tachykinins (Substance P, Neurokinin A, Neuropeptide K) and the Carcinoid Flush. Scand J Gastroenterol 22:99–105, 1987

Creutzfeldt, W., Stöckmann, F.: Carcinoids and Carcinoid Syndrome. Am J Med 82 [Suppl 5 B]:4–16, 1987

Duntas, L., et al: [Malignant Carcinoid Tumor: Dose Dependency of 5-HIAA Secretion on Octreotide (SMS 201-995).] Klin Wochenschr 65 [Suppl IX]:194–195, 1987

Feldman, J. M., O'Dorisio, T. M.: Role of Neuropeptides and Serotonin in the Diagnosis of Carcinoid Tumors. Am J Med 81 [Suppl 6 B]:41–48, 1986

Kvols, L. K., et al: Rapid Reversal of Carcinoid Crisis With a Somatostatin Analogue. N Engl J Med 313 (19):1229–1230, 1985

Kvols, L. K., et al: A Somatostatin Analogue (SOM-AN) (Sandoz 201-995) in Therapy of the Malignant Carcinoid Syndrome. Proc Am Soc Clin Oncol 4:89 (Abstr. No. C 348), 1985

Kvols, L. K.: Metastatic Carcinoid Tumors and the Carcinoid Syndrome: A Selective Review of Chemotherapy and Hormonal Therapy. Am J Med 81 [Suppl 6 B]:49–55, 1986

Kvols, L. K., et al: Treatment of the Malignant Carcinoid Syndrome: Evaluation of a Long-Acting Somatostatin Analogue. N Engl J Med 315:663–666, 1986

Kvols, L., et al: Treatment of Malignant Neuroendocrine Syndromes With a Long-Acting Somatostatin Analogue (SMS 201-995). Can J Physiol Pharmacol [Suppl 10]:10 (Abstr. No. 120), 1986

Marsh, H. M., et al: Carcinoid Crisis during Anesthesia: Successful Treatment With a Somatostatin Analogue. Anesthesiology 66 (1): 89–91, 1987

Moses, A. C., et al: Differential Sensitivity of Growth Hormone Releasing Hormone (GRH) to SMS 201-995 in the Syndrome of Ectopic GRH Secretion. Clin Res 35 (3):399 A, 1987

Norheim, I., et al: Effects of the Somatostatin Analogue SMS 201-995 on Carcinoid Flush. Can J Physiol Pharmacol [Suppl 65]: (Abstr. No. 241), 1986

Oates, J. A.: The Carcinoid Syndrome. N Engl J Med 315:702–704, 1986

Öberg, K., et al: Treatment of the Carcinoid Syndrome with SMS 201-995, a Somatostatin Analogue. Scand J Gastroenterol 21 [Suppl 119]: 191–192, 1986

Öberg, K., et al: Treatment of Malignant Carcinoid Tumors With Human Leukocyte Interferon: Long-term Results. Cancer Treat Rep 70 (11):1297–1304, 1986

Richter, G., Stöckmann, F.: The Effect of Food, Pentagastrin and a Somatostatin Analogue Upon Blood Serotonin Concentration in Healthy Subjects and Patients With Carcinoid Tumours. Acta Endocrinol (Copenh) 108 [Suppl 267]:148 (Abstr. No. 165), 1985

Richter, G., et al: Short-Term Administration of the Somatostatin Analogue SMS 201-995 in Patients with Carcinoid Tumours. Scand J Gastroenterol 21 [Suppl 119]:193–198, 1986

Roy, R. C., et al: Somatostatin, Anaesthesia, and the Carcinoid Syndrome: Peri-Operative Administration of a Somatostatin Analogue to Suppress Carcinoid Tumour Activity. Anaesthesia 42:627–632, 1987

Souquet, J. C., et al: Effects of a Somatostatin Analogue on Symptoms and Amine Secretion in Carcinoid Syndrome. Gastroenterology 90 (5, pt. 2):1643, 1986

Stöckmann, F., Creutzfeldt, W.: SMS 201-995 for Treatment of Patients With Carcinoid Tumors and Zollinger-Ellison-Syndrome. Regul Pept 18:377, 1987

Stöckmann, F., et al: Effect of Short- and Long-Term Treatment With SMS 201-995 in Patients With Carcinoid Tumours. Gastroenterology 90 (5):1650, 1986

Stöckmann, F., et al: Long-Term Treatment of Patients with Endocrine Gastrointestinal Tumours with the Somatostatin Analogue SMS 201-995. Scand J Gastroenterol 21 [Suppl 119]:230–237, 1986

Tsai, S.-T., et al: The Use of a Somatostatin Analogue (SMS 201-995) in the Management of the Flushing Syndrome. Scand J Gastroenterol 21 [Suppl 119]:267–274, 1986

Van Houten, A. A., et al: Successful Symptomatic Treatment of Malignant Carcinoid Syndrome with the Somatostatin Analogue SMS 201-995. Neth J Med 32 (3–4):194–198, 1988

Wiedenmann, B., et al: Tumor Regression of an Ileal Carcinoid Under the Treatment with the Somatostatin Analogue SMS 201-995. Klin Wochenschr 66:75–77, 1988

Ziel, F. H., et al: Biochemical Response of a Growth Hormone Releasing Hormone Producing Carcinoid Tumor to Long Acting Somatostatin Analogue (SMS 201-995). Clin Res 35 (3):405 A, 1987

III. Gastrinoma/Zollinger-Ellison Syndrome

Bonfils, S. S., et al: Long-Term Management of Zollinger-Ellison Syndrome with SMS 201-995, a Long-Lasting Somatostatin Analog. Can J Physiol Pharmacol 64 [Suppl]:63 (Abstr. No. 238), 1986

Bonfils, S. S., et al: Prolonged Treatment of Zollinger-Ellison Syndrome by Long-Acting Somatostatin. Lancet 1 (8480):554–555, 1986

Buck, M., et al: Rebound Hypergastrinemia after Cessation of a Somatostatin Analogue (SMS 201-995) in Malignant Gastrinoma. Am J Med 82 [Suppl 5 B]:92–95, 1987

Campagnolo, D., et al: Effect of Somatostatin Analogue (SMS 201-995) on Molecular Species of Gastrin in Gastrinoma. Surgery 102:982–987, 1987

Ellison, E. C.: Efficacy of Long-Acting Somatostatin Analog (SMS 201-995) in the Ulcerogenic Syndrome. Gastroenterology 88 (5): 1373, 1985

Ellison, E. C., et al: Characterization of the In Vivo and In Vitro Inhibition of Gastrin Secretion from Gastrinoma by a Somatostatin Analogue (SMS 201-995). Am J Med 81 [Suppl 6 B]:56–63, 1986

Ellison, E. C., et al: Long-Acting Somatostatin Analog Inhibits Calcium and Secretion Stimulated Gastrin Release in the Zollinger-Ellison Syndrome. Gastroenterology 90:1405, 1986

Ellison, E. C., et al: Observations on the Effect of a Somatostatin Analog in the Zollinger-Ellison Syndrome: Implications for the Treatment of Apudomas. Surgery 100 (2):437–444, 1986

Ellison, E. C., et al: Suppression of Gastrin and Gastric Acid Secretion in the Zollinger-Ellison Syndrome by Long-Acting Somatostatin (SMS 201-995). Scand J Gastroenterol 21 [Suppl 119]:206–211, 1986

Elouaer-Blanc, L., et al: [Therapeutic Effects of SMS 201-995 in 2 Cases of Hyperprolactinemic Tumors During the Course of Zollinger-Ellison Syndrome (SZE) With Endocrine Neoplasia Type I.] Gastroenterol Clin Biol 11 (2 BIS): 51 A, 1987

Gilsanz-Peral, A., et al: [Use of Somatostatin Analog in the Treatment of Gastrinoma.] (Spanish) Med Clin (Barc) 89:131–132, 1987

Kothary, P. C., Vinik, A. I.: Action of Somatostatin Analogue SMS 201-995 on Gastrin Molecules in Gastrinomas in Culture. Fed Am Soc Exp Biol 2 (4): (Abstr. No. 3303), 1988

Palitzsch, K. D., et al: Protection Against Duodenal Ulceration by Somatostatin. Klin Wochenschr 64 [Suppl VII]:93–96, 1986

Ruszniewski, P., et al: Long-Term Treatment of Zollinger-Ellison Syndrome (ZES) with Long Acting Somatostatin: Efficacy on Gastric Acid and Gastrin Secretions. Gastroenterology 92 (5) (Part 2):1606, 1987

Shepherd, J. J., Senator, G. B.: Regression of Liver Metastases in Patient with Gastrin-Secreting Tumour Treated with SMS 201-995. Lancet 2:574, 1986

Tsai, S. T., et al: Long-Acting Somatostatin Analog for Patients with Gastrinoma Syndrome. Clin Res 33:876 A, 1985

Wilson, D. M., Hoffman, A. R.: Reduction of Pituitary Size by the Somatostatin Analogue SMS 201-995 in a Patient with an Islet Cell Tumour Secreting Growth Hormone Releasing Factor. Acta Endocrinol (Copenh) 113 (1):23–28, 1986

Woermann, B., et al: Treatment of Relapsing Bleeding Peptic Ulcers with the Somatostatin Analogue SMS 201-995 in a Patient with Zollinger-Ellison Syndrome. Hepatogastroenterology 32 (3):152–153, 1985

Woltering, E. A., et al: Sandostatin Decreases Gastrin Release from Acutely Dispersed Gastrinoma Cells. Can J Physiol Pharmacol 64 [Suppl]:61 (Abstr. No. 232), 1986

Woltering, E. A., et al: Somatostatin-Like Peptides Alter Calcium but not Secretin Sensitivity of Gastrinoma Cells. J Surg Res 40 (6):605–610, 1986

IV. Glucagonoma

Altimari, A. F., et al: Use of a Somatostatin Analog (SMS 201-995) in the Glucagonoma Syndrome. Surgery 100 (6):989–996, 1986

Altimari, A. F., et al: Use of Somatostatin Analogue (SMS 201-995) in the Glucagonoma Syndrome. Can J Physiol Pharmacol [Suppl]:65–66, 1986

Bloom, S. R., Polak, J. M.: Glucagonoma Syndrome. Am J Med 82 [Suppl 5 B]:25–36, 1987

Boden, G., et al: Treatment of Inoperable Glucagonoma with the Long-Acting Somatostatin Analogue SMS 201-995. N Engl J Med 314:1686–1689, 1986

Elsborg, L., Glenthoj, A.: Effect of Somatostatin in Necrolytic Migratory Erythema of Glucagonoma. Acta Scand 218:245–249, 1985

Santangelo, W. C., et al: Somatostatin Analog-Induced Remission of Necrolytic Migratory Erythema Without Changes in Plasma Glucagon Concentration. Pancreas 1:464–469, 1986

V. GRFoma

Von Werder, K., et al: Treatment of Metastasizing GRF-Producing Tumour with a Long-Acting Somatostatin Analogue. Lancet 2 (8397):282–283, 1984

Von Werder, K., et al: Long-Term Treatment of a Metastasizing GRFoma with a Somatostatin Analogue (SMS 201-995) in a Gril with Gigantism. Scand J Gastroenterol 21 [Suppl 119]: 238–242, 1986

Wilson, D. M., Hoffman, A. R.: Reduction of Pituitary Size in a Patient with a GRF Secreting Islet Cell Tumor by Continuous Subcutaneous Infusion of a Somatostatin Analog. Endocrinology 116 [Suppl]:39 (Abstr. No. 153), 1985

VI. Insulinoma

Barbetti, F., et al: The Use of the Somatostatin Analogue SMS 201-995 in Insulinoma Patients. Diabetologia 29 (8):515 A (Abstr. No. 24), 1986

Creutzfeldt, W.: Chemotherapeutic Management of Endocrine Tumours of the Gastroentero-Pancreatic Tract. Chemotherapy in Malignant Insulinoma. Dig Dis Sci 31 (10) [Suppl]:511 S (Abstr. No. WS 54), 1986

Diem, P., et al: [Treatment of the Most Severe Hypoglycemia in Inoperable Insulinoma with th Somatostatin Analog SMS 201-995.] (German) Schweiz Med Wochenschr 117 (20) [Suppl 22]:17 (Abstr. No. 40), 1987

Fernandez-Navarro, J. I., et al: [Effects of Intravenous SMS 201-995 Upon Insulin Hormones Stimulated with Arginine in a Case of Insulinoma.] Endocrinologia (Barc) 35 (1):50–54, 1988

Gilsanz-Peral, A., et al: [Malignant Insulinoma: Effects of the Somatostatin Analog in Glycemia and Insulinemia.] Endocrinologia (Barc) 34:158–160, 1987

Kaloustian, E.: [Metabolic Control of an Insulinoma with a Prolonged Action: Agonist of Somatostatin.] (French) Presse Med 15 (37): 1881–1882, 1986

Kvols, L., et al: Treatment of Metastatic Insulin-Producing Islet Cell Carcinomas with a Long Acting Somatostatin Analogue (SMS 201-995). Proc Am Assoc Cancer Res 28:201 (Abstr. No. 799), 1987

O'Dorisio, T. M., et al: Effects of Somatostatin (SMS) Analog (201-995) on Gastrin Releasing Peptide (GRP) and Pancreatic Polypeptide (PP) During Provocative Testings in a Benign Insulinoma. Clin Res 33:877 A, 1985

Osei, K., O'Dorisio, T. M.: Effects of Somatostatin (SMS) Analogue (Compound 201-995) on Serum Glucose, Growth and Gastroenteropancreatic Hormones in a Malignant Insulinoma Patient. Clin Res 33:312 A, 1985

Osei, K., O'Dorisio, T.: Malignant Insulinoma: Effects of a Somatostatin Analog (Compound 201-995) on Serum Glucose, Growth, and Gastro-Entero-Pancreatic Hormones. Ann Intern Med 103 (2):223–225, 1985

Osei, K., et al: Chronic Effects of Somatostatin (SMS) Analog (201-995) May be Independent

of Suppression of Endogenous Insulin Secretion. Clin Res 33:827 A, 1986
Osei, K., et al: Somatostatin Analog SMS 201-995: Long-Term Effects on Endogenous Insulin Secretion in a Malignant Insulinoma Patient. Can J Physiol Pharmacol 68:(Abstr. No. 248), 1986
Osei, K., et al: Somatostatin Analog SMS 201-995: Uncoupling of Effects of Gastrin-Releasing Peptide on Gastrin Release in Man. Can J Physiol Pharmacol [Suppl]:69 (Abstr. No. 250), 1986
Osei, K., et al: Somatostatin (SMS) Analog 201-995: Uncoupling of Effects of Gastrin-Releasing Peptide (GRP) on Gastrin (G) Release in Man. Clin Res 34:444 A, 1986
Sanchez-Garcia-Cervigon, P., et al: [Preoperative Therapy of Hypoglycemia Caused by Insulinoma with the Somatostatin Analogue, SMS 201-995.] (Spanish) Med Clin (Barc) 89 (12):511–513, 1987
Verschoor, L., Lamberts, S. W. J.: [Treatment With Somatostatin Analogs Preventing Hypoglycemia in Patients With Insulinomas.] (Dutch) Ned Tijdschr Geneeskd 131 (6):262, 1987
Verschoor, L., et al: Prevention of Hypoglycemia in Patients with Insulinoma. Diabetes 34 [Suppl 1]:13 A (Abstr. No. 52), 1985
Verschoor, L., et al: On the Use of a New Somatostatin Analogue in the Treatment of Hypoglycaemia in Patients with Insulinoma. Clin Endocrinol (Oxf) 25:555–560, 1986

VII. Medullary Carcinoma of Thyroid (MCT)

Berkelhammer, C. H., et al: Failure of Somatostatin Analogue 201-995 to Reduce Severe Diarrhea in a Patient with Medullary Thyroid Carcinoma. Gastroenterology 90:1344, 1986
Berkelhammer, C. H., et al: Inefficacy of Somatostatin Analogue SMS 201-995 in Reducing Severe Diarrhea in a Patient with Medullary Thyroid Carcinoma. Can J Physiol Pharmacol 64 [Suppl]:67 (Abstr. No. 246), 1986
Jerkins, T. W., et al: Long-Acting Somatostatin Analog (SMS 201-995) Suppresses Elevated Pancreatic Polypeptide (PP) but not Calcitonin (CT) in Medullary Carcinoma of Thyroid. Clin Res 34 (1):196 A, 1986
Jerkins, T. W., et al: Medullary Carcinoma of the Thyroid, Pancreatic Nesidioblastosis and Microadenosis, and Pancreatic Polypeptide Hypersecretion: A New Association and Clinical and Hormonal Response to Long-Acting Somatostatin Analog SMS 201-995. J Clin Endocrinol Metab 64 (6):1313–1319, 1987
Radeke, H., et al: Treatment of Metastatic Medullary Thyroid Carcinoma (MTC) with Somatostatin Analog (SMS 201-995) Resulting in Remission of Diarrhea and Decrease of VIP and GRP Concentrations. Pediatr Res 20 (11):1204 (Abstr. No. 156), 1986
Sacks, H., et al: Medullary Thyroid Carcinoma and Nesidioblastosis with Pancreatic Polypeptide Hypersecretion: A New Association and the Hormonal Response to Somatostatin Analogue SMS 201-995. Can J Physiol Pharmacol [Suppl]:68 (Abstr. No. 247), 1986

VIII. Multiple Endocrine Neoplasia

Souquet, J. C., et al: [Dissociated Effects of a Long-Acting Somatostatin Analogue in a Case of Multiple Endocrine Neoplasia.] Gastroenterology 80:1643, 1986
Toms, G. C., et al: Disseminated Carcinoid in Patients with Multiple Endocrine Neoplasia (Type 1)-Symptomatic Improvement with Somatostatin. Br J Surg 73 (11):936 (Abstr. No. 5), 1986
Toms, G. C., et al: Disseminated Carcinoid in a Patient with Multiple Endocrine Neoplasia (Type I) – Symptomatic Improvement with Somatostatin Analogue (SMS 201-995). J Endocrinol 108 [Suppl]: (Abstr. No. 263), 1986

IX. Pituitary Tumors

Chanson, P.: [Thyrotropic Pituitary Adenoma. Clinical Aspects, Course and Treatment.] (French) Presse Med 16 (33):1644–1648, 1987
Chanson, P., et al: [Pituitary Macroadenoma Secreting Bio-Inactive GH: Effect of SMS 201-995.] (French) Ann Endocrinol (Paris) 48:223, 1987
Comi, R. J., et al: Efficacy of SMS 201-995 in TSH-Secreting Pituitary Adenomas. Clin Res 34 (2):A 714, 1986
Comi, R. J., et al: Response of Thyrotropin-Secreting Pituitary Adenomas to a Long-Acting Somatostatin Analogue. N Engl J Med 317 (1):12–17, 1987
Ducasse, M. C. R., et al: Shrinking of a Growth Hormone-Producing Pituitary Tumor by Continuous Subcutaneous Infusion of the Somatostatin Analog SMS 201-995. J Clin Endocrinol Metab 65:1042–1046, 1987
Duet, M., et al: Gonadotropic Adenoma with Abnormal Secretory Pattern: Case Report. In: Landolt, A. M. (ed) Advances in Pituitary Adenoma Research. Proceedings of the 4th European Workshop, Zurich, 13–16.9.1987. Pergamon Press, Oxford, 1988, pp 433–434 (Advances in Biosciences, Vol 69)

Faglia, G., et al: Inappropriate Secretion of Thyrotropin by the Pituitary. Horm Res 26 (1–4):79–99, 1987

Guillausseau, P. J., et al: Long-Term Efficacy of SMS 201-995 in a TSH-Secreting Pituitary Macroadenoma. In: Jensen, J., Christiansen, C. (eds) 1st European Congress of Endocrinology, Copenhagen (Denmark), June 21–25, 1987. Norhaven, Viborg, 1987, p 8, Abstr. No. 1–23

Guillausseau, P. J., et al: Visual Improvement With SMS 201-995 in a Patient With a Thyrotropin-Secreting Pituitary Adenoma. N Engl J Med 317 (1):53–54, 1987

Houdent, C., et al: [Thyreotropic Adenoma With Somatostatin (SMS 201-995 Sandoz).] (French) Ann Endocrinol (Paris) 48:229, 1987

Kohler, P. O.: Treatment of Pituitary Adenomas. N Engl J Med 317:45–46, 1987

Lamberts, S. W. J.: Somatostatin Analog Treatment of Pituitary Tumors. Eur J Cancer Clin Oncol 22 (6):727, 1986

Lamberts, S. W. J., et al: The Effects of a Long-Acting Somatostatin Analog on Pituitary Tumor Growth and Hormone Secretion in Rat and Man. In: 7th International Congress of Endocrinology, Quebec City (Canada), July 1–7, 1984. Excerpta Medica, Amsterdam Oxford Princeton, 1984, p 847, Abstr. No. 1173 (Int. Congress Series, No. 652)

Landgraf, R., et al: Hormone-Active Intradural Spinal Metastasis of a Prolactinoma. A Case Report. Klin Wochenschr 63:379–384, 1985

Landgraf, R., et al: Hormone-Active Intradural Spinal Metastasis of a Prolactinoma. A Case Report. Acta Endocrinol (Copenh) 108 [Suppl 267]:140–141 (Abstr. No. 158), 1985

Montini, M., et al: Effect of SMS 201-995 in the Treatment of Neoplastic TSH Secretion Syndrome. In: Landolt, A. M. (ed) Advances in Pituitary Adenoma Research. Proceedings of the 4th European Workshop, Zurich, 13–16.9.1987. Pergamon Press, Oxford, 1988, pp 429–430 (Advances in Biosciences, Vol 69)

Reubi, J. C., et al: Visualization of Somatostatin Receptors and Correlation with Immunoreactive Growth Hormone and Prolactin in Human Pituitary Adenomas: Evidence for Different Tumor Subclasses. J Clin Endocrinol Metab 65 (1):65–73, 1987

Von Werder, K., et al: Ectopic Production of Pituitary Hormones and Releasing Hormones. In: Landolt, A. M. (ed) Advances in Pituitary Adenoma Research. Proceedings of the 4th European Workshop, Zurich, 13–16. 9. 1987. Pergamon Press, Oxford, 1988, pp 87–95 (Advances in Biosciences, Vol 69)

Warnet, A., et al: Somatostatin Analog SMS 201-995 (Sandostatin) Can Improve Chiasmatic Compression Due to Nonfunctioning Pituitary Adenoma. In: Jensen, J., Christiansen, C. (eds) 1st European Congress of Endocrinology, Copenhagen (Denmark), June 21–25, 1987. Norhaven, Viborg, 1987, p 16, Abstr. No. 1–54

Wemeau, J. L., et al: Long-Term Treatment of Central Hyperthyroidism With the Somatostatin Analog SMS 201-995. Ann Endocrinol (Paris) 48:93 (Abstr. No. 34), 1987

Wemeau, J. L., et al: Long Term Treatment with the Somatostatin Analog SMS 201-995 in a Patient with a Thyrotropin- and Growth Hormone-Secreting Pituitary Adenoma. J Clin Endocrinol Metab 66:636–639, 1988

X. Tumors (More Than One Kind)

Ahlman, H., Tisell, L. E.: The Use of a Long-Acting Somatostatin Analogue in the Treatment of Advanced Endocrine Malignancies with Gastrointestinal Symptoms. Scand J Gastroenterol 22:938–942, 1987

Anderson, J. V., Bloom, S. R.: Neuroendocrine Tumours of the Gut: Long-Term Therapy with the Somatostatin Analogue SMS 201-995. Scand J Gastroenterol 21 [Suppl 119]:115–128, 1986

Bloom, S. R.: Somatostatin Analogue Treatment of Apudomas and Pancreatic Tumours. Eur J Cancer Clin Oncol 22 (6):727, 1986

Bloom, S. R.: Panel Discussion II. Am J Med 82 [Suppl 5 B]:96–99, 1987

Bonfils, S.: New Somatostatin Molecule for Management of Endocrine Tumours. Gut 26:433–437, 1985

Brennan, F. N., Buchanan, K. D.: Somatostatin (SMS 201-995) Therapy of Diarrhoea Associated with Apudomas. Ir J Med Sci 156 (5):162, 1987

Buchanan, K. D.: Long-Term Control of Endocrine Syndromes by Small, Infrequent Doses of SMS 201-995. Regul Pept 18:355, 1987

Buchanan, K. D., et al: Evaluation of SMS 201-995 in Gastrointestinal APUDomas. Scand J Gastroenterol 21 [Suppl 119]:199–205, 1986

Buchanan, K. D., et al: Neuroendocrine Tumors. A European View. Am J Med 81 [Suppl 6 B]: 14–22, 1986

Buchanan, K. D., et al: Somatostatin (SMS 201-995) Therapy for Gastrointestinal Apudomas. Can J Physiol Pharmacol 65 [Suppl]:64 (Abstr. No. 239), 1986

Ch'ng, J. L. C., et al: Chronic Treatment of Gut Hormone Producing Tumours (Apudomas) with a Long-Acting Somatostatin Analogue. Dig Dis Sci 29 (8) [Suppl 17 S], 1984

Ch'ng, J. L. C., et al: Remission of Symptoms During Long Term Treatment of Metastatic Pancreatic Endocrine Tumours With Long Acting Somatostatin Analogue. Br Med J 292 (6526):981–982, 1986

Ellison, E. C., et al: Modulation of Functional Gastrointestinal Endocrine Tumors by Endogenous and Exogenous Somatostatin. Am J Surg 151:668–675, 1986

Eriksson, B., et al: Treatment of Malignant Endocrine Pancreatic Tumours with Human Leucocyte Interferon. Lancet II (8519):1307–1309, 1986

Fiasse, R., et al: Short-Term Effects of the Long-Acting Somatostatin Analogue SMS 201-995 in Five Cases of APUDoma (Four with Metastases) and in One Case of Systemic Mastocytosis. Scand J Gastroenterol 21 [Suppl 119]: No. 212–216, 1986

Fuessl, H. S., et al: Chronic Administration of a Long Acting Somatostatin Analogue Does Not Lead to Endogenous Antibody Formation. Clin Sci 70 [Suppl 13]:91 P (Abstr. No. 250), 1986

Geelhoed, G. W., et al: Somatostatin Analog: Effects on Hypergastrinemia and Hypercalcitoninemia. Surgery 100:962–970, 1986

Gilsanz, A., et al: Observations on the Hormonal Response of Hormonally Active Pancreatic Tumors With a Somatostatin Analog (SMS 201-995). In: Jensen, J., Christiansen, C. (eds) 1st European Congress of Endocrinology, Copenhagen (Denmark), June 21–25, 1987. Norhaven, Viborg, 1987, p 10, Abstr. No. 1–32

Kaloustian, E., et al: [Mixed Endocrine Tumor of the Pancreas (VIPoma, Glucagonoma). Treatment of Somatostatin Followed by One of Its Long-Acting Analogs.] (French) Presse Med 16 (44):2217–2220, 1987

Kvols, L. K., et al: Treatment of Metastatic Islet Cell Carcinoma with a Somatostatin Analogue (SMS 201-995). Ann Intern Med 107:162–168, 1987

Lamberts, S. W. J., Reubi, J. C.: The Potential Use of Somatostatin Analogs in the Treatment of Cancer. Invest New Drugs 5 (1):102, 1987

Marbet, U. A., et al: [Endocrine Active Stomach-Intestine Tumors: Are There New Therapeutic Possibilities?] Dtsch Med Wochenschr 111: 1120–1123, 1986

O'Dorisio, T. M., et al: Role of Peptide Radioimmunoassay in Understanding Peptide-Peptide Interactions and Clinical Expression of Gastroenteropancreatic Endocrine Tumors. Am J Med 82 [Suppl 5 B]:60–67, 1987

Schrezenmeir, J., et al: Treatment of APUDomas with the Long-Acting Somatostatin Analogue SMS 201-995. Scand J Gastroenterol 21 [Suppl 119]:223–227, 1986

Souquet, J.-C., et al: Biological and Clinical Efficacy of a Long-Acting Somatostatin Analog (SMS 201-995) in Secreting Apudomas. Can J Physiol Pharmacol [Suppl 64]: (Abstr. No. 240), 1986

Souquet, J.-C., et al: [Clinical and Biological Efficacy of the Somatostatin Analog (SMS 201-995) in Treatment of Endocrine Tumors Secretion in Digestion.] Gastroenterol Clin Biol 11 (2 BIS):6 A, 1987

Souquet, J.-C., et al: Clinical and Hormonal Effects of a Long-Acting Somatostatin Analogue in Pancreatic Endocrine Tumors and in Carcinoid Syndrome. Cancer 59 (9):1654–1660, 1987

Tsai, S.-T., et al: Perioperative Use of Long-Acting Somatostatin Analog (SMS 201-995) in Patients With Endocrine Tumors of the Gastroenteropancreatic Axis. Surgery 100 (4):788–795, 1986

Wood, S. M., et al: New Somatostatin Analogue for Home Treatment of Endocrine Tumours. Gut 24:A 984–A 985, 1983

Wood, S. M., et al: Treatment of Patients With Pancreatic Endocrine Tumours Using a New Long-Acting Somatostatin Analogue Symptomatic and Peptides Responses. Gut 26:438–444, 1985

XI. Tumors (Other)

Dorey, F., et al: [Evidence of Partial Resistance of TSH Secretion to the Action of a Somatostatin Analogue (SMS 201-995) in Pituitary Resistance to Thyroid Hormones.] Ann Endocrinol (Paris) 48:203 (Abstr. No. 46), 1987

Favrod-Coune, C. A., et al: [Paraneoplastic Cushing's Syndrome in Metastatic Pancreatic Endocrine Tumour: Control of Hypercortisolism by a Somatostatin Analogue, SMS 201-995.] Ann Endocrinol (Paris) 48:211, 1987

Hearn, P. R., et al: Lung Carcinoid with Cushing's Syndrome: Control of Serum ACTH and Cortisol Levels Using SMS 201-995 (Sandostatin). Clin Endocrinol (Oxf) 28:181–185, 1988

Kung, A. W. C., et al: Prevention of Hypoglycaemia in a Patient with Pancreatic Microadenomatosis by a Long-Acting Somatostatin Analogue SMS 201-995. Clin Endocrinol (Oxf) 27 (4):No. 469–473, 1987

Medri, G., et al: Treatment With Somatostatin Analog SMS 201-995 Restores Euthyroidism in Patients With TSH-Secreting Tumor, But Not in Those With Pituitary Resistance to Thyroid Hormone Action. Ann Endocrinol (Paris) 48:94 (Abstr. No. 35), 1987

Neuroendocrine Tumors with the Long-Acting Somatostatin Analog, SMS 201-995. In: Reichlin, S. (ed) Somatostatin Basic and Clinical Status, Serono Symposia: Proceedings of the International Conference on Somatostatin, Washington, 6–8. 5. 1986. Plenum Press, New York 1987, pp 343–356

Reubi, J. C., et al: High Incidence of Somatostatin Receptors in Human Meningiomas: Biochemical Characterization. J Clin Endocrinol 63:433–438, 1986

Rosak, C., et al: [Influence of a New Somatostatin Analog on the Hormonal Counter Regulation in Insulin Induced Hypoglycemia.] Akt Endokrinol 5:116–117, 1984

Schlauri, H., et al: [Liver Apudomas – Under the Scope of a Cystic Liver.] Dtsch Med Wochenschr 112:1986–1989, 1987

Warnet, A., et al: [A New Female Case of Gonadotropic Adenoma: Response to LRH, TRH, an LRH Agonist (Busarelin), to Bromocriptine and Sandostatin.] Ann Endocrinol (Paris) 48:224, 1987

Wemeau, J. L., et al: [SMS 201-995: New Therapy for Adenoma of Thyroid.] Ann Endocrinol (Paris) 47:248 (Abstr. No. 79), 1986

Williams, G., et al: Clinical Evaluation of SMS 201-995. Long-Term Treatment in Gut Neuroendocrine Tumours, Efficacy of Oral Administration, and Possible Use in Non-Tumoural Inappropriate TSH Hypersecretion. Acta Endocrinol (Copenh) 116 [Suppl 286]:26–36, 1987

Wilson, D. M., Hoffman, A. R.: Suppression of Tumor Secretion of Growth Hormone Releasing Factor (GRF 1–40) and Gastrin by a Somatostatin Analog. Clin Res 33:31 A, 1985

XII. Review

Bloom, S. R., Polak, J. M.: Somatostatin. Br Med J 295:288–290, 1987

Krejs, G. J.: Gastrointestinal Endocrine Tumors. Am J Med 82 [Suppl 5 B]:1–3, 1987

Lamberts, S. W. J.: Non-Pituitary Actions of Somatostatin. A Review on the Therapeutic Role of SMS 201-995 (Sandostatin). Acta Endocrinol (Copenh) 112 [Suppl 276]:41–55, 1986

Lamberts, S. W. J.: A Guide to the Clinical Use of the Somatostatin Analogue SMS 201-995 (Sandostatin). Acta Endocrinol (Copenh) 116 [Suppl 286]:54–66, 1987

Lamberts, S. W. J., et al: Potential Role of Somatostatin Analogue in the Treatment of Cancer. Eur J Clin Invest 17:281–287, 1987

Longnecker, S. M.: Remission of Symptoms of Chemotherapy – Refractory Metastatic Insulinoma Using Octreotide. Drug Intell Clin Pharm 22:136–138, 1988

Longnecker, S. M.: Somatostatin and Octreotide: Literature Review and Description of Therapeutic Activity in Pancreatic Neoplasia. Drug Intell Clin Pharm 22:99–106, 1988

Maton, P. N., et al: The Use of the Long-Acting Somatostatin Analogue SMS 201-995 in Patients With Pancreatic Islet Cell Tumors. Dig Dis Sci: 1–20 (in press)

Moreau, J. P., DeFeudis, F. V.: Pharmacological Study of Somatostatin and Somatostatin-Analogues: Therapeutic Advances and Perspectives. Life Sci 40 (5):419–437, 1987

Müller, M. K., et al: [Gastrointestinal Hormone Producing Tumors and the Therapeutical Possibilities With Somatostatin.] Med Welt 37: 1181–1187, 1986

Mulvihill, S., et al: The Use of Somatostatin and Its Analogs in the Treatment of Surgical Disorders. Surgery 100 (3):467–476, 1986

O'Dorisio, T. M.: Gut Endocrinology: Clinical and Therapeutic Impact. Am J Med 81 [Suppl 6 B]:1–7, 1986

O'Dorisio, T. M., O'Dorisio, M. S.: Endocrine Tumors of the Gastroenteropancreatic (GEP) Axis. In: Mazzaferri, E. L. (ed) Endocrinology, 3rd edn. Elsevier Science, New York, 1986, pp 764–817

Reichlin, S.: Somatostatin (First of Two Parts). N Engl J Med 309 (24):1495–1501, 1983

Reichlin, S.: Somatostatin (Second of Two Parts). N Engl J Med 309 (25):1556–1563, 1983

Vinik, A. I., et al: Somatostatin Analogue (SMS 201-995) in the Management of Gastroenteropancreatic Tumors and Diarrhea Syndromes. Am J Med 81 [Suppl 6 B]:23–40, 1986

Weil, C.: Gastroenteropancreatic Endocrine Tumors. Klin Wochenschr 63:433–459, 1985

XIII. Pharmacology

Anonymous: Somatostatin: Hormonal and Therapeutic Roles. Lancet 2 (8446):77–78, 1985

Babin, T., et al: Long-Term Efficacy of a Continuous S. C. Infusion (CSI) of Somatostatin Analog Sandostatin (SMS 201-995). In: Jensen, J., Christiansen, C. (eds) 1st European Congress of Endocrinology, Copenhagen (Denmark), June 21–25, 1987. Norhaven, Viborg, 1987, p 19, Abstr. No. 1–67

Brazeau, P.: Somatostatin: A Peptide with Unexpected Physiologic Activities. Am J Med 81 [Suppl 6 B]:8–13, 1986

Christiansen, J., et al: Inhibition of Meal-Stimulated Gastric Acid Secretion by an Octapeptide Somatostatin Analogue SMS 201-995. Dig Dis Sci 31 (10) [Suppl 180 S]: (Abstr. No. 710), 1986

Christiansen, J., et al: Inhibition of Meal-Stimulated Gastric Acid Secretion by an Octapeptide Somatostatin Analogue SMS 201-995. Dig Dis Sci 31 (10) [Suppl 229 S]: (Abstr. No. 906), 1986

Creutzfeldt, W., et al: Effect of Somatostatin Analogue (SMS 201-995) on Pancreatic Secretion in Man. Dig Dis Sci 31 (10):1128, 1986

Creutzfeldt, W., et al: Effect of Somatostatin Analogue (SMS 201-995, Sandostatin) on Pancreatic Secretion in Humans. Am J Med 82 [Suppl 5 B]:49–54, 1987

Dammann, H. G., et al: Oral SMS 201-995 – The New Somatostatin Analogue: Influence on Gastric Secretion and Gastrin Release in Man. Gastroenterology 92 (5, pt. 2):1361, 1987

Davies, R. R., et al: Effects of Somatostatin Analogue SMS 201-995 in Normal Man. Clin Endocrinol (Oxf) 24 (6):665–674, 1986

Del Pozo, E., Kutz, K.: SMS 201-995, a New Somatostatin Analog: Pharmacological Profile. Neuroendocrinol Lett 7:111, 1985

Del-Pozo, E., Kutz, K.: Pharmacological Properties and Effect on Glucose Homeostasis of a Somatostatin Derivative (SMS 201-995): Studies in Humans. In: Luedecke, D. K., Tolis, G. (eds) Growth Hormone, Growth Factors, and Acromegaly. Proceedings of the International Symposium, Aegina, April 1985. Raven Press, New York, 1987, pp 207–214 (Progress in Endocrine Research and Therapy, Vol 3)

Del-Pozo, E., et al: Glucose Homeostasis Following Sandostatin Administration to Normal Subjects. J Endocrinol Invest 10 [Suppl 4]:94 (Abstr. No. 146), 1987

Del-Pozo, E., et al: Effect of Sandostatin on Hormonal Homeostasis: Studies in Normal Subjects. In: Landolt, A. M. (ed) Advances in Pituitary Adenoma Research. Proceedings of the 4th European Workshop, Zurich, 13–16.9.1987. Pergamon Press, Oxford, 1988, pp 213–220 (Advances in Biosciences, Vol 69)

Dueno, M. I., et al: Effect of Somatostatin Analog on Water and Electrolyte Transport and Transit Time in the Human Jejunum. Can J Physiol Pharmacol 64 [Suppl]:9 (Abstr. No. 118), 1986

Dueno, M. I., et al: Effect of Somatostatin Analog on Water and Electrolyte Transport and Transit Time in Human Small Bowel. Dig Dis Sci 32:1092–1096, 1987

Editorial: SMS 201-995. Drugs Future 9:342–343, 1984

Escourrou, J., et al: Inhibition of Pancreatic Exocrine Secretion in Man by Somatostatin (s) Comparison of 3 Molecular Forms: S 28, S 14, S 8. Gastroenterology 92 (5, pt. 2):1385, 1987

Fuessl, H. S., et al: The Somatostatin Analogue SMS 201-995 Accelerates Gastric Emptying but Prolongs Intestinal Transit Time. Clin Sci 70 [Suppl 13]:71 P, 1986

Fuessel, H. S., et al: Oral Absorption of the Somatostatin Analogue SMS 201-995: Theoretical and Practical Implications. Clin Sci 72 (2):255–257, 1987

Gyr, K., et al: Effects of Graded Doses of SMS 201-995 on Exocrine Pancreatic Function. Dig Dis Sci 30:974, 1985

Gyr, K. E., et al: Human Pharmacological Effects of SMS 201-995 on Gastric Secretion. Scand J Gastroenterol 21 [Suppl 119]:96–102, 1986

Hashida, S., et al: Serum Concentration of Human Growth Hormone (hGH) After Administration of the Somatostatin Analogue SMS 201-995 in Normal Subjects. Clin Chim Acta 159 (1):93–95, 1986

Jenkins, S. A., et al: Effects of Subcutaneous SMS 201-995 on Exocrine Pancreatic Secretion and Function in Man. Br J Surg 73:1029–1030 (Abstr. No. 22), 1986

Johnston, D. G., et al: Effects of Somatostatin and SMS 201-995 on Carbohydrate Metabolism in Normal Man. Scand J Gastroenterol 21 [Suppl 119]:158–165, 1986

Köhler, E., et al: Effects of Graded Doses of SMS 201-995 on Exocrine and Endocrine Pancreatic Function. Digestion 32:196 (Abstr. No. 85), 1985

Kraenzlin, M. E., et al: Effect of Long-Acting Somatostatin-Analogue, SMS 201-995, on Gut Hormone Secretion in Normal Subjects. Experientia 41 (6):738–740, 1985

Lee, Y. C., et al: the Effects of Somatostatin Analogue SMS 201-995 on Neurotensin Secretion and Intestinal Transit Time in Man. Can J Physiol Pharmacol 64 [Suppl]:73 (Abstr. No. 259), 1986

Lembcke, B., et al: Effect of the Somatostatin Analogue Sandostatin (SMS 201-995) on Gastrointestinal, Pancreatic and Biliary Function and Hormone Release in Normal Men. Digestion 36:108–124, 1987

Lightman, S. L., et al: The Effect of SMS 201-995, a Long-Acting Somatostatin Analogue, on Anterior Pituitary Function in Healthy Male Volunteers. Scand J Gastroenterol 21 [Suppl 119]:84–95, 1986

Londong, W., et al: [Decreasing Responsiveness of Human Parietal Cells to SMS 201-995.] Klin Wochenschr 64 [Suppl V]:42, 1986

Londong, W., et al: Diminishing Sensitivity of Human Parietal Cell Function to SMS 201-995 Treatment. Gut 27 (5):A 613, 1986

Londong, W., et al: Diminishing Sensitivity of Parietal Cell Function to Somatostatin Analogue (SMS 201-995) Treatment in Man. Can J Physiol Pharmacol 64 [Suppl]:72 (Abstr. No. 256), 1986

Maurer, R., et al: Autoradiographic Visualization of Somatostatin Receptors in the Human Brain. J Endocrinol Invest 8 [Suppl 3]:45, 1985

Pless, J., Doepfner, W.: [Somatostatin: Biochemistry, Pharmacology and Therapeutic Aspects.] Dtsch Apoth ZTG 123:1807–1813, 1983

Pless, J., et al: Chemistry and Pharmacology of SMS 201-995, a Long-Acting Octapeptide Analogue of Somatostatin. In: Molinatti, G. M., Martini, L. (eds) Endocrinology '85, Proceedings of the International Congress, Torino (Italy), June 5–8, 1985. Excerpta Medica, Amsterdam Oxford Princeton, 1986, pp 319–333 (Int. Congress Series, No. 683)

Polak, J. M., Bloom, S. R.: Somatostatin Localization in Tissues. Scand J Gastroenterol 21 [Suppl 119]:11–21, 1986

Reubi, J. C., et al: Distribution of Somatostatin Receptors in the Human Brain: An Autoradiographic Study. Neuroscience 18 (2):329–346, 1986

Stoll, R., et al: Effect of the Somatostatin-Analog SMS 201-995 on ATP-Dependent Calcium Transport in Basolateral Vesicles of Human Duodenum. Gastroenterology 90 (5, pt. 2): 1651, 1986

Varga, I., et al: Inhibition of Steroid Biosynthesis by a New Long-Acting Somatostatin Analogue. Acta Physiol Hung 66 (3–4):303, 1985

Verschoor, L., et al: Glucose Tolerance During Long-Term Treatment With a Somatostatin Analogue (Correspondence). Br Med J 294: 177, 1987

Wass, J. A. H.: The Therapeutic Modulation of GH Release. J Endocrinol Invest 10 [Suppl 3]:11 (Abstr. No. S 5), 1987

Whitehouse, I., et al: The Effect of an Octapeptide Somatostatin Analogue (SMS 201-995) and Somatostatin-14 (SST-14) on Pentagastrin-Stimulated Gastric Acid Secretion: A Comparative Study in Man. Hepatogastroenterology 31:227–229, 1984

Whitehouse, I., et al: Inhibition of Pentagastrin-Stimulated Acid Secretion After Subcutaneous Administration of a New Somatostatin Analogue. Gut 27:141–146, 1986

Williams, T. C., et al: Differential Effects of Somatostatin (SRIH) and a SRIH Analog, SMS 201-995, on the Secretion of Growth Hormone and Thyroid-Stimulating Hormone in Man. J Clin Endocrinol Metab 66:39–45, 1988

XIV. Pharmacokinetics

Del Pozo, E., et al: Endocrine Profile of a Long-Acting Somatostatin Derivative SMS 201-995. Study in Normal Volunteers Following Subcutaneous Administration. Acta Endocrinol (Copenh) 111 (4):433–439, 1986

Elkhammas, E. A., et al: Biphasic Response of Hyperplastic G-Cells to Somatostatin Analog. Gastroenterology 90:1405, 1986

Fuessl, H. S., et al: Accelerated Gastric Emptying but Prolonged Mouth-to-Caecum-Transit-Time by a Long-Acting Somatostatin Analogue. Regul Pept 13 (1):101, 1985

Kallivretakis, N., et al: Pharmacokinetics of SMS 201-995 in Normal Subjects and in Patients With Severe Renal Failure. Neuroendocrinol Lett 7:92, 1985

Koehler, E., et al: Effect of a New Somatostatin Analogue on Pancreatic Function in Healthy Volunteers. Pancreas 1 (2):154–159, 1986

Koehler, E., et al: Absorption of an Aqueous Solution of a New Synthetic Somatostatin Analogue Administered to Man by Gavage. Eur J Clin Pharmacol 33:167–171, 1987

Kutz, K., et al: Pharmacokinetics of SMS 201-995 in Healthy Subjects. Scand J Gastroenterol 21 [Suppl 119]:65–72, 1986

Lewin, M. J. M.: Somatostatin Receptors. Scand J Gastroenterol 21 [Suppl 119]:42–46, 1986

Losa, M., et al: Interaction Between Growth Hormone Releasing Factor (GRF) and Somatostatin Analogue (SMS 201-995) in Normal Subjects. Clin Endocrinol (Oxf) 23:715–720, 1985

Reubi, J. C., et al: Distinct Topographical Localization of Two Somatostatin Receptor Subpopulations in the Human Cortex. Brain Res 406:391–396, 1987

Sasaki, Y., et al: Solid-Phase Synthesis and Biological Properties Psi (CH_2NH) Pseudopeptide Analogues of a Highly Potent Somatostatin Octapeptide. J Med Chem 30 (7):1162–1166, 1987

Usadel, K. H., et al: Cytoprotective Properties of Somatostatins. Klin Wochenschr 64 [Suppl VII]:59–63, 1986

Whitehouse, I., et al: SMS 201-995 (A Long Acting, Octapeptide, Somatostatin-Analogue) – Efficacy and Duration of Action After S.C. Administration on Pentagastrin-Stimulated Gastric Acid Secretion in Man. Dig Dis Sci 29 (8) [Suppl 968]:96S, 1984

Wynants, C., et al: Conformational Analysis of Two Somatostatin Analogues by ^1H 500 MHz N.M.R. Spectroscopy. Int J Pept Protein Res 29:90–98, 1987

XV. Acromegaly

Althoff, P. H., et al: Influence of a Long-Acting Somatostatin Analogue (SMS 201-995) in Acromegalic Patients. Acta Endocrinol (Copenh) 105 [Suppl 264]:29 (Abstr. No. 36), 1984

Althoff, P. H., et al: A New Long-Acting Somatostatin Analogue (SMS 201-995): Effects in Acromegalic Patients. In: 7th International Congress of Endocrinology, Quebec City (Canada), July 1–7, 1984. Excerpta Medica, Amsterdam Oxford Princeton, 1984, p 324, Abstr. No. 128 (Int. Congress Series, No. 652)

Althoff, P. H., et al: Results of Long-Term Treatment With the Somatostatin Analogue

SMS 201-995 in Acromegalic Patients: Prognostic Value of Endocrinological Tests. J Endocrinol Invest 10 [Suppl 3]:21 (Abstr. No. P 5), 1987

Arosio, M., et al: Effect of SMS 201-995 Administration in 8 Patients With Active Acromegaly. J Endocrinol Invest 8 [Suppl 3]:192 (Abstr. No. P 203), 1985

Arosio, M., et al: Evaluation of a Long Acting Somatostatin Analogue (SMS 201-995) in Patients with Acromegaly. Eur J Clin Invest 16 (2, pt. 2): A 6, 1986

Astorga, R., et al: [Prolonged Treatment of 5 Acromegalics With an Analog of Somatostatin (SMS 201-995).] (Spanish) Endocrinologia (Barc) 33 [Suppl 1]:5, 1986

Atkinson, A. B., et al: Which Dose of Somatostatin Analogue (SMS 201-995) Best Suppresses Growth Hormone Secretion in Acromegaly? J Endocrinol 117 [Suppl 182], 1988

Babin, T., et al: [Efficacy and Tolerance of Sandostatin Treatment by Continuous Subcutaneous Injection in 12 Acromegalics.] (French) Ann Endocrinol (Paris) 48:229, 1987

Barkan, A., et al: Acromegaly Due to Ectopic Growth Hormone Releasing Hormone Secretion: Treatment With Somatostatin Analogue SMS 201-995. Clin Res 34:908 A, 1986

Barkan, A. L., et al: Acromegaly From Ectopic Growth Hormone-Releasing Hormone Secretion By a Malignant Carcinoid Tumor. Successful Treatment with Long-Acting Somatostatin Analogue SMS 201-995. Cancer 61:221–226, 1988

Barkan, A. L., et al: Treatment of Acromegaly with the Long-Acting Somatostatin Analog SMS 201-995. J Clin Endocrinol Metab 66:16–23, 1988

Barnard, L. B., et al: Treatment of Resistant Acromegaly with a Long-Acting Somatostatin Analogue (SMS 201-995). Ann Intern Med 105 (6):856–861, 1986

Barnard, L. B., et al: Treatment of Resistant Acromegaly With a Somatostatin Analogue (SMS 201-995). Clin Res 34:641 A, 1986

Barnard, L. B., et al: Somatostatin Analog (SMS 201-995) in Acromegaly: Effect on Dynamic Tests of Growth Hormone Release. Clin Res 35 (3):582 A, 1987

Beckers, A., et al: SMS 201-995: Therapeutic Indications for Acromegaly. In: Jensen, J., Christiansen, C. (eds) 1st European Congress of Endocrinology, Copenhagen (Denmark), June 21–25, 1987. Norhaven, Viborg, 1987, p 16, Abstr. No. 1–57

Beckers, A., et al: The Treatment of Acromegaly with SMS 201-995. In: Landolt, A. M. (ed) Advances in Pituitary Adenoma Research. Proceedings of the 4th European Workshop, Zurich, 13–16.9.1987. Pergamon Press, Oxford, 1988, pp 227–228 (Advances in Biosciences, Vol 69)

Besser, G. M., Wass, J. A. H.: Somatostatin Octapeptide in the Medical Treatment of Acromegaly. In: Reichlin, S. (ed) Somatostatin Basic and Clinical Status, Serono Symposia: Proceedings of the International Conference On Somatostatin, Washington, May 6–8, 1986. Plenum Press, New York, 1987, pp 333–336

Besser, G. M., Wass, J. A. H.: Somatostatin Octapeptide Analogue (Octreotide) in the Medical Treatment of Acromegaly. In: Landolt, A. M. (ed) Advances in Pituitary Adenoma Research. Proceedings of the 4th European Workshop, Zurich, 13–16.9.1987. Pergamon Press, Oxford, 1988, pp 221–225 (Advances in Biosciences, Vol 69)

Bloom, S. R.: Acromegaly. Am J Med 82 [Suppl 5 B]:88–91, 1987

Borges, F., et al: Nocturnal Secretion of Growth Hormone During Treatment of Acromegaly With Somatostatin Analogue and Bromocriptine. J Endocrinol 112 [Suppl 188], 1987

Candrina, R., Giustina, A.: Growth Hormone Inhibition After a Standard Dose of SMS 201-995 is Correlated with Paradoxical Stimulation By Non-Specific Releasing Hormones in Acromegalic Patients. J Endocrinol Invest 10 [Suppl 4]:100 (Abstr. No. 157), 1987

Candrina, R., et al: The Long-Acting Somatostatin Analogue SMS 201-995 Does Not Impair Glucose Tolerance After a Mixed Meal in Acromegalic Patients. J Endocrinol Invest 9 [Suppl 1]:257 (Abstr. No. 234), 1986

Candrina, R., et al: Effect of a New Long-Acting Somatostatin Analogue (SMS 201-995) on Glycemic and Hormonal Response to a Mixed Meal in Acromegalic Patients. J Endocrinol Invest 11:21–26, 1988

Chanson, P., et al: Rapid Improvement in Sleep Apnea of Acromegaly After Short-Term Treatment With Somatostatin Analogue SMS 201-995. Lancet I (8492):1270–1271, 1986

Chanson, P., et al: [Rapid Improvement in Sleep Apnea of Acromegaly After Short-Term Treatment With Somatostatin Analogue SMS 201-995.] Lancet (Ed. Esp.) 9:295, 1986

Chanson, P., et al: Long-Term Treatment of Acromegaly By SMS 201-995: Hormonal Improvement and Tumoral Shrinkage. In: Jensen, J., Christiansen, C. (eds) 1st European Congress of Endocrinology, Copenhagen (Denmark), June 21–25, 1987. Norhaven, Viborg, 1987, p 8, Abstr. No. 1–24

Chatterjee, S., et al: High Dose, Long Term, Continuous Subcutaneous Infusion (CSI) of SMS 201-995 in Acromegaly. J Endocrinol 117 [Suppl 124], 1988

Chiodini, P. G., et al: Medical Treatment of Acromegaly: Dopaminergic Agonists and

Long-Acting Somatostatin. J Endocrinol Invest 10 [Suppl 4]:92 (Abstr. No. 141), 1987

Chiodini, P. G., et al: Medical Treatment of Acromegaly with SMS 201-995, a Somatostatin Analog: A Comparison with Bromocriptine. J Clin Endocrinol Metab 64 (3):447–453, 1987

Ch'ng, L. J. C., et al: Long Term Treatment of Acromegaly With a Long Acting Analogue of Somatostatin. Br Med J 290 (6464):284–285, 1985

Christensen, S. E., et al: Continuous Subcutaneous Pump Infusion of Somatostatin Analogue SMS 201-995 Versus Subcutaneous Injection Schedule in Acromegalic Patients. Clin Endocrinol (Oxf) 27:297–306, 1987

Comi, R. J., Gorden, P.: The Response of Serum Growth Hormone Levels to the Long-Acting Somatostatin Analog SMS 201-995 in Acromegaly. J Clin Endocrinol Metab 63 (1): 37–42, 1987

Cozzi, R., et al: Effect of a New Somatostatin Analogue (SMS 201-995) on GH Secretion in Acromegaly. Acta Endocrinol (Copenh) 109 [Suppl 270]:126 (Abstr. No. 231), 1985

Cozzi, R., et al: Medical Treatment of Acromegaly With SMS 201-995, a New Somatostatin Analogue: A Comparison With Bromocriptine. J Endocrinol Invest 8 [Suppl 3]:105 (Abstr. No. OC 103), 1985

Cozzi, R., et al: Comparison Between the Effectiveness of SMS 201-995, a New Somatostatin Analog, and Bromocriptine (BR) in the Medical Treatment of Acromegaly. J Endocrinol Invest 9 [Suppl 1]:225 (Abstr. No. 202), 1986

Cozzi, R., et al: New Approaches to the Medical Treatment of Acromegaly. J Endocrinol Invest 10 [Suppl 3]:26 (Abstr. No. P 15), 1987

Daughaday, W. H.: A New Treatment for an Old Disease. N Engl J Med 313:1604–1605, 1985

Davidson, K., Wass, J. A. H.: The Development of a Radioimmunoassay for Somatostatin Octapeptide (SMS 201-995): Half-Life Studies in Man. J Endocrinol 108 [Suppl]: (Abstr. No. 65), 1986

Dewailly, D., et al: [Twelve Hour Plasma GH Profile After Single Injection of a Somatostatin Analogue (SMS 201-995): Comparison Between the Intravenous and Subcutaneous Routes.] Ann Endocrinol (Paris) 48:228, 1987

Dewailly, D., et al: Twelve Hours Profile of Plasma GH After a Single Bolus of SMS 201-995 in Acromegalic Patients. Comparison Between the I.V. and S.C. Routes. In: Jensen, J., Christiansen, C. (eds) 1st European Congress of Endocrinology, Copenhagen (Denmark), June 21–25, 1987. Norhaven, Viborg, 1987, p 23, Abstr. No. 1–83

Ducasse, M. C. R., et al: [Antisecretory and Antitumor Effects of SMS 201-995 in Acromegaly.] Ann Endocrinol (Paris) 47:240 (Abstr. No. 64), 1986

Garcia-Luna, P. P., et al: [Reduction of a Large Tumor in Acromegaly Chronically Treated With the Somatostatin Analog SMS 201-995.] Endocrinologia (Barc) 33 [Suppl 1]:6, 1986

Gavilan, V. I., et al: [A Study of GH and GRF-29 in 4 Acromegalics Treated With the Analog SMS.] Endocrinologia (Barc) 33 [Suppl 1]:4–5, 1986

Geffner, M. E., et al: Treatment of Acromegaly with a Somatostatin Analog in a Patient with McCune-Albright Syndrome. J Pediatr 111: 740–743, 1987

George, S. R., et al: Prolonged Suppression of Growth Hormone Secretion in Acromegalics By a Long-Acting Somatostatin Analogue. Clin Invest Med 8 (3):A 75 (Abstr. No. C-222), 1985

George, S. R., et al: Suppression of Growth Hormone Secretion in Acromegaly With a Long-Acting Somatostatin Analogue. In: Molinatti, G. M., Martini, L. (eds) Endocrinology '85, Proceedings of the International Congress, Torino (Italy), June 5–8, 1985. Excerpta Medica, Amsterdam Oxford Princeton, 1986, pp 373–376 (Int. Congress Series, No. 683)

George, S. R., et al: Effect of SMS 201-995, a Long-Acting Somatostatin Analogue, on the Secretion and Morphology of a Pituitary Growth Hormone Cell Adenoma. Clin Endocrinol (Oxf) 26 (4):395–405, 1987

George, S. R., et al: The Somatostatin Analogue SMS 201-995 in Acromegaly: Prolonged, Preferential Suppression of Growth Hormone But Not Pancreatic Hormones. Clin Invest Med 10:309–315, 1987

Goday, A., et al: Short-Term Treatment of Active Acromegaly With the Somatostatin Analogue SMS 201-995. In: Jensen, J., Christiansen, C. (eds) 1st European Congress of Endocrinology, Copenhagen (Denmark), June 21–25, 1987. Norhaven, Viborg, 1987, p 17, Abstr. No. 1–60

Hegele, R. A., et al: Suppression of Growth Hormone Secretion in Acromegaly With a Long-Acting Somatostatin Analogue. In: 67th Ann. Meeting, The Endoc. Soc. (Progr. and Abstr.), Baltimore (U.S.A.), 19–21.5.1985. Endocrinology 116 [Suppl]:123 (Abstr. No. 489), 1985

Hildebrandt, G., et al: Another Approach to Medical Treatment of Acromegaly: Continuous Chronic Intravenous Application of SMS 201-995 Via Implantable Pump System. J Endocrinol Invest 10 [Suppl 4]:93 (Abstr. No. 143), 1987

Hildebrandt, G., et al: Continuous Chronic Intravenous Application of SMS 201-995 Via An Implantable Pump System in Therapy-Resistant Acromegaly. Acta Endocrinol (Copenh) 117 [Suppl 287]: 120–121, 1988

Ho, K. Y., et al: Treatment of Acromegaly with the Somatostatin Analogue SMS 201-995. In: Harding, P. E. (ed) Proceedings of the 30th Annual Meeting of the Endoc. Soc. of Australia, Sydney, 23–26.8.1987. Amanda Imprint, Adelaide, 1987, Abstr. No. 1 (Proceedings Vol 30)

Ho, K. Y., et al: Dose and Frequency of SMS 201-995 Administration on Therapeutic Efficacy in Acromegaly. In: Landolt, A. M. (ed) Advances in Pituitary Adenoma Research. Proceedings of the 4th European Workshop, Zurich, 13–16.9.1987. Pergamon Press, Oxford, 1988, pp 231–232 (Advances in Biosciences, Vol 69)

Horikawa, R., et al: Effect of a Single Administration of Somatostatin Analogue (SMS 201-995) on GH, TSH and Insulin Secretion in Patients With Acromegaly. Endocrinol Jpn 33 (6): 743–749, 1986

Jackson, I., et al: Role of a Long-Acting Somatostatin Analogue (SMS 201-995) in the Treatment of Acromegaly. Am J Med 81 [Suppl 6 B]: 94–101, 1986

Lamberts, S. W. J.: The Treatment of Acromegaly With Somatostatin Analogs. J Endocrinol Invest 8 [Suppl 3]: 69 (Abstr. No. S 66), 1985

Lamberts, S. W. J.: Acromegaly: An Update on Therapy. In: Molinatti, G. M., Martini, L. (eds) Endocrinology '85, Proceedings of the International Congress, Torino, June 5–8, 1985. Excerpta Medica, Amsterdam Oxford Princeton, 1986, pp 91–100 (Int. Congress Series, No. 683)

Lamberts, S. W. J.: The Use of Sandostatin Analogs in the Treatment of Acromegaly. J Endocrinol 117 [Suppl 25], 1988

Lamberts, S. W. J., Del Pozo, E.: Acute and Long-Term Treatment of Acromegaly With the Somatostatin Analog SMS 201-995. Neuroendocrinol Lett 7:93, 1985

Lamberts, S. W. J., Del Pozo, E.: Acute and Long-term Effects of SMS 201-995 in Acromegaly. Scand J Gastroenterol 21 [Suppl 119]: 141–148, 1986

Lamberts, S. W. J., Del Pozo, E.: Long-Term Treatment of Acromegaly With the Somatostatin Analogue SMS 201-995 (Correspondence). N Engl J Med 314: 1391–1392, 1986

Lamberts, S. W. J., et al: Long-Term Treatment of Acromegaly With the Somatostatin Analogue SMS 201-995. N Engl J Med 313: 1576–1580, 1985

Lamberts, S. W. J., et al: The Somatostatin Analog SMS 201-995 Induces Long-Acting Inhibition of Growth Hormone Secretion without Rebound Hypersecretion in Acromegalic Patients. Clin Endocrinol Metabol 60 (6): 1161–1165, 1985

Lamberts, S. W. J., et al: A Comparison Among the Growth Hormone-Lowering Effects in Acromegaly of the Somatostatin Analog SMS 201-995, Bromocriptine, and the Combination of Both Drugs. J Clin Endocrinol 63 (1): 16–19, 1986

Lamberts, S. W. J., et al: The Sensitivity of Growth Hormone and Prolactin Secretion to the Somatostatin Analogue SMS 201-995 in Patients With Prolactinomas and Acromegaly. Clin Endocrinol (Oxf) 25 (2): 201–212, 1986

Lamberts, S. W. J., et al: Acute and Long-Term Treatment of Acromegaly with SMS 201-995. In: Luedecke, D. K., Tolis, G. (eds) Growth Hormone, Growth Factors, and Acromegaly. Proceedings of the International Symposium, Aegina, April 1985. Raven Press, New York, 1987, pp 221–227 (Progress in Endocrine Research and Therapy, Vol 3)

Lamberts, S. W. J., et al: A Comparison Between the Effects of SMS 201-995, Bromocriptine and a Combination of Both Drugs on Hormone Release by the Cultured Pituitary Tumour Cells of Acromegalic Patients. Clin Endocrinol (Oxf) 27 (1): 11–23, 1987

Lamberts, S. W. J., et al: Relationship Between Growth Hormone and Somatomedin-C Levels in Untreated Acromegaly After Surgery and Radiotherapy and During Medical Therapy With Sandostatin (SMS 201-995). Eur J Clin Invest 17: 354–359, 1987

Lamberts, S. W. J., et al: SMS 201-995 Induces a Continuous Decline in Circulating Growth Hormone and Somatomedin-C Levels During Therapy of Acromegalic Patients for Over Two Years. J Clin Endocrinol Metab 65 (4): 703–710, 1987

Landolt, A. M., et al: Preoperative SMS 201-995 Treatment: Surgical and Pathological Observations. Neuroendocrinol Lett 7:94, 1985

LeBlanc, H., et al: [Progressive Acromegaly With Normal hGh. Effect of Sandostatin Given as a Continuous Subcutaneous Infusion by Portable Pump.] Ann Endocrinol (Paris) 48: 226, 1987

LeBlanc, H., et al: Effects of An Analog of Somatostatin Administered by Continuous s.c. Infusion on Acromegaly. Presse Med 17 (4): 164, 1988

Liuzzi, A., et al: Hypothalamic Releasing and Inhibiting Hormones in the Control of GH Secretion in Acromegaly. In: Jensen, J., Christiansen, C. (eds) 1st European Congress of Endocrinology, Copenhagen (Denmark), June 21–25, 1987. Norhaven, Viborg, 1987, p 3, Abstr. No. 1–4

Lytras, N., et al: Somatostatin Octapeptide (SMS 201-995) in the Medical Treatment of Acromegaly. J Endocrinol Invest 8 [Suppl 3]: 105 (Abstr. No. OC 104), 1985

Magee, S., et al: Treatment of Refractory Acromegaly With Large Doses of the Somatostatin Analog SMS 201-995. Clin Res 34:428 A, 1986

Martino, I., et al: Treatments for Acromegaly. Rev Fr Endocrinol Clin 28:263–274, 1987

Mayer, G., Tillil, H.: Effect of the Somatostatin Analog SMS 201-995 on GH- and PRL-Secretion in Patients With Acromegaly. Acta Endocrinol (Copenh) 105 [Suppl 264]:30–31, 1984

McHardy, K. C., Pearson, D. W. M.: Glucose Tolerance During Long-Term Treatment With a Somatostatin Analogue. Br Med J 294:176–177, 1987

Micic, D., et al: Suppression of Growth Hormone Secretion in Acromegaly With Long-Acting Somatostatin Analogue Improves the Peripheral Insulin Sensitivity: Sequential Euglycemic Insulin Clamp Studies. J Endocrinol Invest 10 [Suppl 3]:20 (Abstr. No. P4), 1987

Moller, N., et al: High Dose, Long-Term, Continuous Subcutaneous Infusion of SMS 201-995 (Sandostatin) in Acromegaly. In: Landolt, A. M. (ed) Advances in Pituitary Adenoma Research. Proceedings of the 4th European Workshop, Zurich, 13–16.9.1987. Pergamon Press, Oxford, 1988, pp 233–234 (Advances in Biosciences, Vol 69)

Montini, M., et al: Carpal Tunnel Syndrome in Acromegaly: Clinical and Electrophysiological Correlation. J Endocrinol Invest 10 [Suppl 3]: 28 (Abstr. No. P19), 1987

Montini, M., et al: Somatostatin Octapeptide Analogue in the Treatment of Acromegaly: Experience in 16 Patients. J Endocrinol Invest 10 [Suppl 4]:92 (Abstr. No. 142), 1987

Nortier, J. W. R., Croughs, R. J. M.: Medical Therapy of Acromegaly. Neth J Med 28 (7): 299–304, 1985

Oppizzi, G., et al: Relationship Between Somatostatin-C and Growth Hormone Levels in Acromegaly: Basal and Dynamic Evaluation. J Clin Endocrinol 63:1348–1353, 1986

Oliver, C., et al: [Somatostatin and Regulation of GH Secretion.] Ann Endocrinol (Paris) 47: 342–349, 1986

Pagani, G., et al: Effects of a Long Acting Somatostatin Analogue on GH Secretion in Acromegalic Patients. J Endocrinol Invest 8 [Suppl 3]:193 (Abstr. No. P204), 1985

Pagani, G., et al: Chronic Treatment With SMS 201-995 and Glucose Tolerance in Acromegaly. J Endocrinol Invest 10 [Suppl 3]:29 (Abstr. No. P21), 1987

Pagani, G., et al: 1,25-Dihydroxyvitamin D and Calcium Homeostasis Changes in Acromegalic Patients Treated with SMS 201-995. In: Landolt, A. M. (ed) Advances in Pituitary Adenoma Research. Proceedings of the 4th European Workshop, Zurich 13–16.9.1987. Pergamon Press, Oxford, 1988, pp 241–242 (Advances in Biosciences, Vol 69)

Pagani, M. D., et al: SMS 201-995 in Acromegaly: Effect of Chronic Treatment. J Endocrinol Invest 10 [Suppl 3]:28 (Abstr. No. P20), 1987

Page, M. D., et al: The Effect of Long Term Treatment With SMS 201-995 on Clinical, Biochemical and Radiological Parameters in Patients With Acromegaly. J Endocrinol [Suppl 187]:112, 1987

Panagopoulou-Mamalaki, E., et al: Effect of a Cyclic Somatostatin Octapeptide Analogue (SMS 201-995) on Growth Hormone, Insulin and Blood Sugar in Active Acromegaly. Neuroendocrinol Lett 7:109, 1985

Pichl, J., Scheubel, R.: Treatment of Acromegaly With the Somatostatin Analogue SMS 201-995: Dose-Response Relationship. Acta Endocrinol (Copenh) 114 [Suppl 283]:73–74, 1987

Pichl, J., et al: Growth Hormone and Somatomedin C Responsiveness to SMS 201-995 in Acromegalics. J Endocrinol Invest 10 [Suppl 4]: 100 (Abstr. No. 158), 1987

Pieters, G. F. F. M., et al: Kinetics of Growth Hormone in Acromegalics Treated With Minisomatostatin (SMS 201-995). J Endocrinol Invest 8 [Suppl 3]:104 (Abstr. No. OC 102), 1985

Pieters, G. F. F. M., et al: Long-Term Treatment of Acromegaly With the Somatostatin Analogue SMS 201-995. N Engl J Med 314:1391, 1986

Pieters, G. F. F. M., et al: The Effect of Minisomatostatin on Anomalous Growth Hormone Responses in Acromegaly. Acta Endocrinol (Copenh) 114 (4):537–542, 1987

Pieters, G. F. F. M., et al: Long-Term Treatment of Acromegaly with Sandostatin (SMS 201-995). Normalization of Most Anomalous Growth Hormone Responses. Acta Endocrinol (Copenh) 116 [Suppl 286]:9–18, 1987

Plewe, G., et al: Long-Acting and Selective Suppression of Growth Hormone Secretion By Somatostatin Analogue SMS 201-995 in Acromegaly. Lancet 2 (8406):782–784, 1984

Plewe, G., et al: Specific and Long-Acting Suppression of GH Secretion By the Somatostatin Analogue SMS 201-995 in Acromegaly. In: 7th International Congress of Endocrinology, Quebec City (Canada), July 1–7, 1984. Excerpta Medica, Amsterdam Oxford Princeton, 1984, p 1143, Abstr. No. 1765 (Int. Congress Series, No. 652)

Plewe, G., et al: Suppression of GH-Secretion to Normal Values by a Long-Acting Analogue of Somatostatin in Acromegaly. Acta Endocrinol (Copenh) 105 [Suppl 264]:30 (Abstr. No. 37), 1984

Plewe, G., et al: Effect of a New Somatostatin Analog SMS 201-995 on Fat Excretion in Acromegaly After Repeated Administration. Neuroendocrinol Lett 7:110, 1985

Plewe, G., et al: Long-Term Treatment of Acromegaly With the Somatostatin Analogue SMS 201-995. N Engl J Med 314 (21):1390–1391, 1986

Plewe, G., et al: Long-Term Treatment of Acromegaly With the Somatostatin Analogue SMS 201-995 Over 12 Months. Acta Endocrinol (Copenh) 111 [Suppl 274]:25–26, 1986

Plewe, G., et al: Long-term Treatment of Acromegaly with the Somatostatin Analogue SMS 201-995 over 6 Months. Klin Wochenschr 64:389–392, 1986

Ploeckinger, U., Quabbe, H. J.: Treatment of Acromegaly With Somatostatin Analog SMS 201-995: Dose-Response Study and Long-Term Effectiveness. In: Jensen, J., Christiansen, C. (eds) 1st European Congress of Endocrinology, Copenhagen (Denmark), June 21–25, 1987. Norhaven, Viborg, 1987, p 7, Abstr. No. 1–17

Ploeckinger, U., Quabbe, H. J.: Long-Term Effectiveness of the Somatostatin Analog SMS 201-995 in the Treatment of Acromegaly. Acta Endocrinol (Copenh) 117 [Suppl 287]: 107, 1988

Popovic, V., et al: Lymphocyte Subsets in Acromegaly Treated With Long-Acting Somatostatin Analogue. J Endocrinol Invest 10 [Suppl 3]:22 (Abstr. No. P8), 1987

Reubi, J. C., Landolt, A. M.: High Density of Somatostatin Receptors in Pituitary Tumors from Acromegalic Patients. J Clin Endocrinol Metab 59 (6):1148–1151, 1984

Salmoiraghi, M., et al: Insulin and GH Secretion in Acromegalic Patients. Chronic Effects of Somatostatin Octapeptide. In: Jensen, J., Christiansen, C. (eds) 1st European Congress of Endocrinology, Copenhagen (Denmark), June 21–25, 1987. Norhaven, Viborg, 1987, p 11, Abstr. No. 1–37

Salmoiraghi, M., et al: Long-Term Treatment of Acromegaly with SMS 201-995. Gynecol Endocrinol 2 [Suppl 2]:179 (Abstr. No. 201), 1988

Sandler, L. M., et al: Somatostatin Analogue is Effective Long-Term Treatment in Acromegaly. J Endocrinol 107 [Suppl 76], 1985

Sandler, L. M., et al: Symptomatic Improvement with SMS 201-995 in Acromegaly. Scand J Gastroenterol 21 [Suppl 119]:249–250, 1986

Sandler, L. M., et al: Effective Long-Term Treatment of Acromegaly With a Long-Acting Somatostatin Analogue (SMS 201-995). Clin Endocrinol (Oxf) 26:85–95, 1987

Sandler, L. M., et al: Effect of High Dose Somatostatin Analogue on Growth Hormone Concentrations in Acromegaly. Br Med J 296:751–752, 1988

Sandler, L. M., et al: High Dose Somatostatin Analogue Treatment Normalises Growth Hormone in Acromegaly. Clin Sci 74 [Suppl 18]: 67P (Abstr. No. 251), 1988

Schlüter, K. J., et al: Studies in Healthy Volunteers of a New Potent Somatostatin Analogue: SMS 201-995. In: 65th Ann. Meeting, The Endoc. Soc. (Progr. and Abstr.), San Antonio (Tex.), 8–10.5.1983. Endocrinology 112 [Suppl]:212 (Abstr. No. 527), 1983

Schmidt, K., et al: [The Analgesic Activity of the Somatostatin Analog SMS 201-995 in Patients with Acromegaly – a Double-Blind Study.] (German) Klin Wochenschr 64 [Suppl V]:69, 1986

Schmidt, K., et al: Effects of the Somatostatin-Analogue SMS 201-995 on the 'Enteroinsular Axis' in Acromegalic Patients. In: Jensen, J., Christiansen, C. (eds) 1st European Congress of Endocrinology, Copenhagen (Denmark), June 21–25, 1987. Norhaven, Viborg, 1987, p 12, Abstr. No. 1–39

Schmidt, K., et al: [The Results of the Long-term Treatment of Acromegaly by the Somatostatin Analogue SMS 201-995 – Prognostic Value of the Endocrinological Function Test.] (German) Klin Wochenschr 65 [Suppl IX]:203–204, 1987

Spinas, G. A., et al: Pre-Operative Treatment of 5 Acromegalics With a Somatostatin Analogue: Endocrine and Clinical Observations. Acta Endocrinol (Copenh) 114 (2):249–256, 1987

Tauber, J. P., et al: [Treatment With Sandostatin (SMS 201-995) in Acromegaly Secondary to Pancreatic Tumor of GRF.] Ann Endocrinol (Paris) 48:229 (Abstr. No. 97), 1987

Tauber, J. P., et al: Long-Term Treatment of Acromegaly By Continuous Subcutaneous Infusion of the Long-Acting Somatostatin Analogue Octreotide (Sandostatin). In: Landolt, A. M. (ed) Advances in Pituitary Adenoma Research. Proceedings of the 4th European Workshop, Zurich, 13–16.9.1987. Pergamon Press, Oxford, 1988, pp 235–239 (Advances in Biosciences, Vol 69)

Thiel, M., et al: [Difficulties in Treatment of Acromegaly.] Dtsch Med Wochenschr 110: 1512–1513, 1985

Timsit, J., et al: [Sleep Apnea and Acromegaly. Rapid Recovery With Treatment With SMS 201-995.] Ann Endocrinol (Paris) 47:233 (Abstr. No. 49), 1986

Timsit, J., et al: Compared Efficiency of Continuous and Discontinuous Subcutaneous SMS 201-995 Injections in Seven Acromegalic Patients: A Short-Term Trial. In: Jensen, J., Christiansen, C. (eds) 1st European Congress of Endocrinology, Copenhagen (Denmark),

June 21–25, 1987. Norhaven, Viborg, 1987, p 4, Abstr. No. 1–5

Timsit, J., et al: The Effect of Subcutaneous Infusion Versus Subcutaneous Injections of a Somatostatin Analogue (SMS 201-995) on the Diurnal GH Profile in Acromegaly. Acta Endocrinol (Copenh) 116:108–112, 1987

Timsit, J., et al: [SMS 201-995 and Acromegaly: Compared Efficiency of Continuous and Discontinuous Subcutaneous Administration.] Ann Endocrinol (Paris) 48:228 (Abstr. No. 95), 1987

Tolis, G.: SMS 201-995: Long-Term Use in Active Acromegaly. Neuroendocrinol Lett 7:119, 1985

Tolis, G., et al: Therapy of Acromegaly With a Mini-Somatostatin. In: 67th Ann. Meet., The Endoc. Soc. (Progr. and Abstr.), Baltimore (U.S.A.), 19–21.5.1985. Endocrinology 116 [Suppl]:122 (Abstr. No. 488), 1985

Tolis, G., et al: Therapeutic Efficacy of a Somatostatin Analogue (SMS 201-995) in Active Acromegaly. J Neurosurg 65:37–40, 1986

Tolis, G., et al: Therapy of Acromegaly with SMS 201-995: Long-Term Studies. Scand J Gastroenterol 21 [Suppl 119]:149–153, 1986

Tolis, G., et al: Efficacy and Safety of a Somatostatin Analogue in Active Acromegaly. In: Reichlin, S. (ed) Somatostatin Basic and Clinical Status. Serono Symposia: Proceedings of the International Conference on Somatostatin, Washington, 6–8.5.1986. Plenum Press, New York, 1987, pp 337–341

Tolis, G., et al: Treatment of Acromegaly With the Somatostatin Analogue Octreotide (SMS 201-995) for More Than Two Years. In: Jensen, J., Christiansen, C. (eds) 1st European Congress of Endocrinology, Copenhagen (Denmark), June 21–25, 1987. Norhaven, Viborg, 1987, p 12, Abstr. No. 1–41

Tolis, G., et al.: Treatment of Acute Acromegaly with the Long-Acting Somatostatin Analogue SMS 201-995. In: Luedecke, D. K., Tolis, G. (eds) Growth Hormone, Growth Factors, and Acromegaly. Raven Press, New York, 1987, pp 215–219 (Progress in Endocrine Research and Therapy, Vol 3)

Turpin, G., et al: [Study of Somatostatin Analog (SMS 201-995) in Acromegaly.] Ann Endocrinol (Paris) 47:242 (Abstr. No. 68), 1986

Vance, M. L., Thorner, M. O.: Pituitary and Ectopic GRF Mediated Acromegaly Treated With Somatostatin Analog, SMS 201-995. Clin Res 33 (2):575A, 1985

Vance, M. L., et al: SMS 201-995: Studies in Acromegaly and in Normal Men. Scand J Gastroenterol 21 [Suppl 119]:243–248, 1986

Vance, M. L., et al: SMS 201-995 Treatment of Acromegaly: Reduction in Tumor Size and Growth Hormone Secretion. Clin Res 35 (3): 519A, 1987

Verde, G. G., et al: Serum Type III Procollagen Propeptide Levels in Acromegalic Patients. J Clin Endocrinol 63:1406–1410, 1986

Verschoor, L., et al: Glucose Tolerance During Long Term Treatment With a Somatostatin Analogue. Br Med J 293:1327–1328, 1986

Verschoor, L., et al: Glucose Tolerance During Long-Term Treatment With a Somatostatin Analogue (Correspondence). Br Med J 294: 177, 1987

Von Werder, K., et al: Treatment of Therapy-Resistent Acromegaly With the Somatostatin Analog SMS 201-995. Acta Endocrinol (Copenh) 114 [Suppl 283]:202, 1987

Wass, J. A. H., et al: Somatostatin Octapeptide (SMS 201-995) in the Medical Treatment of Acromegaly. Scand J Gastroenterol 21 [Suppl 119]: 136–140, 1986

Wass, J. A. H., et al: The Treatment of Acromegaly By External Pituitary Irradiation and Drugs. In: Luedecke, D. K., Tolis, G. (eds) Growth Hormone, Growth Factors, and Acromegaly. Proceedings of the International Symposium, Aegina, April 1985. Raven Press, New York, 1987, pp 199–206

Williams, G., et al: Effective and Lasting Growth-Hormone Suppression in Active Acromegaly With Oral Administration of Somatostatin Analogue SMS 201-995. Lancet 2 (8510):774–777, 1986

Wilson, D. M., Hoffman, A. R.: Reduction of Pituitary Size in a Patient With a GRF Secreting Islet Cell Tumor by Continuous Subcutaneous Infusion of a Somatostatin Analog. In: 67th Ann. Meeting, The Endoc. Soc. (Progr. and Abstr.), Baltimore (U.S.A.), 19–21.5.1985. Endocrinology 116 [Suppl]:39 (Abstr. No. 153), 1985

XVI. AIDS (Diarrhea)

Cook, D. J., et al: Somatostatin Treatment for Cryptosporidial. Diarrhea in a Patient with the Acquired Immunodeficiency Syndrome (AIDS). Ann Intern Med 108 (5):708–709, 1988

Katz, M. D., et al: Treatment of Severe Cryptosporidium-Related Diarrhea with Octreotide in a Patient with AIDS. Drug Intell Clin Pharm 22:134–136, 1988

Rene, E., et al: Somatostatin and Cryptosporidial Diarrhea During Aids. Can J Physiol Pharmacol [Suppl]:70 (Abstr. No. 252), 1986

XVII. Analgesia

Gennari, C., et al: Calcitonin- and Somatostatin-Induced Analgesia in Pain from Cancer. Gynecol Endocrinol 1 [Suppl 3]:38, 1987

Panconesi, A., et al: Powerful Vasospastic Activity in Man of an Analogue of Somatostatin (SMS 201-995),. a Potential Symptomatic Agent in Cluster Headache. Cephalalgia 5 [Suppl 3]:36–37, 1985

Williams, G., et al: Improvement in Headache Associated with Prolactinoma During Treatment with a Somatostatin Analogue: An "N of 1" Study. N Engl J Med 315 (18):1166–1167, 1986

Williams, G., et al: Analgesic Effect of Somatostatin Analogue (Octreotide) in Headache Associated with Pituitary Tumours. Br Med J 295:247–248, 1987

Williams, G., et al: Analgesic Effect of the Somatostatin Analogue, SMS 201-995, in Headache Associated with Pituitary Tumour. Clin Sci 73 [Suppl 17]:25 (Abstr. No. 90), 1987

XVIII. Cancer (Miscellaneous)

Defeudis, F. V., Moreau, J. P.: Studies on Somatostatin Analogues Might Lead to New Therapies for Certain Types of Cancer. Trends Pharmacol Sci 7:384–386, 1986

Klijn, J. G. M., et al: Effects of Somatostatin Analog (SMS-A) Treatment (Sandostatin) in Experimental and Human Cancer. Eur J Cancer Clin Oncol 22 (6):727 (Abstr. No. V-e), 1986

Setyono-Han, B., et al: Direct Inhibitory Effects of Somatostatin (Analogues) on the Growth of Human Breast Cancer Cells. Cancer Res 47:1566–1570, 1987

XIX. Diabetes

Aarsen, R. S. R., et al: Long-Acting Somatostatin Analogue 201-995 Safely Reduces Late Night Insulinopenic Lipolysis in Diabetic Teenagers. Diabetologia 29 (8):511 A, 1986

Aarsen, R. S. R., et al: Long-Acting Somatostatin Analogue (Sandostatin) Reduces Late Night Insulinopenic Ketogenesis in Diabetic Teenagers. Acta Endocrinol (Copenh) 116 [Suppl 286]:45–53, 1987

Benroubee, M., et al: Improvement of Glycemic Control in Insulin Dependent Diabetics by the Long Acting Somatostatin Analogue Octreotide (SMS 201-995). In: Jensen, J., Christiansen, C. (eds) 1st European Congress of Endocrinology, Copenhagen (Denmark), June 21–25, 1987. Norhaven, Viborg, 1987, p 94, Abstr. No. 10–358

Candrina, R., et al: SMS 201-995 Improves Glucose Tolerance in Insulin-Treated Type II Diabetic Patients. Diabetes Care 10 (4):534–535, 1987

Candrina, R., et al: The Therapeutic Role of the Long-Acting Somatostatin Analogue SMS 201-995 in Type II Diabetes Mellitus. J Endocrinol Invest 10 [Suppl 4]:94 (Abstr. No. 145), 1987

Cantalamessa, L., et al: Improvement of Diabetes After Treatment with Somatostatin Analogue SMS 201-995 in an Acromegalic Patient. Horm Metab Res 18 (11):790–791, 1986

Davies, R. R., et al: Effects of Somatostatin Analogue SMS 201-995 in Non-Insulin-Dependent Diabetes. Clin Endocrinol 25 (6):739–747, 1986

Davies, R. R., et al: The Response of Patients with Type I (insulin-dependent) Diabetes to a Single Night Time Injection of SMS 201-995. Diabetologia 29 (8):53 A (Abstr. No. 118), 1986

Del-Pozo, E., et al: Effect of a Long-Acting Somatostatin Analogue (SMS 201-995) on Glucose Homeostasis in Type I Diabetes and in Acromegaly. In: Reichlin, S. (ed) Somatostatin Basic and Clinical Status, Serono Symposia: Proceedings of the International Conference on Somatostatin, Washington, 6–8.5.1986. Plenum Press, New York, 1987, pp 293–302

Dudl, R. J., et al: Treatment of Diabetic Diarrhea and Orthostatic Hypotension with Somatostatin Analog SMS 201-995. Clin Res 35 (1): 148 A, 1987

Dudl, R. J., et al: Treatment of Diabetic Diarrhea and Orthostatic Hypotension with Somatostatin Analogue SMS 201-995. Am J Med 83:584–588, 1987

Fuessl, H. S., et al: [Metabolic and Endocrine Effects of Various Doses of a Long-Acting Somatostatin Analogue (SMS 201-995) in Non-Insulin-Dependent Diabetes Mellitus.] (German) Klin Wochenschr 64 [Suppl V]:188, 1986

Gil, J., et al.: Hypoglycemia. A Severe Side Effect of Sandostatin in Insulin-Dependent Diabetes Mellitus. J Endocrinol Invest 10 [Suppl 3]:20 (Abstr. No. P 3), 1987

Hadjidakis, D. J., et al: The Effects of Somatostatin Analogue SMS 201-995 on Carbohydrate Homeostasis of Type I Diabetics as Assessed by the Artificial Endocrine Pancreas (AEP). Diabetes 36 [Suppl 1]:124 (Abstr. No. 489), 1987

Harris, A., et al: [Amelioration of Metabolism of Gluco-Lipids With Evening Administration of Somatostatin Analog SMS 201-995 in Adolescents With Diabetes Type I.] Ann Endocrinol (Paris) 47:210 (Abstr. No. 3), 1986

Haupt, E., et al: The Effect of the Octapeptide Somatostatin Analogue Sandostatin in Type-2 (Non-Insulin-Dependent) Diabetes. Diabetes 30:538–529 (Abstr. No. 207), 1987

Hyer, S. L., et al: Growth Hormone Suppression in Diabetic Retinopathy. Diabetologia 30 (7):534 A (Abstr. No. 238), 1987

Johnston, D. G., et al: Effects of SMS 201-995 on Intermediary Metabolism and Endocrine Status in Normal and Diabetic Humans. Am J Med 81 [Suppl 6 B]:88–93, 1986

Karamanos, B., et al: Effect of the Long-Acting Somatostatin Analogue SMS 201-995 on the Glycaemic Control in Insulin-Treated Diabetics. Scand J Gastroenterol 21 [Suppl 119]:262–266, 1986

Karamanos, B., et al: Effect of Pump-Infused Somatostatin Analogue SMS 201-995 on Glycemic Control in Insulin Dependent Diabetics. In: Jensen, J., Christiansen, C. (eds) 1st European Congress of Endocrinology, Copenhagen (Denmark), June 21–25, 1987. Norhaven, Viborg, 1987, p 94, Abstr. No. 10–357

Mohan, V., et al: Effects of a Somatostatin Analogue (SMS 201-995) on Insulin Induced Hypoglycaemia – A Randomized Double Blind Crossover Study. Diabetologia 29 (8):572 A (Abstr. No. 344), 1986

Murat, A., et al: A Single Injection of 50 mg of Somatostatin (SMS) at Bed-Time Does Not Prevent the Dawn-Phenomenon. In: Jensen, J., Christiansen, C. (eds) 1st European Congress of Endocrinology, Copenhagen (Denmark), June 21–25, 1987. Norhaven, Viborg, 1987, p 94, Abstr. No. 10–356

Navasues, I., et al: Effect of SMS 201-995 in Type 1 (Insulin-Dependent) Diabetes Mellitus Assessed by the Artificial Pancreas. Diabetologia 29 (8):575 A (Abstr. No. 361), 1986

Noelken, G., et al: [Lowering of Insulin Need and Growth Hormone Secretion With the Long Acting Somatostatin Analog SMS 201-995 in Type I Diabetics With Retinopathy.] Endocrinology 5:111, 1984

Ordonez, A., et al: Somatostatin Analog (SMS 201-995) Decreases Meal Induced Glucagon Secretion in Type I Diabetic Patients. J Endocrinol Invest 8 [Suppl 3]:129 (Abstr. No. P 127), 1985

Phillips, R. E., et al: Effectiveness of SMS 201-995, a Synthetic, Long-Acting Somatostatin Analogue, in Treatment of Quinine-Induced Hyperinsulinaemia. Lancet 1 (8483):713–716, 1986

Plewe, G., et al: Reduction of Growth Hormone and Somatomedin C Secretion by Long-Acting Somatostatin Analogue SMS 201-995 in Type I Diabetics. Diabetes 33 [Suppl 1]:25 A (Abstr. No. 97), 1984

Plewe, G., et al: Suppression of Growth Hormone and Somatomedin C Secretion by Long-Acting Somatostatin Analogue (SMS 201-995) in Type 1 (Insulin-Dependent) Diabetes. Diabetologia 27:320 A (Abstr. No. 419), 1984

Plewe, G., et al: Somatostatin Analogue SMS 201-995 in Type I Diabetes Mellitus. Initial Experience After Repeated Administration. Scand J Gastroenterol 21 [Suppl 119]:166–169, 1986

Plewe, G., et al: Suppression of Growth Hormone and Somatomedin C by Long-Acting Somatostatin Analog SMS 201-995 in Type I Diabetes Mellitus. Horm Res 27 (1):7–12, 1987

Rodier, M., et al: Effect of a Long-Acting Somatostatin Analog Sandostatin (SMS 201-995) on Glycemic Control in Type I Diabetes (IDDM). In: Jensen, J., Christiansen, C. (eds) 1st European Congress of Endocrinology, Copenhagen (Denmark), June 21–25, 1987. Norhaven, Viborg, 1987, p 80, Abstr. No. 10–302

Rodier, M., et al: Long Acting Somatostatin Analogue (SMS 201-995) Lowers Endogeneous Insulin Secretion in Type 2 Diabetics Without Worsening Blood Glucose Control. In: Jensen, J., Christiansen, C. (eds) 1st European Congress of Endocrinology, Copenhagen (Denmark), June 21–25, 1987. Norhaven, Viborg, 1987, p 116, Abstr. No. 14–442

Rodier, M., et al: Long Acting Somatostatin Analogue SMS 201-995 Lowers Endogenous Insulin in Type 2 (Non-Insulin-Dependent) Diabetic Patients Without Worsening Blood Glucose Control. Diabetologia 30 (7):574 A–575 A (Abstr. No. 469), 1987

Rohr, G., et al: [Effect of the Somatostatin Analog, SMS 201-995, on Diabetes. Regulation Quality in Type II Diabetics.] (German) Klin Wochenschr 65 [Suppl IX]:77 (Abstr. No. 172), 1987

Rosak, C., et al: [Changes of Hormonal Counter Regulation Following Insulin Induced Hypoglycemia under Concomitant Administration of the Somatostatin Analogue SMS 201-995.] (German) Med Klin 81 (24):773–778, 1986

Rosak, C., et al: Importance of Epinephrine and Cortisol Secretion Following Altered Hormonal Counterregulation by the Somatostatin Analogue SMS 201-995 in Insulin Induced Hypoglycemia. Diabetes 35 [Suppl 1]:160 A, 1986

Sadoul, J. L., et al: [Effects of Somatostatin Analog on Glycemic Equilibrium and the Insulin Requirements in Diabetes Type I.] Ann Endocrinol (Paris) 47:214 (Abstr. No. 11), 1986

Scheen, A. J., et al: Attempt to Prevent the Dawn Phenomenon by a Bedtime Subcutaneous Injection of a Somatostatin Analogue (SMS 201-995) in Type 1 (Insulin-Dependent) Diabetic

Patients. Diabetologia 29 (8): 590 A–591 A (Abstr. No. 450), 1986

Scheen, A. J., et al: Clinical Use of a New Analogue of Somatostatin SMS 201-995, in Type-1 Diabetes Mellitus. Acta Clin 42 (3): 222, 1987

Schlueter, K. J., et al: Receptor Binding of a New Modified Potent and Selective Somatostatin (SMS 201-995). Diabetes 32 [Suppl 1]: 135 A (Abstr. No. 517), 1983

Serrano Riosi, M. S., et al: Somatostatin Analog SMS 201-995 and Insulin Needs in Insulin-Dependent Diabetic Patients Studied by Means of an Artificial Pancreas. J Clin Endocrinol 63: 1071–1074, 1986

Serrano Riosi, M. S., et al: Dawn Phenomenon: Suppression by a Single Nightly Dose of Somatostatin Analog SMS 201-995. Diabetes 36 [Suppl 1]: 134 A (Abstr. No. 522), 1987

Serrano Riosi, M. S., et al: Effects of SMS 201-995 on Dawn Phenomenon in Type I Diabetic Patients. In: Jensen, J., Christiansen, C. (eds) 1st European Congress of Endocrinology, Copenhagen (Denmark), June 21–25, 1987. Norhaven, Viborg, 1987, p 93, Abstr. No. 10–354

Sharp, P. S., et al: Somatostatin Analogue and Diabetic Retinopathy. J Endocrinol 112 [Suppl]: Abstr. No. 124, 1987

Shumak, S. L., et al: The Effect of Growth Hormone Suppression on Established Preproliferative Diabetic Retinopathy. Diabetes 36 [Suppl 1]: 42 A, 1987

Spinas, G. A., et al: Reduction of Postprandial Hyperglycaemia and Suppression of Gastrointestinal Hormones after s.c. Administration of a New Somatostatin Analogue in Type I Diabetics. Eur J Clin Invest 14 (2) (Part 2): 24 (Abstr. No. 142), 1984

Spinas, G. A., et al: Reduced Postprandial Hyperglycemia After Subcutaneous Injection of a Somatostatin-Analogue (SMS 201-995) in Insulin-Dependent Diabetes Mellitus. Diabetes Care 8 (5): 429–435, 1985

Tauber, J. P., et al: SMS 201-995 Treatment in Diabetic Proliferative Retinopathy. In: Jensen, J., Christiansen, C. (eds) 1st European Congress of Endocrinology, Copenhagen (Denmark), June 21–25, 1987. Norhaven, Viborg, 1987, p 85, Abstr. No. 10–320

Tsai, S. T., Vinik, A. I.: Diabetic Diarrhea and Somatostatin. Ann Intern Med 104: 894, 1986

Tsai, S., et al: Management of Refractory 'Diabetic Diarrhea' Using a Somatostatin Analogue (SMS 201-995). Diabetes 35 [Suppl 1]: 141 A (Abstr. No. 547), 1986

Williams, G., et al: Postprandial Effects of SMS 201-995 on Gut Hormones and Glucose Tolerance. Scand J Gastroenterol 21 [Suppl 119]: 73–83, 1986

Williams, G., et al: Somatostatin Analogue (SMS 201-995) and Glycaemic Control in Acromegaly and Noninsulin-Dependent Diabetes Mellitus. Can J Physiol Pharmacol [Suppl]: 65 (Abstr. No. 242), 1986

Williams, G., et al: Post-Prandial Effects of the Long-Acting Somatostatin Analogue, SMS 201-995, in Non-Insulin Dependent Diabetes Mellitus (NIDDM). Clin Sci 72 [Suppl 16]: 14 P, 1987

Williams, G., et al: Postprandial Glycaemic Effects of a Long-Acting Somatostatin Analogue (Octreotide) in Non-Insulin Dependent Diabetes Mellitus. Horm Metab Res 20 (3): 168–170, 1988

Willms, B., et al: Effects of a Single Nocturnal Administration of a Long Acting Somatostatin Analogue, SMS 201-995 on Blood Glucose Profile During the Night, Human Growth Hormone and Cortisol Secretion in Type 1 (Insulin-Dependent) Diabetic Patients. Diabetologia 30 (7): 597 A (Abstr. No. 594), 1987

XX. Dumping Syndrome

Donald, R. A., et al: Treatment of Acromegaly with the Somatostatin Analogue SMS 201-995. In: Harding, P. E. (ed) Proceedings of the Annual Scientific Meeting of the New Zealand Society of Endocrinology, Canterbury, 18–20.5.1987. Amanda Imprint, Adelaide, 1987, Suppl 2, Abstr. No. 34 (Proceedings Vol 30)

Donald, R. A., et al: Treatment of Acromegaly with the Somatostatin Analogue SMS 201-995. In: Landolt, A. M. (ed) Advances in Pituitary Adenoma Research. Proceedings of the 4th European Workshop, Zurich, 13–16.9.1987. Pergamon Press, Oxford, 1988, pp 229–230 (Advances in Biosciences, Vol 69)

Hopman, W. P. M., et al: Treatment of the Dumping Syndrome with the Somatostatin Analogue SMS 201-995. Gastroenterology 92 (5) (Part 2): 1440, 1987

Hopman, W. P. M., et al: Treatment of the Dumping Syndrome with the Somatostatin Analogue SMS 201-995. Ann Surg 207 (2): 155–159, 1988

Kapoor, A., et al: Use of a Long-Acting Somatostatin Analog (Sandostatin, SMS 201-995) in the Treatment of Refractory Postgastrectomy Hypoglycemia. Clin Res 35 (3): 507 A, 1987

Parr, N., et al: Somatostatin Analogue (SMS 201-995) Inhibitis Early Rapid Gastric Emptying After Truncal Vagotomy and Drainage. Gut 27: A 1272–A 1273 (Abstr. No. T 94), 1986

Primrose, J. N., Johnston, D.: Somatostatin Analogue SMS 201-995 is an Effective Treatment for the Post Gastric Surgery-Dumping Syndrome Provoked by Hypertonic Glucose. Gastroenterology 92 (5) (Part 2): 1580, 1987

Primrose, J. N., Johnston, D.: Somatostatin Analogue SMS 201-995: A Solution to the Dumping-Diarrhea Syndrome After Gastrectomy or Vagotomy? Br J Surg 74 (6):527, 1987

Primrose, J. N., et al: Somatostatin Analogue SMS 201-995 in the Dumping Syndrome: Effect on Packed Cell Volume (PCV), Blood Glucose (BG) and Plasma GI Peptides. Gut 28 (10):A 1396, 1987

Santangelo, W. C., et al: Clinical Efficacy of the Somatostatin Analogue 201-995 in the Post-Gastrectomy Dumping Syndrome. Gastroenterology 92 (5) (Part 2):1613, 1987

XXI. Fistula

Ellison, E. C., et al: The Effect of Long-Acting Somatostatin Analog (SMS 201-995) on Basal Pancreatic Exocrine Secretion in Man. Gastroenterology 88:1371, 1985

Faroux, R., et al: [Treatment of a Postoperative External Pancreatic Fistula by Somatostatin Retard.] (French) Presse Med 16 (28):1379, 1987

Goodgame, R., et al: Pancreatic Secretion in Man: Effects of Drugs, Somatostatin, Porcine Pancreatic Supplements, or Intraduodenal Infusion of Pure Human Pancreatic Juice. Gastroenterology 90:1433, 1986

Heij, H. A., et al: A Comparison of the Effects of Two Somatostatin Analogues in Patient with an External Pancreatic Fistula. Pancreas 1 (2):188–190, 1986

Lewis, E., et al: The Role of a Long-Acting Somatostatin Analogue (SMS 201-995) in the Management of a Patient with Benign Insulin-Secreting Adenoma of the Pancreas and a Postoperative Pancreatic Fistula. Scand J Gastroenterol 21 [Suppl 119]:217–222, 1986

Nubiola-Calonge, P., et al: Blind Evaluation of the Effect of Octreotide (SMS 201-995), a Somatostatin Analogue, on Small-Bowel Fistula Output. Lancet 2 (8560):672–674, 1987

Nubiola-Calonge, P., et al: [Blind Evaluation of the Effect of Octreotide (SMS 201-995), a Somatostatin Analogue, on Small-Bowel Fistula Output.] Lancet 12 (2):120–121, 1988

Prinz, R. A., et al: Treatment of Pancreatic Cutaneous Fistulas with a Somatostatin Analog. Am J Surg 115 (1):36–42, 1988

Rosenberg, L., et al: Administration of Somatostatin Analog (SMS 201-995) in the Treatment of a Fistula Occurring After Pancreas Transplantation: Interference with Cyclosporine Immunosuppresion. Transplantation 43 (5):763–766, 1987

Tulchinsky, M., et al: Successful Treatment of Enterocutaneous Fistula with Somatostatin Analog (SMS 201-995). Clin Res 35 (5):798 A, 1987

XXII. GI Bleeding

Baxter, J. N., et al: SMS 201-995 and Variceal Haemorrhage. Acta Endocrinol (Copenh) 116 [Suppl 286]:37–44, 1987

Burroughs, A. K., et al: Effect of a Long Acting Analogue of Somatostatin (SMS 201-995) on Hepatic Venous Pressures and Azygous Blood Flow in Cirrhotics. Gut 26:A 562 (Abstr. No. F 28), 1985

Christiansen, J., Yotis, A.: The Role of Somatostatin and a Long-Acting Analogue, SMS 201-995, in Acute Bleeding Due to Peptide Ulceration. Scand J Gastroenterol 21 [Suppl 119]: 109–114, 1986

Eriksson, L. S., et al: Effect of SMS, a Long-Acting Somatostatin Analogue, on Hepatic Hemodynamics and Metabolism in Patients with Liver Cirrhosis. Scand J Gastroenterol 20 [Suppl 113]:68 (Abstr. No. 116), 1985

Eriksson, L. S., et al: Haemodynamic Effects of a Long-Acting Somatostatin Analogue in Patients with Liver Cirrhosis. Scand J Gastroenterol 22:919–925, 1987

Gaginella, T. S., O'Dorisio, T. M.: Octreotide: Entering the New Era of Peptidomimetic Therapy. Drug Intell Clin Pharm 22:154–155, 1988

Jenkins, S. A., et al: Effects of a Long Acting Analogue of Somatostatin (SMS 201-995) on Hepatic Haemodynamics in the Pig and on Intravariceal Pressure in Cirrhotic Patients. Gut 26:A 1102 (Abstr. No. W 9), 1985

Jenkins, S. A., et al: Effects of a Somatostatin Analogue SMS 201-995 on Hepatic Haemodynamics in the Pig and on Intravariceal Pressure in Man. Br J Surg 72 (12):1009–1012, 1985

McKee, R. K., et al: SMS 201-995 in the Management of Variceal Bleeding. Gut 28 (10):A 1380, 1987

Mortensen, P. E., et al: Effect of a Somatostatin Analogue on 133-Xenon Clearance from Colonic Mucosa in Unanaesthetized Man. Gastroenterology 92 (5) (Part 2):1542, 1987

Olsen, J. A., et al: Inhibition of Meal Stimulated Gastric Acid Secretion by an Octapeptide Somatostatin Analogue SMS 201-995. Gut 28 (4): 464–467, 1987

Stalder, G. A., et al: [Somatostatin in Gastroenterological Therapy.] (German) Schweiz Med Wochenschr 115 (35) [Suppl 19]:30–36, 1985

Wahren, J., Eriksson, L. S.: The Influence of a Long-Acting Somatostatin Analogue on Splanchnic Haemodynamics and Metabolism in Healthy Subjects and Patients with Liver Cirrhosis. Scand J Gastroenterol 21 [Suppl 119]:103–108, 1986

Wolfe, M. M., et al: Zollinger-Ellison-Syndrome (=Gastrinoma): A Review. N Engl J Med 317:1200–1209, 1987

XXIII. Ileostomy

Cooper, J. C., et al: Use of a Somatostatin Analogue in the Treatment of Severe Ileostomy Diarrhoea. Br J Surg 72 (5):404 (Abstr. No. 29), 1985

Cooper, J. C., et al: Effects of a Long-Acting Somatostatin Analogue in Patients with Severe Ileostomy Diarrhoea. Br J Surg 73 (2):128–131, 1986

Mueller, M. K., et al: [Treatment of Chronic Diarrhea After Ileostomy with Somatostatin SMS 201-995.] (German) Klin Wochenschr 64 [Suppl V]:63–64, 1986

Mueller, M. K., et al: Treatment of Chronic Diarrhea Following Ileostomy by Somatostatin SMS 201-995. Z Gastroenterol 26 (3):166–168, 1988

Ohlbaum, P., et al: Use of a Long-Acting Somatostatin Analogue (SMS 201-995) in Controlling a Significant Ileal Output in a 5-Year-Old Child. J Pediatr Gastroenterol Nutr 6 (3):466–470, 1987

Williams, N. S., et al: Use of a Long-Acting Somatostatin Analogue in Controlling Life Threatening Ileostomy Diarrhoea. Br Med J 289 (6451):1027–1028, 1984

XXIV. Nesidioblastosis

Bruining, G. J., et al: Normalization of Glucose Homeostasis by a Long-Acting Somatostatin Analog SMS 201-995 in a Newborn with Nesidioblastosis. Acta Endocrinol (Copenh) 113 [Suppl 279]:334–339, 1986

Delemarre, H. A., et al: Long-Term Treatment of an Infant with Nesidioblastosis Using the Somatostatin Analogue. N Engl J Med 316 (4): 222–223, 1987

Hindmarsh, P., Brook, C. G. D.: Short-Term Management of nesidioblastosis Using the Somatostatin Analogue SMS 201-995. N Engl J Med 316 (4):221–222, 1987

Jackson, J. A., et al: Long-Term Treatment of Refractory Neonatal Hypoglycemia with a Long-Acting Somatostatin Analog. Clin Res 35 (3):506 A, 1987

Jackson, J. A., et al: Long-Term Treatment of Refractory Neonatal Hypoglycemia with Long-Acting Somatostatin Analog. J Pediatr 111: 548–551, 1987

XXV. Psoriasis

Camisa, C., et al: Treatment of Psoriasis with Somatostatin Analog 201-995. Clin Res 34 (4): 907 A, 1986

Camisa, C., et al: Improvement of Psoriasis with Chronic Use of Somatostatin (SMS) Analog 201-995. Clin Res 35 (3):673 A, 1987

Camisa, C., et al: Improvement of Psoriasis with Chronic Use of Somatostatin (SMS) Analog 201-995. J Invest Dermatol 88 (4):480, 1987

XXVI. Secretory Diarrhea

Edwards, C. A., et al: Effect of Somatostatin Analogue SMS 201-995 on Fluid and Electrolyte Transport in a Patient with Secretory Diarrhoea. Gut 26 (10):A 1115, 1985

Edwards, C. A., et al: The Effect of Somatostatin Analogue SMS 201-995 on Fluid and Electrolyte Transport in a Patient with Secretory Diarrhoea. Scand J Gastroenterol 21 [Suppl 119]:259–261, 1986

Edwards, C., et al: Effect of Two New Antisecretory Drugs on Fluid and Electrolyte Transport in a Patient with Secretory Diarrhoea. Gut 27:581–586, 1986

Hunziker, U. A., et al: Effects of the Long Acting Somatostatin Analogue SMS 201-995 in an Infant with Intractable Diarrhea. Eur J Pediatr 144 (5):523, 1986

Jaros, W., et al: Successful Treatment of Idiopathic Secretory Diarrhea of Infancy with a Somatostatin Analogue SMS 201-995. Gastroenterology 88:1432, 1985

Jaros, W., et al: Successful Treatment of Idiopathic Secretory Diarrhea of Infancy with the Somatostatin Analogue SMS 201-995. Gastroenterology 94:189–193, 1988

Marinier, E., et al: [Action of Somatostatin With Long Term Therapy in Prolonged Diarrhea. Effects on Glucidic Tolerance, Secretion of Growth Hormone, of VIP and Gastrin.] Gastroenterol Clin Biol 11 (2 BIS):107 A, 1987

Mueller, M. K., et al: [Treatment of Chronic Diarrhea Following Ileostomy With Somatostatin SMS 201-995.] Klin Wochenschr [Suppl V]:63–64 (Abstr. No. 131), 1986

Santangelo, W. C., et al: Pseudopancreatic Cholera Syndrome: Effect of a Synthetic Somatostatin Analogue, SMS 201-995. Am J Med 82 [Suppl 5 B]:84–87, 1987

Shulman, D., et al: Enlarged Pancreas, Secretory Diarrhea and Elevated Vasoactive Intestinal Peptide (VIP) Levels in an Infant: Poor Response to a Somatostatin Analogue. Clin Res 34 (1):239 A, 1986

XXVII. Other

Bannister, R., et al: The Somatostatin Analogue SMS 201-995 Reduces Oral Glucose-Induced Hypotension in Human Autonomic Failure. J Physiol 396:90P, 1988

Bauer, W., et al: Rational Drug Design of Long-Acting Somatostatin Analogues. In: 7th International Congress of Endocrinology, Quebec City (Canada), July 1–7, 1984. Excerpta Medica, Amsterdam Oxford Princeton, 1984, p 330, Abstr. No. 139 (Int. Congress Series, No. 652)

Bonfils, S., et al: [Somatostatin – Inhibitory Actions of Exocrine and Endocrine Secretions in the Digestive Tract – Therapeutic Implications.] Med Hyg (Geneve) 44:256–258, 261–262, 1986

Dunne, M. J., Lightman, S. L.: The Vasopressin and Oxytocin Response to Hypoglycaemia: Effect of the Somatostatin Analogue SMS 201-995. J Endocrinol Invest 8 [Suppl 3]:134 (Abstr. No. P138), 1985

Ellison, E. C., et al: Successful Treatment of Pancreatic Ascites with Somatostatin Analog (SMS 201-995). Gastroenterology 90 (5, pt. 2): 1405, 1986

Escourrou, J., et al: [Comparative Study in Man of Action of 3 Molecular Forms of Somatostatin on Exocrine Stimulated Pancreatic Secretion.] Gastroenterol Clin Biol 11 (2BIS):17A, 1987

Florio, T., et al: Sandostatin Reverts the Impairment of Cognitive Functions Induced by Cysteamine Depletion of Brain Somatostatin. J Endocrinol Invest 10 [Suppl 3]:56 (Abstr. No. P47), 1987

Foote, R. W., Niemerich, G.: Weakening of Naloxone Antagonism In Vitro and In Vivo with Octreotide (SMS 201-995). Eur J Pharmacol 141 (3):325–330, 1987

Fuessl, H. S., et al: [The Somatostatin Analog SMS 201-995 Accelerates Gastric Emptying, but Prolongs the Intestinal Transit Time.] (German) Klin Wochenschr 64 [Suppl V]:41–42, 1986

Fuessl, H. S., et al: Chronic Administration of the Somatostatin Analogue SMS 201-995 Does Not Lead to Endogenous Antibody Formation. Aliment Pharmacol Ther 1:45–50, 1987

Glaser, B., et al: Treatment of G-I/Pancreatic Hormone Hypersecretion Syndromes With the Long-Acting Somatostatin Analogue SMS 201-995. In: Jensen, J., Christiansen, C. (eds) 1st European Congress of Endocrinology, Copenhagen (Denmark), June 21–25, 1987. Norhaven, Viborg, 1987, p 96, Abstr. No. 11–365

Gomez, P. A., et al: Advances in Somatostatin Research. In: Del Pozo, E., Flueckinger, E. (eds) Dopamine and Neuroendoc. Active Substances. Proceedings of the 1st Symposium of European Neuroendocrine Association, Basle (CH), 4–7. 3. 1984. Academic Press, New York, 1985, pp 223–238

Hanisch, E., et al: Reduction of Urinary Calcium Excretion by a Long-Acting Somatostatin Analogue: Results of a Study Using Human Parathyroid Tissue Transplanted to Athymic Nude Mice. In: Jensen, J., Christiansen, C. (eds) 1st European Congress of Endocrinology, Copenhagen (Denmark), June 21–25, 1987. Norhaven, Viborg, 1987, p 20, Abstr. No. 1–72

Harris, A. G.: [Role of Somatostatin in Clinical Human Studies. Recent Findings and Perspectives in Therapy.] Med Hyg (Geneve) 44:1457–1458, 1460, 1986

Hindmarsh, P. C., et al: The Role of Somatostatin Analogue (SMS 201-995) in the Management of Children with Tall Stature. J Endocrinol 117 [Suppl]: Abstr. No. 120, 1988

Hoeldtke, R., Boden, G.: Treatment of Autonomic Neuropathy with a Somatostatin Analogue. Clin Res 34:683A, 1986

Hoeldtke, R., et al: Treatment of Autonomic Neuropathy with a Somatostatin Analogue SMS 201-995. Lancet 2:602–607, 1986

Hoeldtke, R. D., et al: Treatment of Postprandial Hypotension with a Somatostatin Analogue (SMS 201-995). Am J Med 81 [Suppl 6B]:83–87, 1986

Hoeldtke, R. D., et al: Treatment of Severe Orthostatic Hypotension: Comparison of a Somatostatin Analogue and Dihydroergotamine-Caffeine. Clin Res 35 (3):443A, 1987

Jenkins, S. A., et al: The Effects of Somatostatin and SMS 201-995 on Experimentally-Induced Pancreatitis and Endotoxaemia in Rats and on Monocyte Activity in Patients with Cirrhosis and Portal Hypertension. Klin Wochenschr 64 [Suppl VII]:100–106, 1986

Junker, M., et al: Alterations of Phagocytosis by Somatostatin and SMS in Patients With Crohn's Disease. Eur J Clin Invest 17 (2, pt. II):A62 (Abstr. No. 353), 1987

Krejs, G. J.: Panel Discussion I. Am J Med 82 [Suppl 5B]:55–59, 1987

Kusterer, K., et al: Gastric Mucosal Protection by Somatostatins. Klin Wochenschr 64 [Suppl VII]:97–99, 1986

Kutz, M., et al: [Decreasing Claim of the Human Parietal Cell on SMS 201-995.] Klin Wochenschr 64 [Suppl V]:42 (Abstr. No. 84), 1986

Lamberts, S. W. J.: [New Therapeutic Possibilities With Growth Hormone Releasing Hormone and Somatostatin.] Ned Tijdschr Geneesk 130:904–908, 1986

Marbach, P., et al: Clinical Applications of Somatostatin Analogs. In: Patel, Y. C., Tannen-

baum, G. S. (eds) Somatostatin. Proceedings of the Satellite Symposium, 7th International Congress of Endocrinology, Montreal (Canada), 29–30.5.1984. Plenum Press, New York, 1985, pp 339–353
Maurer, R., et al: Somatostatin Receptors. JAMA 253 (18):2741, 1985
McHardy, K. C., Pearson, D. W. M.: Glucose Tolerance During Long-Term Treatment With a Somatostatin Analogue (Correspondence). Br Med J 294:176–177, 1987
Munger, R., et al: [Effect of a New Analog of Somatostatin (SMS 201-995) on the Secretion of GH During Sleep in Healthy Volunteers.] (French) Schweiz Med Wochenschr 117 (20) [Suppl 22]:20, 1987
Reubi, J. C., Palacios, J.: Somatostatin and Alzheimer's Disease: A Hypothesis. J Neurol 233:370–372, 1986
Reubi, J. C., et al: Different Ionic Requirements for Somatostatin Receptor Subpopulations in the Brain. Regul Pept 14:301–311, 1986
Reubi, J. C., et al: Distribution of Somatostatin Receptors in the Human Brain: An Autoradiographic Study. Neuroscience 18:329–346, 1986
Schlueter, K. J., et al: [In-Vivo and In-Vitro Studies With a New Mini Somatostatin (SMS 201-995).] Akt Endokrinol 5:120, 1984
Sieber, C., et al: Effect of a New Somatostatin Analogue SMS 201-995 (Sandostatin) on the Renin-Aldosterone Axis. Clin Endocrinol (Oxf) 28:25–32, 1988
Southgate, H. J., et al: Ectopic Release of GHRH and ACTH From an Adenoid Cystic Carcinoma Resulting in Acromegaly and Complicated by Pituitary Infarction. Postgrad Med J 64:145–148, 1988
Tauber, M. T., et al: Effect of a Long-Acting Somatostatin Analogue (SMS 201-995) on the Growth Velocity of 8 Tall Adolescents: Preliminary Results. J Endocrinol Invest 10 (4):93 (Abstr. No. 144), 1987
Tortosa, F., Pou, J. M.: [SMS 201-995: An Analog of Somatostatin With Multiple Therapeutic Efficacies.] Endocrinologia (Barc) 34 (3): 71–73, 1987
Tortosa, F., et al: [Biological Effect of a New Analog of Somatostatin With Low Molecular Weight.] Endocrinologia (Barc) 31:85, 1984
Von Werder, K., et al: Pulsatile GRF Administration Depletes the Releasable GH-Pool in Normal Subjects. In: 67th Ann. Meeting, The Endoc. Soc., Baltimore (U.S.A.), 19–21.5.1985. Endocrinology 116 [Suppl]:36 (Abstr. No. 141), 1985
Williams, G., et al: Hyperthyroidism Due to Non-Tumoural Inappropriate TSH Secretion. Effect of a Long-Acting Somatostatin Analogue (SMS 201-995). Acta Endocrinol (Copenh) 113 (1):42–46, 1986
Zdon, M. J., et al: Somatostatin Analogue Inhibition of Isolated Parietal Cell Secretion. Surgery 102:967–973, 1987

XXVIII. Preclinical

Altimmari, A. F., et al: Comparison of a Long-Acting Somatostatin Analogue and Trasylol for Treatment of Experimental Pancreatitis. Can J Physiol Pharmacol 64 [Suppl]:72 (Abstr. No. 257), 1986
Arnold, R.: [Is There a Sensible Use of Somatostatin in Gastroenterology?] Internist (Berlin) 27:697–703, 1986
Arosio, M., et al: Long-Term Treatment of Acromegaly With SMS 201-995 (Sandostatin). J Endocrinol Invest 10 [Suppl 3]:23 (Abstr. No. P 10), 1987
Bauer, A. J., et al: Non-Adrenergic, Non-Cholinergic (NANC) Inhibitory Innervation of the Canine and Opossum Sphincter of Oddi. Gastroenterology 92 (5, pt. 2):1311, 1987
Bauer, W., et al: SMS 201-995: A Very Potent and Selective Octapeptide Analogue of Somatostatin With Prolonged Action. Life Sci 31 (11): 1133–1140, 1982
Bauer, W., et al: Structure-Activity Relationships of Highly Potent and Specific Octapeptide Analogues of Somatostatin. In: Blaha, K., Malon, P. (eds) Peptides 1982. Proceedings of the 17th European Peptide Symposium, Prague (Czechoslovakia), Aug. 29–Sept. 3, 1982. De Gruyter, Berlin, 1983, pp 583–588
Baxter, J. N., et al: Effects of a Somatostatin Analogue (SMS 201-995) on Hepatic and Splenic Reticulo-Endothelial Function in the Rat. Br J Surg 72:1005–1008, 1985
Baxter, J. N., et al: Effects of Somatostatin and a Long-Acting Somatostatin Analogue on the Prevention and Treatment of Experimentally Induced Acute Pancreatitis in the Rat. Br J Surg 72 (5):382–385, 1985
Baxter, J. N., et al: Effects of a Somatostatin Analogue SMS 201-995 on Endotoxaemia in the Rat. Gut 27:A-1247–A-1248 (Abstr. No. W 56), 1986
Beal, M. F., Martin, J. B.: The Effect of Somatostatin on Striatal Catecholamines. Neurosci Lett 44:271–276, 1984
Beal, M. F., Martin, J. B.: Effects of Somatostatin on Striatal Dopamine. Neurology (NY) 34 [Suppl 1]:98, 1984
Blei, A. T.: Somatostatin Analogues: Treatment for Portal Hypertension? Hepatology 6:1432–1433, 1986
Brand, S. J., Stone, D.: Omeprazole Stimulates Gastrin Gene Expression Through a Decrease in Somatostatin Gene Expression. Gastroenterology 92 (5, pt. 2):1326, 1987

Brazeau, P., et al: Hypothalamic Polypeptide That Inhibits the Secretion of Immunoreactive Pituitary Growth Hormone. Science 179:77–79, 1973

Bueno, L., et al: [Original Central Action of Somatostatin and Structural Analogs on Profile of Gastrointestinal Motion in the Dog.] Gastroenterol Clin Biol 11 (2 BIS):245 A, 1987

Cadiot, G., et al: [Effects of Somatostatin Long Acting (SMS 201-995) on Gastric Acid Secretion Stimulated by Pentagastrin or Inhibited by Omeprazole. Study in the Rat.] Gastroenterol Clin Biol 11 (2 BIS):232 A, 1987

Cadiot, G., et al: Long-Acting Somatostatin Analog (SMS 201-995) Partly Antagonizes the Trophic Effect Due to Omeprazole in Rat Gastric Mucosa. Gastroenterology 92 (5, pt. 2):1336, 1987

Cadiot, G., et al: [Long-Acting Somatostatin Analog (SMS 201-995) Partly Effects the Trophic Effect Due to Omeprazole in the Rat Gastric Mucosa.] Gastroenterol Clin Biol 11 (2 BIS):235 A, 1987

Cambria, R. P., et al: Somatostatin and Analogues Fail to Decrease Splanchnic Blood Flow in Anesthetized Pigs. Gastroenterology 90: 1363, 1986

Cerini, R., et al: Circulatory Effects of Somatostatin Analogue in Two Conscious Rat Models of Portal Hypertension. Gastroenterology 94: 703–708, 1988

Danguir, J.: Food Intake in Rats is Increased by Intracerebroventricular Infusion of the Somatostatin Analogue SMS 201-995 and is Decreased by Somatostatin Antiserum. Peptides 9 (1):211–213, 1988

Dashwood, M. R., et al: An Etorphine-Evoked Vagal Reflex in Rats is Inhibited by Naloxone, N-Methylnaloxone, and SMS 201-995. Arch Int Pharmacodyn 266:77–82, 1983

Doepfner, W., et al: Effects on Blood Glucose in Rats and Rhesus Monkeys of a New Highly Active Analogue of Somatostatin: SMS 201-995. Acta Endocrinol (Copenh) 103 [Suppl 256]:79 (Abstr. No. 144), 1983

Doepfner, W., et al: Regression of Oestrogen-Induced Pituitary Hyperplasia After Chronic Treatment With Sandostatin (SMS 201-995) in the Rat. Eur J Cancer Clin Oncol 22 (6):749, 1986

Florio, T., et al: Depletion of Brain Somatostatin (SRIF) by Cysteamine (CSH) Induces Impairment of Cognitive Functions in Rat: Reversal by Administration of Exogenous SRIF or Its Analogue SMS 201-995. Pharm Res Commun 20 (3):241–242, 1988

Gärtner, R., et al: Involvement of Cyclic AMP, Iodide and Metabolites of Arachidonic Acid in the Regulation of Cell Proliferation of Isolated Porcine Thyroid Follicles. Mol Cell Endocrinol 42 (2):145–155, 1985

Greenberg, R. N., et al: Inhibition of *Escherichia Coli* Heat-Stable Enterotoxin by Somatostatin Analog SMS 201-995. Can J Physiol Pharmacol 64 [Suppl]:70 (Abstr. No. 251), 1986

Hirning, L. D., et al: Opioid Antagonist Action of Conformationally Constrained Somatostatin Analogues In Vitro. Fed Proc 44 (3):611 (Abstr. No. 1171), 1985

Iversen, J.-G., et al: On the Functional Relationship Between $^{45}Ca^{2+}$ Release and Prolactin Secretion in Cultured Rat Pituitary Tumour (GH_3) Cells. Acta Physiol Scand 127:249–255, 1986

Jenkins, S. A., et al: Effects of a Long Acting Somatostatin Analogue (SMS 201-995) on the Activity of the Reticuloendothelial System (RES) in Rats. Gut 26:A 1138 (Abstr. No. T 8), 1985

Jenkins, S. A., et al: The Effects of a Somatostatin Analogue SMS 201-995 on Hepatic Haemodynamics in the Cirrhotic Rat. Br J Surg 72:864–867, 1985

Jenkins, S. A., et al: Effects of SMS 201-995 on Reticuloendothelial System (RES) Activity in Rats With Acute Pancreatitis. Gut 28 (10): A 1381, 1987

Kiang, J. G., Wei, E. T.: Inhibition of an Opioid-Evoked Vagal Reflex in Rats by Naloxone, SMS 201-995 and ICI 154,129. Regul Pept 6 (3):255–262, 1983

Kiang, J. G., et al: Inhibition of an Opiate-Induced Vagal Reflex in Rats by Naloxone, N-Methylnaloxone, SMS 201-995 and ICI 154,129. Fed Proc 42 (3):358 (Abstr. No. 391), 1983

Konturek, S. J., et al: Comparison of Somatostatin and Its Highly Potent Hexa- and Octapeptide Analogs on Exocrine and Endocrine Pancreatic Secretion. Proc Soc Exp Biol Med 187:241–249, 1988

Koper, J. W., et al: Direct Growth Inhibitory Action of Somatostatin and Its Analog Sandostatin on Rat Pituitary 7315 A Tumor Cells In Vitro. J Endocrinol Invest 10 [Suppl 3]:38 (Abstr. No. OC 8), 1987

Krulich, L., et al: Stimulatory and Inhibitory Effects of Purified Hypothalamic Extracts on Growth Hormone Release from Rat Pituitary *in Vitro*. Endocrinology (United States): 783–790, 1968

Lamberts, S. W. J., et al: Studies on the Mechanism of Action of the Inhibitory Effect of the Somatostatin Analog SMS 201-995 on the Growth of the Prolactin/Adrenocorticotropin-Secreting Pituitary Tumor 7315 a. Endocrinology 118 (6):2188–2194, 1986

Lamberts, S. W. J., et al: The Effect of the Somatostatin Analog SMS 201-995 on Normal

Growth Hormone Secretion in the Rat. A Comparison With the Effect of Bromocriptine on Normal Prolactin Secretion. Acta Endocrinol (Copenh) 115 (2):196–202, 1987

Lemaire, M., et al: Disposition of Sandostatin (SMS 201-995) in the Rat. Pharm Weekbl [Sci] 10 (1):52, 1988

Limberg, B., Kommerell, B.: Influence of Somatostatin on Galactosamine-induced Liver Injury. Klin Wochenschr 64 [Suppl VII]:64–65, 1986

Maurer, R., Reubi, J. C.: Brain Somatostatin Receptor Subpopulation Visualized by Autoradiography. Brain Res 333 (1):178–181, 1985

Maurer, R., Reubi, J. C.: Distribution and Coregulation of Three Peptide Receptors in Adrenals. Eur J Pharmacol 125:241–247, 1986

Maurer, R., Reubi, J. C.: Somatostatin Receptors in the Adrenal. Mol Cell Endocrinol 45:81–90, 1986

Maurer, R., et al: Opiate Antagonistic Properties of an Octapeptide Somatostatin Analog. Proc Natl Acad Sci USA 79 (15):4815–4817, 1982

Misumi, A., et al: Effect of SMS 201-995, a Somatostatin Analogue, on the Exocrine Pancreatic Secretion in Dogs. Dig Dis Sci 31 (10): 1142, 1986

Misumi, A., et al: Effects of SMS 201-995, a Somatostatin Analogue, on the Exocrine Pancreatic Secretion and Gut Hormone Release in Dogs. Surgery 103 (4):450–455, 1988

Mountokalakis, T., Levy, M.: Effect of a Selective Octapeptide Analogue of Somatostatin on Renal Water Excretion in the Dog. Metabolism 34:408–409, 1985

Murphy, W. A., et al: Octapeptide Analogs of Somatostatin Exhibiting Greatly Enhanced In Vivo and In Vitro Inhibition of Growth Hormone Secretion in the Rat. Biochem Biophys Res Commun 132:922–928, 1985

Myren, J., et al: The Effect of the Somatostatin Analogue (Sandoz) on the Liver Injury Following Single Injections of Carbon Tetrachloride in Mice. Can J Physiol Pharmacol [Suppl 73]: Abstr. No. 258, 1986

Nagasawa, H., et al: Inhibition by SMS 201-995 of Normal Mammary Gland Growth in Mice. Experientia 43 (4):417–419, 1987

Nakamura, H., et al: Identification of Lymphoid Cell Lines Bearing Receptors for Somatostatin. Immunology 62:655–658, 1987

Nott, D. M., et al: Effect of SMS 201-995 on the Growth and Development of Hepatic Metastases. Gut 28 (10):A 1350, 1987

Oosterom, R., et al: Studies on Insulin Secretion by Monolayer Cultures of Normal and Tumorous Human Pancreatic Cells. Effects of Glucose, Sandostatin and SMS 201-995. J Endocrinol Invest 10 (6):547–552, 1987

Palacios, J. M., et al: Somatostatin Receptors in Rat Hippocampus: Localization to Intrinsic Neurons. Neurosci Lett 67:169–174, 1986

Palitzsch, K. D., et al: Protection Against Duodenal Ulceration by Somatostatin. Klin Wochenschr 64 [Suppl VII]:93–96, 1986

Palitzsch, K. D., et al: "Low-T3-Syndrome" in Cysteamine-Induced Peptic Ulcer in the Rat: Prevention by the Somatostatin Analog SMS 201-995. Acta Endocrinol (Copenh) 114 [Suppl 283]:164–165, 1987

Peeters, T. L., et al: Changes in Small Intestinal Motility Provoked by the Long-Acting Somatostatin Analogue SMS 201-995 (Sandostatin) in Dog. Gastroenterology 92 (5, pt. 2): 1570, 1987

Peterson, L. J., et al: A Comparison of the Opioid Antagonist Properties of Novel Somatostatin Analogs *In Vitro*. Proc West Pharmacol Soc 28:165–167, 1985

Pless, J., et al: Chemistry and Pharmacology of SMS 201-995, a Long-Acting Octapeptide Analogue of Somatostatin. Scand J Gastroenterol 21 [Suppl 119]:54–64, 1986

Polak, J. M., et al: Growth-Hormone Release-Inhibiting Hormone in Gastrointestinal and Pancreatic D Cells. Lancet *i*: 1220–1222, 1975

Primi, M. P., Bueno, L.: Influence of Centrally Administered Somatostatin and Two Related Peptides on Intestinal Absorption of Water and Electrolytes in Conscious Dogs. Peptides 8: 619–623, 1987

Reubi, J. C.: Evidence for Two Somatostatin-14 Receptor Types in Rat Brain Cortex. Neurosci Lett 49:259–263, 1984

Reubi, J. C.: Novel Selective Radioligand for One Subpopulation of Rat Cortex Somatostatin Receptors. Br J Pharmacol 83 [Proc Suppl]:428 P, 1984

Reubi, J. C.: New Specific Radioligand for One Subpopulation of Brain Somatostatin Receptors. Life Sci 36 (19):1829–1836, 1985

Reubi, J. C.: A Somatostatin Analogue Inhibits Chondrosarcoma and Insulinoma Tumour Growth. Acta Endocrinol (Copenh) 109 (1): 108–114, 1985

Reubi, J. C., Maurer, R.: Autoradiographic Mapping of Somatostatin Receptors in the Rat Central Nervous System and Pituitary. Neuroscience 15 (4):1183–1193, 1985

Reubi, J. C., Maurer, R.: Different Ionic Requirements for Somatostatin Receptor Subpopulations in the Brain. Regul Pept 14:301–311, 1986

Reubi, J. C., et al: Hormone-Producing Gastrointestinal Tumors Contain a High Density of Somatostatin Receptors. J Clin Endocrinol Metab 65:1127–1134, 1987

Roberts, W. G., et al: In Vitro Effects of Somatostatin 201-995 on Intestinal Ion Transport:

Comparison of Antisecretory Effects With SRIF-14 and Alpha-2 Agonists. Gastroenterology 90:1606, 1986

Savage, A. P., et al: Effect of a Long-Acting Analogue of Somatostatin, SMS 201-995, on the Development of Intestinal Tumours in Azoxymethane-Treated Rats. Carcinogenesis (London) 8 (4):561–563, 1987

Schally, A. V., et al: Isolation and Structure of Somatostatin from Porcine Hypothalami. Biochemistry 15 (3):509–514, 1976

Singh, P., et al: A Long-Acting Somatostatin Analog (SRIF) (201-995) and Proglumide (PGL) Inhibit the Trophic and Gastrin Receptor (GR) Regulatory Effects of Pentagastrin (PG) on Mouse Colon Cancer (MC-26) Cells In Vivo. Gastroenterology 90 (5, pt. 2):1636, 1986

Sninsky, C. A., Lynch, D. F.: Which Component of Opiate Withdrawal Causes Diarrhea, Intestinal Motility or Secretion? Clin Res 1 (36):14A, 1988

Stöckmann, F., et al: The Effect of Proglumide and SMS 201-995 on Camostate Induced Pancreatic Hypertrophy. Dig Dis Sci 31 (10):1150, 1986

Stöckmann, F., et al: Influence of SMS 201-995, a Long Acting Somatostatin Analogue, in Exocrine Pancreatic Secretion in the Rat. Dig Dis Sci 31 (10):1151, 1986

Stoll, R., et al: Effect of the Somatostatin Analogue SMS 201-995 on ATP-Dependent Calcium Transport of Basolateral Vesicles From Human Duodenum. Scand J Gastroenterol 22 (10):1200–1204, 1987

Takemura, J., Brown, J. C.: Comparison of the Effect of Somatostatin and a Somatostatin Analogue (SMS 201-995) on Insulin Secretion in the Isolated Perfused Rat Pancreas. Can J Physiol Pharmacol [Suppl 69]: Abstr. No. 249, 1986

Takemura, J., et al: Comparison of the Effect of Somatostatin and an Analogue, SMS 201-995, on Gastrin and Insulin Secretion from Isolated Perfused Rat Stomach and Pancreas. Am J Med 81 [Suppl 6B]:65–73, 1986

Tran, V. T., et al: Two Types of Somatostatin Receptors Differentiated by Cyclic Somatostatin Analogs. Science 228:492–495, 1985

Upp, J. R., Jr., et al: Inhibition of Growth of Two Human Pancreatic Adenocarcinomas In Vivo By Somatostatin Analog SMS 201-995. Am J Surg 155 (1):29–35, 1988

Van Wimersma-Greidanus, T. B., et al: Excessive Grooming Induced by Somatostatin or Its Analog SMS 201-995. Eur J Pharmacol 144: 277–285, 1987

Verchere, C. B., et al: Inhibition of Insulin Secretion in the Isolated, Perfused Rat Pancreas by Somatostatin and a Somatostatin Analog (SMS 201-995). Gastroenterology 92 (5, pt. 2): 1806, 1987

Weber, C. J., et al: Passage of Somatostatin Analogue Across Human and Mouse Skin. Surgery 102:974–981, 1987

Weightman, D. R., Kendall-Taylor, P.: The Effect of SMS 201-995 and Mg^{++} on the Binding of ^{125}I-[Leu^8, D Trp^{22}, Tyr^{25}]- Somatostatin in Rat Brain. J Endocrinol 108 [Suppl 324], 1986

Werz, M. A., et al: Actions of *Mu, Delta and Kappa* Opioid Agonists and Antagonists on Mouse Primary Afferent Neurons in Culture. J Pharmacol Exp Ther 243:258–263, 1987

Whitford, C. A., et al: Autoradiographic Visualization of Binding Sites for [^{3}H]Somatostatin in the Rat Brain. Eur J Pharmacol 138:327–333, 1987

Williams, G., et al: Hypothalamic VIP and Neuromedin B Levels are Increased in Streptozotocin-Diabetic Rats. Clin Sci 2 [Suppl 16]:14P (Abstr. No. 37), 1987

Wynants, C., et al: Hexapeptide Analogue of Somatostatin, Sandoz 201-456. Int J Pept Protein Res 25 (6):622–627, 1985

Wynants, C., et al: SMS 201-995, an Octapeptide Somatostatin Analogue. Int J Pept Protein Res 25 (6):615–621, 1985

Wynants, C., et al: SMS 201-995, a Very Potent Analogue of Somatostatin. Int J Pept Protein Res 25 (6):608–614, 1985

Wynants, C., et al: Conformational Study of a Somatostatin Analogue by High-Field n.m.r. Spectroscopy, in Aqueous Solution. Int J Pept Protein Res 30 (4):541–547, 1987